AF735923

2014 YEAR BOOK OF SURGERY®

The 2014 Year Book Series

Year Book of Endocrinology®: Drs Schott, Apovian, Clarke, Eugster, Khaodhiar, Meikle, Oetgen, Petersenn, Toth, and Willenberg

Year Book of Hand and Upper Limb Surgery®: Drs Yao, Adams, and Rizzo

Year Book of Medicine®: Drs Barker, DeVault, Garrick, Gold, Khardori, Lawton, LeRoith, and Pearson

Year Book of Neonatal and Perinatal Medicine®: Drs Fanaroff, Benitz, Donn, Neu, Papile, and Van Marter

Year Book of Ophthalmology®: Drs Rapuano, Fudemberg, Gupta, Hammersmith, Milman, Nagra, Nelson, Penne, Pyfer, Sergott, Shields, and Talekar

Year Book of Orthopedics®: Drs Morrey, Huddleston, Rose, Swiontkowski, and Trigg

Year Book of Pathology and Laboratory Medicine®: Drs Raab and Bissell

Year Book of Pediatrics®: Dr Cabana

Year Book of Plastic and Aesthetic Surgery™: Drs Miller, Gutowski, and Smith

Year Book of Pulmonary Disease®: Drs Barker, Jones, Maurer, Spradley, Tanoue, and Willsie

Year Book of Surgery®: Drs Behrns, Daly, Fahey, Hines, Howe, Huber, Klodell, Mozingo, and Pruett

Year Book of Urology®: Drs Andriole and Coplen

Year Book of Vascular Surgery®: Drs Gillespie, Bush, Passman, Starnes, and Watkins

2014

The Year Book of SURGERY®

Editor-in-Chief

Kevin E. Behrns, MD

Chairman, Edward R. Woodward Professor, Department of Surgery, University of Florida, Gainesville, Florida

ELSEVIER
MOSBY

ELSEVIER
MOSBY

Vice President, Global Medical Reference: Mary E. Gatsch
Acquisitions Editor: John Vassallo
Developmental Editor: Susan Showalter
Production Supervisor, Electronic Year Books: Donna M. Skelton
Electronic Article Manager: Mike Sheets
Illustrations and Permissions Coordinator: Dawn Vohsen

2014 EDITION
Copyright 2014, Mosby, Inc. All rights reserved.

No part of this publication may be reproduced, stored in a retrieval system, or transmitted, in any form or by any means, electronic, mechanical, photocopying, recording, or otherwise, without prior written permission from the publisher.

Permission to photocopy or reproduce solely for internal or personal use is permitted for libraries or other users registered with the Copyright Clearance Center, provided that the base fee of $35.00 per chapter is paid directly to the Copyright Clearance Center, 21 Congress Street, Salem, MA 01970. This consent does not extend to other kinds of copying, such as copying for general distribution, for advertising or promotional purposes, for creating new collected works, or for resale.

Composition by TNQ Books and Journals Pvt Ltd, India

Editorial Office:
Elsevier
1600 John F. Kennedy Blvd.
Suite 1800
Philadelphia, PA 19103-2899

International Standard Serial Number: 0090-3671
International Standard Book Number: 978-0-323-26489-1

Editorial Board

Editor-in-Chief

Kevin E. Behrns, MD

Chairman, Edward R. Woodward Professor, Department of Surgery, University of Florida, Gainesville, Florida

Associate Editors

John M. Daly, MD, FACS, FRCSI (hon)

Harry C. Donohoo Professor of Surgery and Dean Emeritus, Temple University School of Medicine; Temple University Hospital; Fox Chase Cancer Center, Philadelphia, Pennsylvania

Thomas J. Fahey III, MD

Professor of Surgery, Weill Cornell Medical College and Chief, Endocrine Surgery, The New York Presbyterian Hospital – Weill Cornell Medical Center, New York, New York

O. Joe Hines, MD, FACS

Professor and Chief, Division of General Surgery, Robert and Kelly Day Chair in General Surgery; Director, Surgery Residency Program, Department of Surgery, David Geffen School of Medicine at the University of California, Los Angeles, Los Angeles, California

James R. Howe, M.D.

Professor of Surgery, Director, Surgical Oncology and Endocrine Surgery, Roy J. and Lucille A. Carver University of Iowa College of Medicine, Iowa City, Iowa

Thomas S. Huber, MD, PhD

Professor and Chief, Division of Vascular Surgery and Endovascular Therapy, University of Florida College of Medicine, Gainesville, Florida

Charles T. Klodell, Jr, MD

Associate Professor, Thoracic and Cardiovascular Surgery, University of Florida College of Medicine, Gainesville, Florida

David W. Mozingo, MD

Professor of Surgery and Anesthesiology, Department of Surgery, University of Florida College of Medicine; Director, UF Health Shands Burn Center, Gainesville, Florida

Timothy L. Pruett, MD

Chief of Transplantation, John S. Najarian Clinical Professor of Transplantation, Professor of Surgery and Internal Medicine, University of Minnesota, Minneapolis, Minnesota

Table of Contents

Journals Represented

Journals represented in this YEAR BOOK are listed below.

Air Medical Journal
AJR American Journal of Roentgenology
American Journal of Clinical Nutrition
American Journal of Respiratory and Critical Care Medicine
American Journal of Surgery
American Journal of Transplantation
Annals of Surgery
Annals of Surgical Oncology
Annals of the American Thoracic Society
Annals of Thoracic Surgery
Annals of Vascular Surgery
Archives of Disease in Childhood
British Journal of Anaesthesia
British Journal of Surgery
British Medical Journal
Burns
Cancer
Cancer Epidemiology, Biomarkers & Prevention
Chest
Circulation
Circulation Cardiovascular Interventions
Clinical Nuclear Medicine
Clinical Pediatrics
Clinical Toxicology
Critical Care Medicine
Digestive Diseases and Sciences
Diseases of the Colon and Rectum
European Journal of Surgical Oncology
Gastroenterology
Gut
Health Affairs
Intensive Care Medicine
Journal of Burn Care & Research
Journal of Clinical Endocrinology & Metabolism
Journal of Clinical Oncology
Journal of Drugs in Dermatology
Journal of Emergency Medicine
Journal of Pediatrics
Journal of Surgical Oncology
Journal of Surgical Research
Journal of the American College of Cardiology
Journal of the American College of Surgeons
Journal of the American Medical Association
Journal of the American Medical Association Dermatology
Journal of the American Medical Association Internal Medicine
Journal of the American Medical Association Surgery
Journal of the American Society of Nephrology

Journal of Thoracic and Cardiovascular Surgery
Journal of Trauma and Acute Care Surgery
Journal of Vascular Surgery
Journal of Vascular Surgery. Venous and Lymphatic Disorders
JPEN Journal of Parenteral and Enteral Nutrition
Lancet
Lancet Oncology
Neurology
New England Journal of Medicine
Surgery
Transplantation Proceedings
World Journal of Surgery
World Neurosurgery
Wound Repair and Regeneration

Standard Abbreviations

The following terms are abbreviated in this edition: acquired immunodeficiency syndrome (AIDS), cardiopulmonary resuscitation (CPR), central nervous system (CNS), cerebrospinal fluid (CSF), computed tomography (CT), deoxyribonucleic acid (DNA), electrocardiography (ECG), health maintenance organization (HMO), human immunodeficiency virus (HIV), intensive care unit (ICU), intramuscular (IM), intravenous (IV), magnetic resonance (MR) imaging (MRI), ribonucleic acid (RNA), and ultrasound (US).

Note

The Year Book of Surgery is a literature survey service providing abstracts of articles published in the professional literature. Every effort is made to assure the accuracy of the information presented in these pages. Neither the editors nor the publisher of the Year Book of Surgery can be responsible for errors in the original materials. The editors' comments are their own opinions. Mention of specific products within this publication does not constitute endorsement.

To facilitate the use of the Year Book of Surgery as a reference tool, all illustrations and tables included in this publication are now identified as they appear in the original article. This change is meant to help the reader recognize that any illustration or table appearing in the Year Book of Surgery may be only one of many in the original article. For this reason, figure and table numbers appear to be out of sequence within the Year Book of Surgery.

Introduction

There were three seminal articles selected for this year's YEAR BOOK OF SURGERY, and all merit full review. The IMPROVE and Amsterdam Acute Aneurysm Trial both compared open and endovascular repair for *ruptured* abdominal aortic aneurysms in a randomized, controlled fashion. They found no difference in outcome despite the fairly strongly held bias that the endovascular approach is superior. Notably, the mortality rates for both approaches were lower than predicted, emphasizing the importance of a system-wide approach with the concentration of the repairs in centers of excellence. The CORAL Trial was a randomized, controlled trial that compared medical management with angioplasty and intraluminal stenting for patients with renal artery stenosis and hypertension or chronic kidney disease. Despite the widespread application of endovascular treatment in this setting, the study failed to demonstrate and benefit for these interventions in terms of either the cardiovascular or renal endpoints.

The articles selected among the aortic and aneurysm subsections document the continued evolution of the endovascular therapies and the natural history of aneurysmal disease while calling attention to the potential complications. A comparison of fenestrated endovascular aneurysm repair (FEVAR) with the open, juxtarenal approach demonstrated that the fenestrated approach may be superior, reminiscent of the early EVAR trials. The long-term outcome of the INSTEAD trial, comparing medical management with TEVAR for uncomplicated type B aortic dissections, reported a decrease in aortic-related mortality and a trend toward a decrease in all-cause mortality, unlike the initial report. Notably, the benefits of TEVAR were noted between 2 – 5 years after the index dissection and were associated with thrombosis of the false lumen. A meta-analysis of the small aneurysm trials (ie, 3.0 – 5.4 cm) documented the growth rate and defined surveillance intervals. Notably, the growth rates were comparable for men and women, although the rupture risk was higher for women per specific aneurysm diameter, suggesting that women should be repaired at a smaller threshold. Similarly, the Low Frequency Consortium attempted to define the natural history of femoral artery aneurysms, suggesting that a diameter of 3.5 cm may be the optimal threshold for repair. The limitations of the EVAR and TEVAR approaches were emphasized by reports documenting the limited follow-up and potential for retrograde Type A dissection, respectively. The "lost to follow-up" rate after EVAR in the paper selected was 56%, but, unfortunately, no predictors were identified for the "at risk" patients. Retrograde Type A dissection is an uncommon but known complication of TEVAR; strategies to prevent the complication were identified in the selected manuscript. The role of volume resuscitation for patients with ruptured aneurysms was examined in a retrospective study. The authors reported that the volume of fluid resuscitation was the only independent predictor of mortality, suggesting that permissive hypotension may be protective. Lastly, patients who were identified to be on a statin agent at the onset of the DREAM Trial (ie, open AAA repair vs EVAR) were found to have better long-term survival, underscoring the importance of these agents for all vascular patients.

The focus of the peripheral arterial occlusive disease subsection was the continued application of the endovascular therapies. Intraluminal stents appear to be effective for patients with isolated popliteal artery occlusive disease, despite the clinical impression that they are contraindicated in this location. The endovascular treatment of tibial vessels for patients with critical limb ischemia was associated with reasonable patency and limb salvage rates. However, the presence of gangrene was associated with lesion recurrence, and there was a subset of patients who were initially open revascularization candidates who progressed to limb loss. Similarly, the comparison of bare metal and covered stents for patients with femoropopliteal artery occlusive disease found that stent graft failure was associated with acute lower extremity ischemia and loss of infrageniculate targets for potential open revascularization. The outcomes for most vascular surgical procedures, including those for peripheral arterial occlusive disease, appear to be compromised in patients with end stage renal disease (ESRD), suggesting that the threshold for procedures performed for "prophylactic" indications (ie, asymptomatic carotid stenosis, asymptomatic aneurysm) may need to be redefined. A small, randomized trial comparing the vacuum-assisted dressing with topical wound products for patients with complex femoral wounds was stopped prematurely because of the favorable outcomes in the vacuum group. Lastly, the outcomes after infrainguinal percutaneous procedures appear to be related to platelet responsiveness to clopidogrel and seem to justify some type of "point of care" testing when/if these technologies become more available.

The selected venous articles address clinically relevant problems encountered by most vascular surgeons. The endovascular treatment of patients with the May-Thurner syndrome (ie, compression of left iliac vein by right iliac artery) appears to be well-tolerated and associated with excellent long-term outcome. A nice randomized, controlled trial from Europe comparing treatments for varicose veins (ie, stripping vs laser ablation vs foam sclerotherapy) reported that the treatment options were largely equivalent from a clinical standpoint, although the ultrasound-based outcome measures were inferior in the foam sclerotherapy group. Unfortunately, radiofrequency ablation was not examined in the trial, largely because its use wasn't very prevalent at the onset of the study. A systematic review of the literature and meta-analysis compared percutaneous inserted central catheters (PICCs) and central venous lines, reporting that the incidence of deep venous thromboses was more than two-fold higher for PICC lines with the highest incidence among ICU patients. The interventional treatment for iliofemoral DVT in pregnant women was reported to be both safe and effective in terms of long-term patency and fetal survival. Notably, a nice description of the treatment algorithm was provided in the Methods section of the manuscript.

The balance of the articles selected deal with a variety of topics that round out the spectrum of care provided by vascular surgeons. A nice review of the literature and consensus statement addressing the management of cerebrovascular disease in women was included. Notably, women appear to have slightly worse outcomes for both carotid endarterectomy (CEA) and carotid angioplasty/stenting (CAS), although the treatment recommendations are largely the same as those for men. A meta-analysis of the European CEA vs CAS trials reported that early CAS (ie, 0 – 7 days after index neurologic event) was associated with a higher incidence of stroke or death. Although this was a secondary analysis, it raises some concerns about the timing of CAS after a transient ischemic attack or stroke. This is particularly relevant given the national guidelines that emphasize intervention within 14 days. A study examining survival among elderly hemodialysis patients reported that survival was worse if the first access was a catheter, but found no difference between autogenous (ie, fistula) or prosthetic (ie, grafts) accesses. These data argue for a "personalized" approach to the elderly dialysis patient and suggest that the "fistula first" approach may not be ideal. Lastly, a prospective study reported that the use of dual antiplatelet agents (ie, aspirin + clopidogrel) was safe across a range of peripheral vascular surgical procedures, including aneurysm repair. Importantly, the dual therapy was not associated with an increased incidence of bleeding.

Thomas S. Huber, MD, PhD

1 General Considerations

General Surgery Residency Inadequately Prepares Trainees for Fellowship: Results of a Survey of Fellowship Program Directors

Mattar SG, Alseidi AA, Jones DB, et al (Indiana Univ School of Medicine, Indianapolis; Virginia Mason Med Ctr, Seattle, WA; Beth Israel Deaconess Med Ctr, Boston, MA; et al)

Ann Surg 258:440-449, 2013

Objective.—To assess readiness of general surgery graduate trainees entering accredited surgical subspecialty fellowships in North America.

Methods.—A multidomain, global assessment survey designed by the Fellowship Council research committee was electronically sent to all subspecialty program directors. Respondents spanned minimally invasive surgery, bariatric, colorectal, hepatobiliary, and thoracic specialties. There were 46 quantitative questions distributed across 5 domains and 1 or more reflective qualitative questions/domains.

Results.—There was a 63% response rate (n = 91/145). Of respondent program directors, 21% felt that new fellows arrived unprepared for the operating room, 38% demonstrated lack of patient ownership, 30% could not independently perform a laparoscopic cholecystectomy, and 66% were deemed unable to operate for 30 unsupervised minutes of a major procedure. With regard to laparoscopic skills, 30% could not atraumatically manipulate tissue, 26% could not recognize anatomical planes, and 56% could not suture. Furthermore, 28% of fellows were not familiar with therapeutic options and 24% were unable to recognize early signs of complications. Finally, it was felt that the majority of new fellows were unable to conceive, design, and conduct research/academic projects. Thematic clustering of qualitative data revealed deficits in domains of operative autonomy, progressive responsibility, longitudinal follow-up, and scholarly focus after general surgery education.

► Since the inception of duty hour regulations and increased supervision of general surgery residents, there is a prevailing sentiment that general surgery trainees lack the skills and confidence to practice independently after completion of their residency. This survey of fellowship program directors was conducted by Mattar et al under the auspices of the Fellowship Council. The response rate was 63%, and questions across several domains, including professionalism, preparedness, technical skills, and academic interest, were assessed. The results showed that fellowship directors opined that general surgery residents lacked ownership of patients, could not operate independently for 30 minutes in a major operation, had inadequate laparoscopic skills, and had little interest in scholarly activities. Are these findings the natural evolution of decreased duty hours and increased supervision? I suspect not. Moreover, with fewer surgeons receiving National Institutes of Health funding and decreased resources for research, is it any wonder that residents, who likely have limited exposure to research, have limited interest in conducting research? Furthermore, with the popularity of fellowships, the senior or chief residents may be pushed downstream for cases and thus have decreased operating exposure. These findings support the concept of "fixing the five" and making the general surgery training program the priority over fellowship programs. Perhaps it is time to limit fellowships and focus our efforts on the general surgery residents.

K. E. Behrns, MD

Characteristics of Highly Ranked Applicants to General Surgery Residency Programs

Stain SC, Hiatt JR, Ata A, et al (Albany Med College, NY; Univ of California at Los Angeles; et al)

JAMA Surg 148:413-417, 2013

Importance.—With duty hour debates, specialization, and sex distribution changes in the applicant pool, the relative competitiveness for general surgery residency (GSR) is undefined.

Objective.—To determine the modern attributes of topranked applicants to GSR.

Design.—Validation cohort, survey.

Setting.—National sample of university and community-based GSR programs.

Participants.—Data were abstracted from Electronic Residency Application Service files of the top 20–ranked applicants to 22 GSR programs. We ranked program competitiveness and blinded review of personal statements.

Main Outcomes and Measures.—Characteristics associated with applicant ranking by the GSR program (top 5 vs 6-20) and ranking by highly competitive programs were identified using t and χ^2 tests and modified Poisson regression.

Results.—There were 333 unique applicants among the 440 Electronic Residency Application Service files. Most applicants had research experience (93.0%) and publications (76.8%), and 28.4% had Alpha Omega Alpha membership. Nearly half were women (45.2%), with wide variation by program (20.0%-75.0%) and a trend toward fewer women at programs in the South and West (38.0% and 37.5%, respectively). Men had higher United States Medical Licensing Examination Step 1 scores (238.0 vs 230.1; $P < .001$) but similar Step 2 scores (245.3 vs 244.5; $P = .54$). Using bivariate analysis, highly competitive programs were more likely to rank applicants with publications, research experience, Alpha Omega Alpha membership, higher Step 1 scores, and excellent personal statements and those who were male or Asian. However, the only significant predictors were Step 1 scores (relative risk [RR], 1.36 for every 10-U increase), publications (RR, 2.20), personal statements (RR, 1.62), and Asian race (RR, 1.70 vs white). Alpha Omega Alpha membership (RR, 1.62) and Step 1 scores (RR, 1.01) were the only variables predictive of ranking in the top 5.

Conclusions and Relevance.—This national sample shows GSR is a highly competitive, sex-neutral discipline in which academic performance is the most important factor for ranking, especially in the most competitive programs. This study will inform applicants and program directors about applicants to the GSR program.

▶ Annually, general surgery training programs seek to identify the best medical students as surgical trainees for their institution. Much effort goes into establishing criteria to determine the best applicants and individuals who have the right fit for the medical center. Although medical centers may strive to identify the best general surgery trainees for their program, the best candidates obviously look more alike than different. Stain et al studied the top 20 applicants to 22 general surgery residency programs. The 22 programs were ranked as highly competitive, very competitive, and competitive. To determine the attributes of contemporary applicants, they examined race, the United States Medical Licensing Examination (USLME) scores, research, publications, honor society membership, and applicants' personal statements. Notably, the candidate interviews with the faculty or residents at the training program were not assessed. The results showed, not surprisingly, that predictors of top 5 applicants were honor society membership and USLME Step I scores. Highly competitive programs were more likely to rank top 5 applicants by honor society membership and Step I scores. Thus, despite machinations of ranking candidates at many institutions, the best-ranked applicants in the best programs are assessed by academic performance determined by honor society ranking, a surrogate of good academic performance throughout medical school, and high USMLE scores. However, the good news from this work is that 333 unique applicants were identified and deemed worthy of top 20 ranking at the 22 institutions. These students could occupy nearly one-third of the 1108 categorical surgical training positions available each year. Indeed, the applicant pool to general surgery training programs is strong! Perhaps we should work on identifying the middle third of the applicants and those that might be at risk at our various institutions.

K. E. Behrns, MD

Accelerating Physician Workforce Transformation Through Competitive Graduate Medical Education Funding

Goodman DC, Robertson RG (Dartmouth Inst for Health Policy and Clinical Practice, Lebanon, NH; Chicago Med School, IL)

Health Aff (Millwood) 32:1887-1892, 2013

Graduate medical education (GME) has fallen short in training physicians to meet changes in the US population and health care delivery systems. The shortfall in training has happened despite a consensus on the need for accelerated change. This article discusses the varied causes of GME inertia and proposes a new funding mechanism coupled to a competitive peer-review process. The result would be to reward GME programs that are aligned with publicly set priorities for specialty numbers and training content. New teaching organizations and residency programs would compete on an equal footing with existing ones. Over a decade, all current programs would undergo peer review, with low review scores leading to partial, but meaningful, decreases in funding. This process would incentivize incremental and continual change in GME and would provide a mechanism for funding innovative training through special requests for proposals.

▶ Funding for graduate medical education (GME) has been a frequently discussed topic here—of late because of the $13 billion annual price tag. Although these costs may appear high to the uninitiated observer, it is not an accurate assessment of the true costs, as many GME programs are well over the cap of trainees and self-fund additional, needed positions. Therefore, before we encourage a substantial change in GME funds distribution, we should thoroughly understand the number of trainees and how these individuals are compensated—through funding by Center for Medicare and Medicaid Services or through local graduate medical education programs, usually the affiliated hospital. Goodman and Robertson propose an innovative model of funding GME that includes the formation of a publically oriented federal advisory committee that would set the direction for GME funding by aligning funding with specialty needs and awarding both direct and indirect funding in a competitive fashion. They envision a review system that functions much like the National Institutes of Health study sections in which experts review proposals and score them, and dollars are awarded on a competitive basis. In the absence of issues, funding for a program would be 10 years in duration before a competitive renewal would occur. The authors contend that these changes are necessary, because the current system is inflexible and does not account for training needed largely in outpatient venues. The recommendations for change in GME funding may be innovative, but would they lead to real change in GME? The first assertion that GME funding and change are inflexible is accurate, but this is the byproduct of a stagnant system that has been in place for nearly 17 years—since the Balanced Budget Act of 1997. Is it any wonder that the system is not innovative or flexible when health care leaders must fund new positions through hospital revenues? Furthermore, how does the proposed system work in concert with the Accreditation Council for Graduate Medical Education, the Residency Review Committees, and the American

Board of Medical Specialties? An entirely new system is not required, but improved communication and coordination through the existing system and organizations are required. Importantly, the current product is well trained and disruption of the system should come only after a careful and thorough assessment.

K. E. Behrns, MD

The Residency Mismatch

Iglehart JK

N Engl J Med 369:297-299, 2013

Background.—The supply of practicing physicians in the United States fluctuates from too few to too many and back generation after generation. The physician shortage was tackled in 2006 with a recommendation that medical school enrollments be increased by 30% over the next decade, and we are on track to achieve that expansion. However, the number of residency posts available to medical graduates has not kept pace, and there are now too few to meet the demand. As a result, the number of practicing physicians may remain well below the need.

Federal Barriers.—The federal government has been the major source of funding for the increased number of medical schools in the past but did not lend direct financial support to the recent expansion. In addition, the increase in graduate medical education (GME) programs, which are also largely federally funded, has been extremely slow, with an annual growth rate of 0.9% between 2001 and 2010. The major barrier has been the payment cap placed by Congress on Medicare's funding of advanced training in the balanced Budget Act of 1997. Medicare is the primary supporter of GME programs, with about two thirds of its support through a payment adjustment for patient care, also mandated by Congress. However, efforts to persuade Congress to increase Medicare GME support and fund an additional 15,000 GME positions have been thwarted by debate over the Affordable Care Act (ACA) and the move to constrain government spending. In addition, for the 2014 budget the Obama administration has called on a reduction in Medicare GME spending by $11 billion over the next decade. The American Academy of Family Physicians (AAFP) is especially concerned that the administration's cuts could adversely affect family-medicine residency programs. The 2013 results of the National Residency Matching Program demonstrate an ongoing trend of just small increases in applicants choosing family medicine, even though some of the best medical students are now applying for primary care residency positions.

State Barriers.—In the 2009-2010 academic year 27 states still had more GME positions than they had undergraduate medical and osteopathic students to fill them. Usually governors and state legislators see in-state medical schools, whether public or private, as mechanisms by which physicians will be created who will practice in their state. However, where new physicians do their GME training is now recognized as being more determinative of where they will practice. Florida and Texas face the situation of

TABLE.—Growth of First-Year Enrollment in U.S. Schools of Medicine and Osteopathy since 2002*

	2002 Base	2012 Current			2017 Projected		
	Enrollment	Enrollment	Increase Since 2002		Enrollment	Increase Since 2002	
Degree	*no.*	*no.*	*no.*	%	*no.*	*no.*	%
M.D.	16,488	19,517	3029	18	21,434	4946	30
D.O.	2,968	5,804	2836	96	6,675	3707	125
Total	19,456	25,321	5865	30	28,109	8653	44

*Data are from Association of American Medical Colleges and the American Association of Colleges of Osteopathic Medicine.

having added new medical schools but very few advanced training posts. Barriers specific to states include declines in state GME support and an unwillingness of large community hospitals to create training programs because of costs and staff reluctance to take on teaching roles. In addition, state support is a fraction of the amount by which Medicaid patient care reimbursements for state teaching hospitals have been reduced.

Conclusions.—Unless the number of accredited residency-training posts increases dramatically, it may soon be impossible for all the graduates of US medical and osteopathic colleges to find GME slots. The large number of international medical school graduates who seek positions in the United States is in even greater jeopardy. Inadequate or absent planning for a sufficient health workforce has created physician shortages that will become even more apparent once the ACA's coverage expansion is fully implemented (Table).

▶ For several years we have heard of the workforce shortage in general surgery, and with increased access to care through the Affordable Care Act many are concerned about how we will care for an additional 35 million potential patients. In this Perspective paper in the *New England Journal of Medicine*, Iglehart reviews the nation's response to the need for an increased number of physicians. Of course, we cannot train more physicians if we do not increase the number of medical school seats available. As Iglehart highlights, we have greatly increased not only the number of medical students but also doctors of osteopathy (Table). Furthermore, the number of foreign medical graduates continues to increase at an accelerated rate. Even though the number of positions in medical school has increased dramatically, the rate-limiting point is the number of graduate medical education (GME) training positions. The funding for these positions has been capped for 15 years since the passage of the Balanced Budget Act of 1997. With the current proposed budget cut of $11 billion to GME over 10 years, the future for training additional physicians does not look bright. Even now, many large teaching hospitals are well over the cap of trainees, and these teaching hospitals carry the financial burden of, on occasion, more than 100 trainees over the institutional cap. These costs mount quickly when considering the entire workforce needed to care for an increasing number of patients. Hospital administrators are unlikely to willingly add more dollars to the existing financial commitment. Without an increase in the number of GME training positions, administrators and educators will likely have to make decisions about the types of trainees they wish to include in their GME programs. We may not be far from some residency programs being eliminated at major teaching hospitals. As noted in the article, family medicine training programs have seen decreasing numbers and are at risk at some institutions. Clearly, not all teaching institutions can house every program, but the elimination or major downsizing of some programs will hurt the overall teaching environment of major teaching centers. These decisions should be weighed carefully at the national and local levels before we take drastic approaches to dealing with decreased funding for GME.

K. E. Behrns, MD

Projecting Surgeon Supply Using a Dynamic Model

Fraher EP, Knapton A, Sheldon GF, et al (Univ of North Carolina at Chapel Hill; Natl Health Service Workforce Review Team, Winchester, England, UK)

Ann Surg 257:867-872, 2013

Objective.—To develop a projection model to forecast the head count and fulltime equivalent supply of surgeons by age, sex, and specialty in the United States from 2009 to 2028.

Summary Background Data.—The search for the optimal number and specialty mix of surgeons to care for the United States population has taken on increased urgency under health care reform. Expanded insurance coverage and an aging population will increase demand for surgical and other medical services. Accurate forecasts of surgical service capacity are crucial to inform the federal government, training institutions, professional associations, and others charged with improving access to health care.

Methods.—The study uses a dynamic stock and flow model that simulates future changes in numbers and specialty type by factoring in changes in surgeon demographics and policy factors.

Results.—Forecasts show that overall surgeon supply will decrease 18% during the period form 2009 to 2028 with declines in all specialties except colorectal, pediatric, neurological surgery, and vascular surgery. Model simulations suggest that none of the proposed changes to increase graduate medical education currently under consideration will be sufficient to offset declines.

Conclusions.—The length of time it takes to train surgeons, the anticipated decrease in hours worked by surgeons in younger generations, and the potential decreases in graduate medical education funding suggest that there may be an insufficient surgeon workforce to meet population needs. Existing maldistribution patterns are likely to be exacerbated,

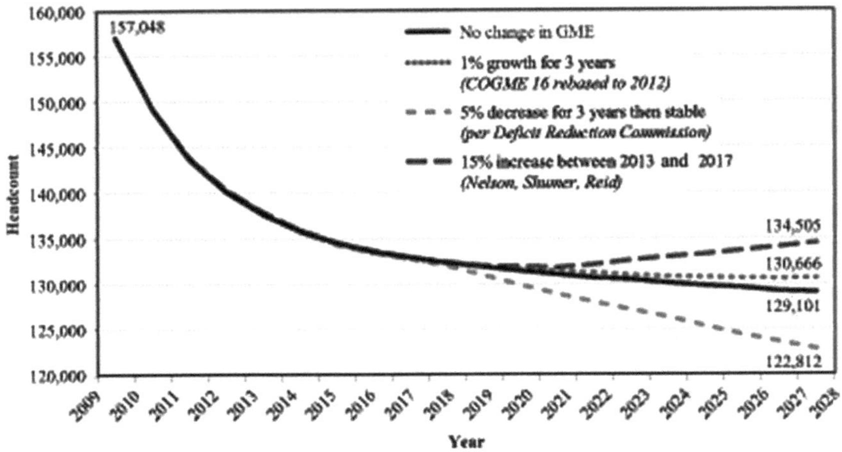

FIGURE 3.—Graduate medical education scenarios. (Reprinted from Fraher EP, Knapton A, Sheldon GF, et al. Projecting surgeon supply using a dynamic model. *Ann Surg*. 2013;257:867-872, © 2013, Southeastern Surgical Congress.)

leading to delayed or lost access to time-sensitive surgical procedures, particularly in rural areas (Fig 3).

▶ Over the last 15 to 20 years, multiple investigators have performed workforce assessments in surgery. Most of the published studies indicate the potential for a significant shortage of surgeons. Although a deficit of working surgeons has always been an important topic, the Affordable Care Act has placed renewed emphasis on the surgical workforce, as an infusion of several million potential patients into the health care system is anticipated. Most of the models of surgeon supply do not look at surgeon inflow and outflow in the system. However, Fraher et al have addressed this criticism by applying a dynamic model that takes these considerations into account. Using this model, they found that over the next 20 years, the number of surgeons would decrease 18%, with a 16% reduction in full-time equivalents. The shortage would be most severe in cardiothoracic surgery, with a 25% reduction in the workforce. In addition to a reduction in the number of surgeons, the geographic maldistribution of surgeons will be exacerbated, as fewer surgeons are choosing careers in rural surgery given the economic considerations and the pressure to provide services to a large number of patients with too few surgeons. Moreover, the number of surgery training slots allocated through the Residency Review Committee has not changed appreciably over the years. The lack of foresight to increase training slots has potentially created significant access issues for patients. Finally, there is a relatively high likelihood that funding for graduate medical education will decrease substantially and place further pressure, limiting training spots (Fig 3). Collectively, these findings suggest that the surgical workforce will be insufficient to care for an increasing number of patients and that regulatory bodies and the government do not intend to actively seek timely solutions.

K. E. Behrns, MD

Pilot Testing of a Model for Insurer-Driven, Large-Scale Multicenter Simulation Training for Operating Room Teams

Arriaga AF, for the Harvard Surgical Safety Collaborative (Brigham and Women's Hosp, Boston, MA; et al)

Ann Surg 259:403-410, 2014

Objective.—To test the feasibility of implementing a standardized teamwork training program with full operating room teams in multiple institutions, driven by malpractice insurer support and incentives.

Background.—Failures in intraoperative teamwork are among the leading causes of preventable patient injury and death in surgical patients. Teamwork training , particularly using simulation, can be an effective intervention but is difficult to scale.

Methods.—A malpractice insurer convened a collaborative with 4 Harvard-affiliated simulation programs to develop a standardized operating room teamwork training curriculum, including principles of communication, assertiveness, and use of the World Health Organization Surgical Safety Checklist. Participant teams were compensated for lost operative time via malpractice premium discounts, continuing education credits, and compensation for lost wages. The course was delivered through a simulation program involving the management of intraoperative emergency scenarios. Participants were surveyed for their perceptions of the program and of its impact on clinical practice.

Results.—A total of 221 active operating room staff members participated in the program. Each team contained at least 1 attending surgeon, 1 attending anesthesiologist, and 1 operating room nurse (mean size per team: 7 ± 2 participants). No study dates were cancelled because of lack of attendance. The survey response rate was 99% (218/221). Overall, the vast majority of participants found the scenarios realistic [94% (95% confidence interval: 90.9%, 97.2%)], appropriately challenging [95.4% (92.6%, 98.2%)], relevant to their practice [96.3% (93.8%, 98.8%)], and found the training would help them provide safer patient care [92.6% (89.1%, 96.1%)]. Surgeons reported their greatest personal deficit as communication skills. Operating room nurses and anesthesiologists reported a greater need than surgeons to work on personal assertiveness.

Conclusions.—A standardized multicenter team training program involving full operative teams is feasible with high-fidelity simulation and modest compensation for lost time. The vast majority of the multidisciplinary participants believed the course to have had a meaningful impact on their approach to clinical practice (Fig 3).

► The institution of surgical checklists in the operating room has undoubtedly improved communication and reduced errors. The checklists are designed to foster communication between operating room personnel and should engage the patient in the process. However, despite the widespread use of validated checklists, such as the World Health Organization Surgical Safety Checklist, these tools are too often used as rote lists that are quickly accomplished without

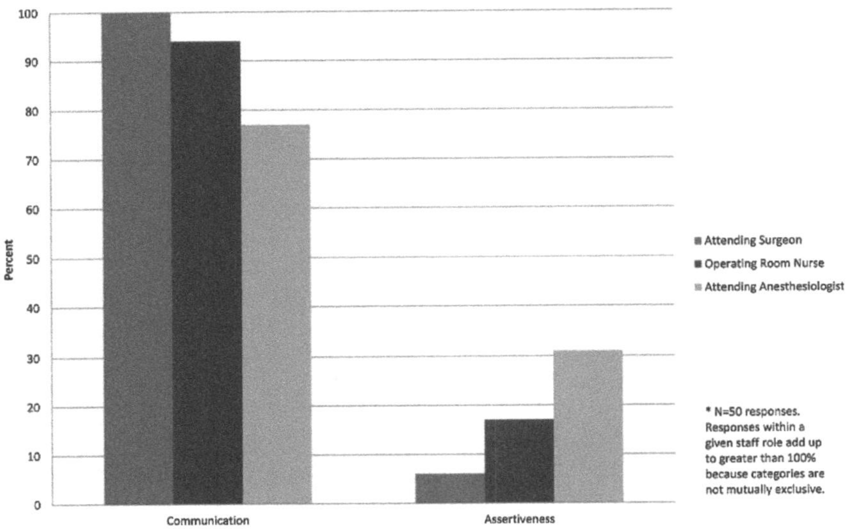

FIGURE 3.—Responses from attending surgeon, operating room nurses, and attending anesthesiologists regarding personal communication and/or assertiveness skills to improve. N = 50 responses. Responses within a given staff role add up to more than 100% because categories are not mutually exclusive. (Reprinted from Arriaga AF, for the Harvard Surgical Safety Collaborative. Pilot testing of a model for insurer-driven, large-scale multicenter simulation training for operating room teams. *Ann Surg.* 2014;259:403-410, Copyright 2014, with permission from Southeastern Surgical Congress.)

communication of patient-specific issues. Checklists alone will not foster teamwork in the operating room. To this end, Arriaga et al report an innovative approach to fostering teamwork in the operating room. Although team training has long been discussed, implementation for entire operating room teams has been infrequent. This study is intriguing in that it was largely driven and supported by the self-insurance program, and surgeon participants received a discount on the malpractice insurance premium. Additional incentives were offered to the surgeons, anesthesiologists, and operating room staff. As noted in the Results section, the engagement of the participants was spectacular. Also, not surprisingly, the results demonstrated that surgeons need to improve communication, whereas anesthesiologists and operating room personnel should be encouraged to be more assertive (Fig 3). The results of this study were so impressive that the institutional leaders and insurance providers have committed to a multimillion-dollar project to train more than 400 surgeons in the system. This is a model program for all institutions. The focus of teamwork in the operating room should be a primary impetus to improve patient care. The habit of superior teamwork will not evolve without practice, and team training is a must for all operating room teams.

K. E. Behrns, MD

The Value of Sharing Treatment Decision Making With Patients: Expecting Too Much?

Katz SJ, Hawley S (Univ of Michigan, Ann Arbor)

JAMA 2013 [Epub ahead of print]

Background.—Shared decision making (SDM) with patients is being emphasized to more fully engage patients and their families in determining the course of treatment. SDM is designed to fully inform patients and their families about treatment options and the risks and benefits that attend each one, while incorporating the patient's values and preferences into the final decision. The influence of SDM on the outcomes of clinical encounters must be understood to fully appreciate the implications of this course of action. Clinicians are ethically required to facilitate patient involvement in treatment decisions because patients and families are ultimately the ones who will be most affected. In addition, more engaged patients tend to be more informed, more likely to fully consider the risks and benefits of the various treatment options, and eventually more satisfied with the outcome. Recently SDM has been touted as a way to reduce overtreatment and excessive costs based on the view that more informed patients may be less likely to choose treatment more extensive than that which is recommended. Whether this is a reasonable expectation for SDM remains to be seen.

Evidence for SDM Reducing Overtreatment and Costs.—Analysis of the literature concerning the potential of SDM to reduce excessive treatment and cost factors shows several discrepancies. Seldom do studies pay sufficient attention to disentangling patient- from clinician-level effects in studies of interventions. Lack of clarity about patient versus clinician influences on utilization of treatment can lead to inaccurate conclusions. In addition, the complexity of how patients construct and express their preferences for treatment has not been considered sufficiently. A key objective of SDM is ensuring patients express their values, understand their values and incorporate those values into decisions regarding therapy. However, preference construction is a complex interplay between intuitive and deliberative mental processes. The stability of values and preferences over time when patients face various treatment experiences and choices is also unknown. There is no evidence supporting the view that patient preferences will inherently favor less extensive treatments than those recommended by physicians. Some studies even indicate that patients have unrealistically high standards that may prompt them to choose more extensive treatments. Finally, there is a wide variability in the clinical management context. Contributing factors include variations in evaluative test strategies with respect to patient preferences.

Challenges to SDM.—It can be difficult to achieve the goals of SDM. Patients have different preferences for their involvement in decision-making processes, and not much information indicates how to incorporate a desire for greater participation. Some patients may see the decision-making process as a burden, whereas others may seek increasingly more information. In addition, many clinicians are inadequately prepared to elicit patient values and preferences for treatment, so they cannot sufficiently implement SDM.

Conclusions.—Promoting SDM as a way to control overtreatment and rising health costs may be an improper direction to pursue. An "overselling" of SDM may produce expectations that cannot be met, undermining the adoption of SDM for effects that are supported by evidence.

▶ Patient-centric care is a major emphasis of numerous quality programs, and although it has many implications and meanings to different providers, a central tenet is patient engagement in the health care process. Traditionally, especially in surgical practices, decisions were rendered "top-down" from the surgeon to the patient with too little room for discussion. Fortunately, this has changed over the years as we have emphasized patient satisfaction and engagement. In this piece by Katz and Hawley, we learn about patient engagement and shared decision making as a mechanism to control costs. The assumption that patient involvement in decision making about expensive or invasive treatments will lead to enhanced patient scrutiny and increased likelihood that expensive treatments will not occur is not supported by a critical evaluation of the literature. Is this surprising? No; as surgeons who deal with critical and high-stakes decision making on a daily basis, we recognize the inherent difficulties in shared decision making. Although this process is laudable, we need to consider the patient with a new or recent diagnosis of severe disease. First, these patients are not equipped with the medical knowledge to make an informed decision, and no clinic visit of any duration will replace the surgeon's experiences in medical school, surgical training, and practice. Indeed, medical knowledge is a core competency for physicians, not patients. Second, a patient with a new diagnosis of a significant illness likely cannot emotionally separate the terrifying diagnosis from the proper treatment. Given these facts, how can we reasonably expect a patient to be an equal partner in shared decision making regarding an invasive treatment? Having said that, patient involvement and education are obviously necessary before embarking on a treatment with significant risks. This is why we have informed consent. The patient should feel completely comfortable providing written consent if they have appropriate involvement and education about the process. Although shared decision making is a goal of surgeon-patient interactions, we should not expect this process to be a cost-saving measure.

K. E. Behrns, MD

Impact of Medical Malpractice Environment on Surgical Quality and Outcomes

Minami CA, Chung JW, Holl JL, et al (Northwestern Univ, Chicago, IL)
J Am Coll Surg 218:271-278.e1-e9, 2014

Background.—The medical malpractice system was designed to spur practitioners to deliver excellent care and thereby avoid the threat of a malpractice suit. However, the system appears to generate many unintended consequences, such as defensive medicine, that leave the patient with poorer outcomes and unnecessary testing or treatment costs and inconveniences. Perceived high malpractice risk may lead practitioners to leave particular fields of medicine, which affects access to care and potentially patient outcomes as well. Surgical specialties are among those with higher proportions of malpractice claims. A systematic review was done to determine if there is an association between the malpractice environment and surgical specialty outcomes.

Methods.—A literature search of Medline, PubMed, and the Cochrane Database of Reviews of Effectiveness focused on original research articles written in English that were published between 1980 and 2012 in peer-reviewed journals, with the study performed in the United States. All had to demonstrate some link or lack thereof between the malpractice environment and physician practice or patient outcomes. Using the Preferred Reporting Items for Systematic Reviews and Meta-Analyses (PRISMA) checklist, the 29 studies selected were divided into those addressing the intended consequences of malpractice liability on physician practice or on patient outcomes and those focused on the unintended consequences of malpractice liability on physician practice or on patient outcomes.

Results.—None of the studies directly tested whether malpractice risk was associated with physician adherence to standards of care or changes in national measures of quality of care or patient safety. Physicians' perception of malpractice pressures produced a measurable effect on their treatment decisions. Defensive medicine tactics were often chosen in certain specialties, such as obstetrics, that had a high risk of malpractice suits. In obstetrics, physicians tended to intervene sooner or more often and encouraged women not to deliver vaginally after a previous cesarean delivery. It was difficult to compare studies because there tended to be surveys and empirical assessments focused on specific subsets of physicians.

No studies addressed the intended consequences of the malpractice system increasing adherence to standards of care. In addition, it was unclear whether there was any beneficial effect on patient outcomes.

Conclusions.—Some evidence indicates that physicians may allow the malpractice system to influence their clinical choices. However, there is no evidence supporting the assumption that working under the threat of a malpractice suit increases the physician's adherence to quality care indicators or improves patient outcomes.

▶ Conscientious surgeons, likely more than 95% of all surgeons, require few incentives to provide the best care to each patient. Through rigorous training and long-held practices of morbidity and mortality presentations and peer review, surgeons are imprinted with the desire to optimize patient care. However, for 5% of the population of surgeons, we have a medical malpractice system that greatly influences surgeon and patient approaches to care. Is medical malpractice a deterrent to bad medicine? Minami et al attempt to answer this question through a systematic review of the literature. Of note, it appears that their preference would have been to address their research questions by conducting a meta-analysis through pooling of data. However, the heterogeneity of the reports in the literature precluded such an analysis. This deviation from the desired approach is the most important message in the report; we have too little data and poorly orchestrated information related to our medical malpractice system to thoroughly study it. Thus, the lessons learned from this report, although important, need to be put into the context of limited information on the subject. Indeed, the authors highlight the absence of reliable information and emphasize the need for further investigation. However, this work does contain several important messages. First, there is a paucity of evidence that medical malpractice acts as a sufficient deterrent to improve patient care. Second, the perception, by physicians, that medical malpractice alters the approach to care, creating a defensive approach, is real. Our entire health care system suffers from the current approach of medical malpractice. Patients, physicians, and payers should work together with our legal system to adequately study malpractice and devise a system that is centered on excellent outcomes at reasonable costs.

K. E. Behrns, MD

It's Big Surgery: Preoperative Expressions of Risk, Responsibility, and Commitment to Treatment After High-Risk Operations

Pecanac KE, Kehler JM, Brasel KJ, et al (Univ of Wisconsin, Madison; Med College of Wisconsin, Milwaukee; et al)

Ann Surg 259:458-463, 2014

Objective.—To identify the processes, surgeons use to establish patient buy-in to postoperative treatments.

Background.—Surgeons generally believe they confirm the patient's commitment to an operation and all ensuing postoperative care, before surgery. How surgeons get buy-in and whether patients participate in this agreement is unknown.

Methods.—We used purposive sampling to identify 3 surgeons from different subspecialties who routinely perform high-risk operations at each of 3 distinct medical centers (Toronto, Ontario; Boston, Massachusetts; Madison, Wisconsin). We recorded preoperative conversations with 3 to 7 patients facing high-risk surgery with each surgeon ($n = 48$) and used content analysis to analyze each preoperative conversation inductively.

Results.—Surgeons conveyed the gravity of high-risk operations to patients by emphasizing the operation is "big surgery" and that a decision to proceed invoked a serious commitment for both the surgeon and the patient. Surgeons were frank about the potential for serious complications and the need for intensive care. They rarely discussed the use of prolonged life-supporting treatment, and patients' questions were primarily confined to logistic or technical concerns. Surgeons regularly proceeded through the conversation in a manner that suggested they believed buy-in was achieved, but this agreement was rarely forged explicitly.

Conclusions.—Surgeons who perform high-risk operations communicate the risks of surgery and express their commitment to the patient's survival. However, they rarely discuss prolonged life-supporting treatments explicitly and patients do not discuss their preferences. It is not possible to determine patients' desires for prolonged postoperative life support on the basis of these preoperative conversations alone.

▶ Few points in time in the care of a patient are more important than the preoperative discussion about the risks of an operation. For all its importance, we do not teach this well or even discuss it much in our training programs. It's not a surprise that patients sometimes feel poorly informed, and families are surprised when complications arise and significant interventions are necessary to treat these untoward events. However, Pecanac et al have shed light on this subject with an ingenious, technologic approach to determining the content and structure as well as the important tenets of the preoperative discussion. The preoperative discussion is a delicate discussion that should provide evidence-based information in language that is readily understood by the patient; thus, the statement "big surgery." Although this report makes huge strides in bringing this discussion into focus, it is surprising that many of the quotes depict a much generalized discussion. Why are we not using data and quoting national or personal mortality rates? We should tell patients undergoing a Whipple procedure that the complication rate is approximately 50%. The patient and family should be presented the best- and worst-case scenarios. We need to give patients and families realistic expectations about the outcomes, and we have plenty of data. In my experience, patients understand these numbers, although the surgeon must phrase these statistics several ways. Finally, the authors' orientation as critical care specialists places appropriate emphasis on the discussion of life support, but other equally important, nonlethal unanticipated consequences, such as life-altering changes in gastrointestinal function and diet, should be considered and discussed. The preoperative discussion of risks is much more than a process of informed consent—it is the time to develop a bond of trust between the patient and surgeon.

K. E. Behrns, MD

Bridging the Gap from T to K: Integrated Surgical Research Fellowship for the Next Generation of Surgical Scientists

Moore HB, Moore EE, Nehler MR, et al (Univ of Colorado, Aurora)

J Am Coll Surg 218:279-282, 2014

Background.—Fewer than 2% of physicians choose research as their primary pursuit. The numbers of physician-scientists have been declining, leading the National Institutes of Health (NIH) and academic medical societies to seek ways to recruit and train more of them. A restructuring of surgical research fellowships was proposed to bridge the gap between aspiring academicians and independently funded surgical scientists. This requires recognizing the barriers to training in addition to coming up with new ways to entice clinicians to take on this area of specialization.

Barriers.—To understand disease processes and develop the technical skills to provide patient care requires intense, prolonged commitments of time. With the increasing numbers of older patients, advanced disease and more comorbidities are being seen. Technologic advances, increased specialization to manage complex clinical care demands, and the explosion of medical knowledge have created the need for multidisciplinary research teams. New faculty members want and require the ability to become independently comfortable with their clinical and surgical skills while earning a salary. As a result, the time to devote to research becomes scarcer, with the distinct possibility that the research will be interrupted or suspended. Senior faculty tend to spend more time in administrative tasks and compete for research efforts. Academic surgeons struggle to establish and maintain independent funding for their projects. As a result, it seems logical that training residents to balance clinical and research activities will help prepare for these real-life situations.

Training.—Currently surgeons train clinically for 5 years with 2 to 3 years of interruption to provide protected research time. Trainees often do not achieve research independence in this structure, it is difficult to stay current, and juggling clinical and research endeavors becomes a significant challenge. This research education tends to be unstructured and informal, and no board certification examinations test research skills. Internationally, residents are expected to obtain an advanced degree during their time away from clinical duties, and those who do so tend to have higher productivity and academic achievements. Continuous protected research would maximize scientific study, but does not teach the skills of grantsmanship or juggling clinical and research duties.

Alternatives have been proposed. One suggestion is to recognize that there are differences in the interests of surgical residents who are pursuing research fellowships and structure programs accordingly. The characteristics and ambitions of the candidate should be matched to the specific branch of academic pursuit early in the process. The training for surgical scientists should emphasize core grantsmanship training, integration with clinical duties, collaboration, and continuity of research. Two residents alternative between the basic science laboratory and clinical rotations in 12-month blocks over the course of a 4-year fellowship. They work collaboratively with the same principal investigator on the same projects to ensure research continuity and develop team skills. Both complete their American Board of Surgery-n-required clinical rotations, complete research projects and publishable papers, and obtain a Master of Science in Clinical Science (MSCS) degree. A development grant must be submitted within 1 year of completing the fellowship, but it is not expected to be successful on the first try. However, the feedback from the process provides educational insight.

Conclusions.—Surgical scientists are becoming older and fewer in number, making recruitment of young men and women to academia an important goal. Research guided by surgeons who have few research skills can risk the development of "paralyzed academic investigator disease syndrome," with no creative approach to solving problems and an inability to form and establish a highly functioning interdisciplinary team–which is essential to manage the complex health care scenarios of patients. Training surgeon scientists during residency training seems to be a logical step.

▶ Academic surgery departments and their faculty face many pressures, many of which are economic in origin, and in response to these financial pressures, the focus has been on the revenue-generating clinical practice. Unfortunately, the research and education missions tend to take a back seat, with the research mission often neglected because regulatory agencies do not review academic research programs like educational agencies scrutinize surgical training programs. The lack of focus on research has resulted in decreased research training and, subsequently, research funding. To address integration of research training into clinical programs, Moore et al propose a new training program in a research fellowship. The concept of integration of research training and clinical training is a novel and needed paradigm shift. Research-intensive universities must train the next generation of surgical scientists if clinical translational research is a major goal of institutional academic practices. Obviously, the necessary resources must be invested in surgical research training programs regardless of the needs of other research-intensive departments at academic medical centers. Although surgeons must compete for these resources, surgery departments must be funded to reach the full potential not only of the surgery department but also the university. It is no surprise that the best research universities generally have well-funded surgery departments. To continue to grow academically, we must forge new models of research training, and this model, although potentially institutionally unique, is a major step in the right direction.

K. E. Behrns, MD

Comparison of Registered and Published Primary Outcomes in Randomized Clinical Trials of Surgical Interventions

Hannink G, Gooszen HG, Rovers MM (Radboud Univ Nijmegen Med Ctr, The Netherlands)
Ann Surg 257:818-823, 2013

Objective.—To assess the proportion of registered surgical trials with results published in journals with high-impact factors; compare the primary outcomes specified in trial registries with those reported in the published papers; and determine whether primary outcome-reporting bias favored significant outcomes.

Background.—Outcome-reporting bias, that is, the selective reporting of a subset of the original registered outcome measures based on their results, has not yet been studied specifically for surgical trials.

Methods.—We searched PubMed for reports of surgical randomized controlled trials (RCTs) indexed between 2007 and 2012 in 10 general medical journals and 10 surgical journals with the highest impact factors.

TABLE 4.—Discrepancies Between Primary Outcomes in Trial Registration and Published Studies With Trial Registration Mentioned in Paper, and Discrepancies Favoring Significant Outcomes of the 152 Papers Registered Before the End the Trial

	All	General Medical Journals	Surgical Journals
No. papers, n (%)	152 (100)	88 (57.9)	64 (42.1)
Number of papers with discrepancies between trial registration and publication, n (%)	75 (49.3)	36 (40.9)	39 (60.9)
Registered primary outcome reported as secondary outcome in text*	8 (5.3)	1 (1.1)	7 (10.9)
Registered primary outcome omitted in text*	32 (21.1)	18 (20.5)	14 (21.9)
New primary outcome introduced in text*	24 (15.8)	14 (15.9)	10 (15.6)
Published primary outcome described as secondary outcome in registry*	14 (9.2)	5 (5.7)	9 (14.1)
Different timing of assessment of primary outcome*	9 (5.9)	4 (4.5)	5 (7.8)
Papers with discrepancies in primary outcome favoring statistically significant results, n (%)	21 (28.0)	9 (25.0)	12 (30.8)

*Numbers represent the number of papers with at least 1 primary outcome with a discrepancy. Note that some papers reported more than one primary outcome (Table 3). Percentages were calculated from the total number of papers registered before the end of the trial.

For each article included, we obtained the trial registration information using a standardized data extraction form.

Results.—Of the 327 evaluated surgical trials, registration was lacking for 109 (33%) published papers. Two (2%) of these papers were published in general medical journals and 107 (98%) in surgical journals. Twelve (6%) of the trials were still recruiting patients, and 48 (22%) were registered after completion of the study. A total of 152 trials were registered before the end of the trial with the primary outcome clearly specified. Among these papers, 49% (75 of 152) showed some evidence of discrepancies between outcomes registered and the outcomes published, most often related to omitting or introducing a primary outcome. These discrepancies favored statistically significant results in 28% of the papers.

Conclusions.—The quality of registration of surgical trials published in surgical journals was inferior to those published in general medical journals. Comparison of the primary outcomes of surgical RCTs registered with their subsequent publication indicated that selective outcome reporting is prevalent and appears to be higher than in general medical trials (Table 4).

► Meticulously performed clinical trials in medicine are the Holy Grail for determining effective treatments for patients. As such, substantial rigor has been placed around the conduct of clinical trials, including registering the trial before initiation as a precondition to publication. These rules were adopted by medical and surgical journals shortly after their inception in 2005. Compliance with these rules, however, has been a subject of debate. In this study, Hannink et al reviewed compliance with the policies of publishing clinical trials in each of the top 10 journals in the disciplines of medicine and surgery and found several deficiencies in the system. First, one-third of the studies were not registered, with nearly all of these missed registrations published in surgical journals. In addition, 22% of the trials were registered after the trial was conducted, which, again, is a more common occurrence in surgical journals. Most importantly, an astonishing 49% of the trials showed some evidence of outcome reporting bias—that is, the results reported in the study were not necessarily those outcomes that were intended to be reported at the time of trial registration (Table 4). Again, this finding was more common in surgical rather than medical journals. The authors concluded that despite widespread acceptance of the policies related to publication of clinical trials, surgical journals aren't as effective as medical journals in registration of trials, and, importantly, selective outcome reporting is prevalent, especially in surgical journals. This report is a bit sobering, but it offers the challenge of improving compliance and transparency. Investigators conducting clinical trials and reviewers and editors alike should take heed of this publication and work diligently for accurate reporting of results. It is not surprising that the results of a clinical trial may not be as predicted; however, we need to present the trial results as registered so that we can conduct further studies with the appropriate primary outcome variables.

K. E. Behrns, MD

The randomized registry trial—the next disruptive technology in clinical research?

Lauer MS, D'Agostino RB Sr (Natl Heart, Lung, and Blood Inst, Bethesda, MD; Boston Univ, MA)

N Engl J Med 369:1579-1581, 2013

The randomized trial is one of the most powerful tools clinical researchers possess, a tool that enables them to evaluate the effectiveness of new (or established) therapies while accounting for the effects of unmeasured confounders and selection bias by indication. Randomized trials, especially huge megatrials, have transformed medical practice. Thanks to randomized trials, we no longer, for example, treat acute myocardial infarction with lidocaine and nitrates. Instead we use rapid revascularization, anticoagulants, and antiplatelet agents, and during long-term follow-up we routinely prescribe statins, beta-blockers, and angiotensin-converting—enzyme inhibitors. But the reputation of randomized trials has suffered of late, 1 owing to reasonable concern about excess complexity, expense, and time required to recruit study participants, as well as inadequate representativeness. What good are trials if the results aren't applicable to real-world patients and if, because of excessive expense, they can be used to answer only a tiny fraction of our important clinical questions?

▶ Lauer and D'Agostino provide an outstanding review of a new approach to clinical research—a randomized registry trial. As the authors point out, the gold standard for clinical research—the randomized trial—has nearly priced itself out of existence. Certainly, most investigators or institutions do not have the wherewithal to conduct first-rate randomized clinical trials, which may cost several hundred thousand or even millions of dollars. Even the National Institutes of Health, with its limited dollars, must be selective about the clinical trials that are funded, and this is in the era of comparative effectiveness research! It seems counterintuitive that clinical researchers cannot harness the power of big data that are collected during the course of patient care. However, the article by Fröbert et al[1] published in the *New England Journal of Medicine* discusses the use of registry data. This approach substantially reduced the costs of this megatrial and allowed rapid dissemination of important data related to the care of patients with myocardial infarction. It is important to note that use of registries is becoming commonplace not only in clinical research but also in clinical care. The American College of Surgeons' development of the Surgeon Specific Registry to track quality outcomes for individual practitioners is an example of a clinical care and quality registry. As the electronic medical record is further disseminated across medical practices and software development permits culling of the medical record for data points, registries will become more common. As clinical practitioners we will need to be forward thinking about development and use of the medical record and disciplined about entry of information so the output of registry data is complete and accurate.

K. E. Behrns, MD

Reference

1. Fröbert O, Lagerqvist B, Olivecrona GK, et al. Thrombus aspiration during ST-segment elevation myocardial infarction. *N Engl J Med.* 2013;369:1587-1597.

Black patients more likely than whites to undergo surgery at low-quality hospitals in segregated regions

Dimick J, Ruhter J, Sarrazin MV, et al (Univ of Michigan, Ann Arbor)
Health Aff (Millwood) 32:1046-1053, 2013

Research has shown that black patients more frequently undergo surgery at low-quality hospitals than do white patients. We assessed the extent to which living in racially segregated areas and living in geographic proximity to low-quality hospitals contribute to this disparity. Using national Medicare data for all patients who underwent one of three high-risk surgical procedures in 2005-08, we found that black patients actually tended to live closer to higher-quality hospitals than white patients did but were 25-58 percent more likely than whites to receive surgery at low-quality hospitals. Racial segregation was also a factor, with black patients in the most segregated areas 41-96 percent more likely than white patients to undergo surgery at low-quality hospitals. To address these disparities, care navigators and public reporting of comparative quality could steer patients and their referring physicians to higher-quality hospitals, while quality improvement efforts could focus on improving outcomes for high-risk surgery at hospitals that disproportionately serve black patients. Unfortunately, existing policies such as pay-for-performance, bundled payments, and nonpayment for adverse events may divert resources and exacerbate these disparities.

▶ The Affordable Care Act has sharpened the focus on the availability of health care and the necessity to have access to care before patients can receive high-quality care. Often, it is presumed that patients who receive no care or low-quality care have limited access. However, Dimick et al show that the issue is more complex. In a study designed to determine if black patients undergoing surgery have access to and use high-quality health care centers, they showed that black patients are more likely than white patients to have surgery at low-quality hospitals. Surely, this must be related to poor access to high-quality hospitals, right? Surprisingly, black patients live closer to high-quality hospitals than white patients, but they chose to drive past these high-quality hospitals to have surgery at low-quality hospitals. While education of the patient and the referring physician regarding the quality of surgical care may impact the use of high- vs low-quality hospitals, likely this strategy would result in little change. Policy changes are also unlikely to favor low-quality hospitals. What are the solutions? First, as a medical community we should strive to convert low-quality surgical hospitals to at least average-quality hospitals. In addition, high-quality hospitals should have a sense of community within their walls that welcomes black patients. We need to recognize the uniqueness of our varying populations of patients and address their needs so that all patients choose to access high-quality surgical hospitals.

K. E. Behrns, MD

Distributions of Industry Payments to Massachusetts Physicians

Kesselheim AS, Robertson CT, Siri K, et al (Brigham and Women's Hosp and Harvard Med School, Boston, MA; Kyruus, Boston, MA; Edmond J. Safra Ctr for Ethics at Harvard Univ, Cambridge, MA)

N Engl J Med 368:2049-2052, 2013

Some states have mandated systematic public disclosure of payments made by drug- and device-makers to health care practitioners. We used Massachusetts data to characterize the distribution of payment types and the variation among medical specialties. The 30 months' of data included 32,227 reported payments to 11,734 Massachusetts physicians, for a total of $76.7 million. The most common form of payment was food. Compensation for bona fide services was the payment type with the highest value. We found that 25% of currently licensed Massachusetts physicians received at least one payment during the study period. Prevalence ranged by specialties from pediatricians (12%) and family practitioners (21%) to urologists (61%) and gastroenterologists (57%). The highest average per-physician amounts were received by orthopedic surgeons ($18,446) and

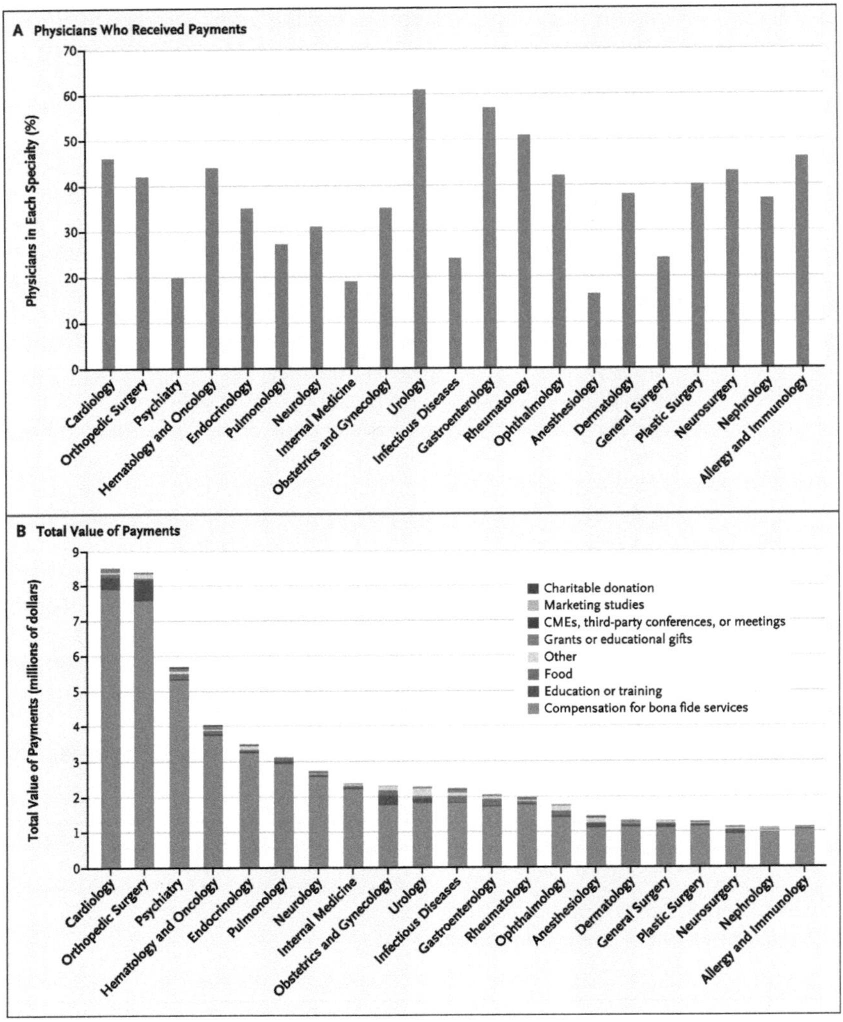

FIGURE.—Percentages of All Licensed Massachusetts Physicians in Each Specialty Who Received Payments (Panel A) and Total Value of Payments Received by Such Physicians, According to Specialty (Panel B), 2009–2011. Data include only those specialties registering total payments of more than $1 million. (Reprinted from Kesselheim AS, Robertson CT, Siri K, et al. Distributions of Industry payments to Massachusetts physicians. *N Engl J Med.* 2013;368:2049-2052, © 2013, Massachusetts Medical Society.)

physicians in various specialties within internal medicine, including endocrinology ($17,407), infectious diseases ($15,922), and pulmonology ($13,027). The policy implications are briefly discussed (Fig).

▶ The last decade has seen a marked increase in awareness of industry payments to physicians, and most academic institutions have developed conflict-of-interest programs that tightly monitor the association between industry and faculty members. In many cases, these efforts were warranted as physicians received exorbitant payments for services that were either nonexistent or had value far less than the reimbursement. However, relationships between physicians and biomedical scientists and industry have much to offer in terms of new discoveries and the conduct of clinical trials. Thus, conflict should be managed rather than avoided. Transparency of relationships between industry and physicians is important, and the federal Physician Payment Sunshine Act began with industry collecting data on August 1, 2013, and reporting it to the Center for Medicare and Medicaid Services by March 31, 2014. This database will identify physicians that have received payments from industry, perhaps as little as $50. What might this database reveal? Kesselheim et al provide a snapshot of industry involvement with physicians when they reviewed the Massachusetts database. The information in this database details the physicians by specialty, the payment, and the reason for the reimbursement. Trends over time are also noted; that is, for example, reimbursement for meals has decreased recently because most physicians are not allowed to accept food from industry. Nonetheless, the Fig in the article shows that most of the services rendered by physicians were bona fide but that the money involved is real—nearly $77 million in 30 months. About 25% of general surgeons received money from industry, and this figure appears to be about the mean across medical specialties. However, the dollars paid to general surgeons was relatively low and nearly all for bona fide services. Surgeons should be aware of the Federal Sunshine Act because all industry spending on physicians will be publicly reported.

K. E. Behrns, MD

An Interactive Individualized Intervention to Promote Behavioral Change to Increase Personal Well-Being in US Surgeons

Shanafelt TD, Kaups KL, Nelson H, et al (Mayo Clinic, Rochester, MN; Univ of California, San Francisco Fresno; et al)

Ann Surg 259:82-88, 2014

Objective.—Evaluate the utility of a computer-based, interactive, and individualized intervention for promoting well-being in US surgeons.

Background.—Distress and burnout are common among US surgeons. Surgeons experiencing distress are unlikely to seek help on their own initiative. A belief that distress and burnout are a normal part of being a physician and lack of awareness of distress level relative to colleagues may contribute to this problem.

Methods.—Surgeons who were members of the American College of Surgeons were invited to participate in an intervention study. Participating surgeons completed a 3-step, interactive, electronic intervention. First, surgeons subjectively assessed their well-being relative to colleagues. Second, surgeons completed the 7-item Mayo Clinic Physician Well-Being Index and received objective, individualized feedback about their well-being relative to national physician norms. Third, surgeons evaluated the

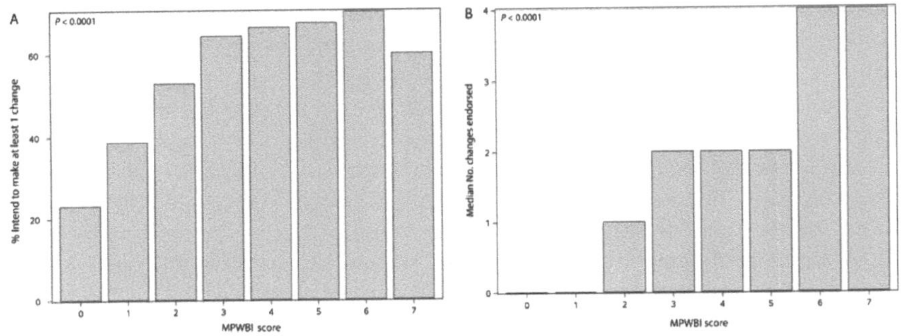

FIGURE 4.—MPWBI score and intent to make changes. MPWBI scores are shown on the x axis (higher scores indicate greater levels of distress) of each figure. A, The proportion of surgeons who indicated they were considering making changes in at least 1 of the 4 dimensions assessed (Fig. 3) as a direct result of the individualized feedback they received is shown on the y axis. B, The median number of changes (range = 1–4) being considered is shown on the y axis. MPWBI indicates Mayo Physician Well-Being Index. (Reprinted from Shanafelt TD, Kaups KL, Nelson H, et al. An interactive individualized intervention to promote behavioral change to increase personal well-being in US surgeons. *Ann Surg.* 2014;259:82-88, Copyright 2014, with permission from Southeastern Surgical Congress.)

usefulness of the feedback and whether they intended to make specific changes as a result.

Results.—A total of 1150 US surgeons volunteered to participate in the study. Surgeons' subjective assessment of their well-being relative to colleagues was poor. A majority of surgeons (89.2%) believed that their well-being was at or above average, including 70.5% with scores in the bottom 30% relative to national norms. After receiving objective, individualized feedback based on the Mayo Clinic Physician Well-Being Index score, 46.6% of surgeons indicated that they intended to make specific changes as a result. Surgeons with lower well-being scores were more likely to make changes in each dimension assessed (all Ps < 0.001).

Conclusions.—US surgeons do not reliably calibrate their level of distress. After self-assessment and individualized feedback using the Mayo Clinic Physician Well-Being Index, half of participating surgeons reported that they were contemplating behavioral changes to improve personal well-being (Fig 4).

▶ Surgeon well-being has been a topic of keen interest in recent years because a series of studies supported by the American College of Surgeons suggests that the level of surgeon distress is significant. Up to 45% of surgeons experience burnout, or the syndrome of emotional exhaustion and depersonalization that leads to decreased effectiveness at work, which, not surprisingly, may lead to medical errors. Likely, much of the increased surgeon distress is related to the pressure to have increased productivity to compensate for the decreased reimbursement per unit of work. Although surgeon burnout has been studied in aggregate through relatively complex assessments, the opportunities to study burnout through a straightforward mechanism have been limited. However, Shanafelt et al used the Mayo Physician Well-Being Index in 1150 US surgeons to provide an assessment of distress and to determine the likelihood that the findings of the assessment would be addressed through intervention. The results showed that surgeons are poor self-judges of distress. Over two-thirds of surgeons with scores indicating significant distress thought that their well-being was above average. In addition, after feedback from the computerized assessment, nearly one-half of surgeons indicated that they would contemplate changes in behavior (Fig 4). This is the surprise of the study—less than one-half of surgeons would make changes even though the assessment indicated distress! One has to ask if the surgeons who were not contemplating changes were so despondent that they deemed changes hopeless. Clearly, as a surgical community, we need to look after one another and ask each other how we can be of assistance. Please accept the challenge of looking after your colleagues.

K. E. Behrns, MD

2 Trauma

Laparoscopic radiofrequency ablation for traumatic splenic rupture
Li Y, Cui L, Zhang W, et al (Suining Central Hosp, Sichuan, China)
J Surg Res 185:711-716, 2013

Background.—Laparotomy was formerly the routine approach for treating traumatic splenic rupture. Traumatic splenic rupture has traditionally been treated with open splenectomy. The advent of laparoscopy and radiofrequency ablation (RFA) has ushered in new approaches to this surgical problem. The purpose of this study was to evaluate the use of laparoscopic RFA to treat traumatic splenic rupture.

Methods.—Four patients with traumatic splenic ruptures underwent laparoscopic RFA-assisted spleen-preserving surgery between September 2011 and April 2012. RFA electrodes were used for traumatic rupture repair or partial splenectomies using classic laparoscopic procedures. Safety and efficacy parameters were documented, including surgery time, intraoperative blood loss, postoperative drainage quantities, and recovery conditions.

Results.—Three patients received laparoscopic splenic rupture repair and one patient received a partial splenectomy. Three surgeries were successful, based on 1-mo follow-up with computerized tomography and ultrasound examinations that indicated the restoration of satisfactory splenic blood supply. The fourth patient received a laparotomy for a total splenectomy because of massive postoperative bleeding 24 h after surgery.

Conclusions.—Laparoscopic RFA-assisted spleen-preserving surgery is another modality that may be considered in the management of splenic trauma. This small sample size and limited clinical experience does not justify its use on a routine basis and requires additional clinical research to fully evaluate its efficacy in certain critical traumatic scenarios compared with traditional open splenectomy.

► Partial splenectomy is considered to be preferable to total splenectomy when feasible, and preservation of at least 25% of the spleen may ensure adequate splenic function. Therefore, spleen-preserving surgeries are of clinical significance for maximizing patient safety. This selection was chosen, as it represents a novel approach to dealing with splenic injury. The authors showed the feasibility of radiofrequency ablation (RFA)-assisted laparoscopic splenectomy for selected patients with traumatic splenic rupture. Laparoscopic RFA-assisted spleen-preserving surgery is another modality that may be considered in the management of splenic trauma. Splenic salvage is preferred, and this method adds another minimally invasive technique to accomplish this goal.

The small sample size and limited clinical experience does not justify its use on a routine basis and requires additional clinical research to fully evaluate its efficacy in certain critical traumatic scenarios compared with that of traditional open splenectomy. One would need to compare results of this technique with those of selective embolization to determine if a benefit exists.

D. W. Mozingo, MD

Clinical Outcome After Vertebral Artery Injury Following Blunt Cervical Spine Trauma

Mitha AP, Kalb S, Ribas-Nijkerk JC, et al (St. Joseph's Hosp and Med Ctr, Phoenix, AZ)

World Neurosurg 80:399-404, 2013

Objective.—Imaging after blunt cervical trauma is being used increasingly to screen patients for injury of the vertebral artery (VA). There are no guidelines for imaging of the VA for nonpenetrating cervical trauma. The purpose of this study was to determine the effect of VA injury on clinical outcome after blunt cervical trauma.

Methods.—Sixty-six patients who underwent computed tomographic angiography (CTA) and magnetic resonance angiography (MRA) after blunt cervical trauma were reviewed. Medical records were reviewed for clinical status, including the presence of a neurologic deficit or pain related to spine or vascular injury. Any suggested brain injury was evaluated with diffusion-weighted MR imaging. Both clinical and radiographic data were analyzed to determine the incidence of VA abnormalities and their association with clinical outcome.

Results.—VA abnormalities were present in 19.7% of cases. Two patients had symptomatic brain sequelae from VA injury. There was no significant association between VA abnormalities and the presence of symptoms and/or cervical spine fractures at presentation. The presence of a fracture and neurologic symptoms at presentation predicted a significantly worse outcome at a mean follow-up of 5 months. However, the presence of VA abnormalities did not predict a worse clinical outcome.

Conclusions.—The clinical outcome of patients with blunt cervical trauma was not associated with the presence of VA abnormalities. Given the rare but potentially devastating consequences of a VA injury, however, screening may still be worthwhile.

▶ Arterial injury in the setting of blunt cervical spine injury is common, and vertebral artery injury is more common than injury to the carotid arteries. Angiographically, vertebral artery injury can manifest as dissections, pseudoaneurysms, and arterial occlusions. Because of the potential for devastating neurologic injury related to these lesions and because access to noninvasive angiographic imaging techniques and faster imaging protocols has improved, screening for vertebral artery injury in the setting of blunt cervical trauma has increased. The utility of screening for injury, however, is questionable, partly because the incidence of vertebral artery injury is unclear. Furthermore, vertebral artery injuries are rarely symptomatic. Even selecting patients with a high clinical suspicion of vertebral artery injury and subjecting them to a radiographic evaluation yields meager results. Even more controversial is whether screening patients with cervical spine trauma for vertebral artery injury improves their overall outcome. This uncertainty is primarily because the natural history of traumatic vertebral artery injury has not been established. Similarly, the benefit of treatment for traumatic cervical arterial injuries is not well studied. In recent years, the prophylactic use of antiplatelet agents for the treatment of asymptomatic vertebral artery dissections and systemic anticoagulation for ischemic symptoms has been advocated, largely based on empirical evidence. The major impetus for screening patients with these injuries, however, has been to avoid unexpected deterioration along with its associated medicolegal implications in those patients who might otherwise have had an excellent functional outcome.

D. W. Mozingo, MD

Triage of Elderly Trauma Patients: A Population-Based Perspective

Staudenmayer KL, Hsia RY, Mann NC, et al (Stanford Univ, CA; Univ of California San Francisco; Univ of Utah, Salt Lake City; et al)

J Am Coll Surg 217:569-576, 2013

Background.—Elderly patients are frequently undertriaged. However, the associations between triage patterns and outcomes from a population perspective are unknown. We hypothesized that triage patterns would be associated with differences in outcomes.

Study Design.—This is a population-based, retrospective, cohort study of all injured adults aged 55 years or older, from 3 counties in California and 4 in Utah (2006 to 2007). Prehospital data were linked to trauma registry data, state-level discharge data, emergency department records, and death files. The primary outcome was 60-day mortality. Patients treated at trauma centers were compared with those treated at nontrauma centers. Undertriage was defined as an Injury Severity Score (ISS) >15, with transport to a nontrauma center.

Results.—There were 6,015 patients in the analysis. Patients who were taken to nontrauma centers were, on average, older (79.4 vs 70.7 years, $p < 0.001$), more often female (68.6% vs 50.2%, $p < 0.01$), and less often had an ISS >15 (2.2% vs 6.7%, $p < 0.01$). There were 244 patients with an ISS >15 and the undertriage rate was 32.8% (n = 80). Overall 60-day mortality for patients with an ISS >15 was 17%, with no difference between trauma and nontrauma centers in unadjusted or adjusted analyses. However, the median per-patient costs were $21,000 higher for severely injured patients taken to trauma centers.

Conclusions.—This is the first population-based analysis of triage patterns and outcomes in the elderly. We have shown high rates of undertriage that are not associated with higher mortality, but are associated with higher costs. Future work should focus on determining how to improve outcomes for this population.

▶ As geriatric injuries are increasing in frequency, there is evidence that care could be improved for these patients. Even with minor injuries, it is well known that there is at least a 2- to 5-fold increase in mortality compared with the younger population with similar injury severity. Although some of this is likely because of the higher rate of comorbidities in the elderly, it also may be because elderly patients with severe injuries are frequently undertriaged and less frequently referred to trauma centers. Age has been found to be inversely correlated with admission to a trauma center, even when controlling for injury, patient, and geographic factors. With the country's aging population, it is important to understand and address the patterns of injury and outcomes of these patients. The current body of literature and this study certainly suggest opportunities for improvement in care of the injured elderly population. Further study is required to determine what interventions may be beneficial to the elderly, such as specialized geriatric hospitalist services. We also need to better understand the determinants of mortality in the less severely injured older patient. Future work exploring this topic will require the use of databases designed to capture functional status, frailty, and comorbidities in this population.

D. W. Mozingo, MD

Analysis of remote trauma transfers in South Central Texas with comparison with current US combat operations: Results of the RemTORN-I study

Gerhardt RT, Koller AR, Rasmussen TE, et al (Brooke Army Med Ctr, Fort Sam Houston, TX; Univ of North Texas Med Ctr, Fort Worth, TX; US Army Inst of Surgical Res, San Antonio, TX; et al)

J Trauma Acute Care Surg 75:S164-S168, 2013

Background.—This study aimed to analyze demographic, epidemiologic, temporal, and outcome data from an integrated trauma registry of patients undergoing initial stabilization and transfer within a mature domestic trauma network; compare data with a companion subset from the Department of Defense Trauma Registry. Texas Trauma Service Area-P is composed of 25 counties, 15 rural Level IV trauma centers (no acute care surgery), and two Level I trauma centers.

Methods.—This study has a retrospective cohort design. We hypothesize that Injury Severity Scores (ISSs), time intervals, and other clinical indicators would be complimentary to contemporary combat casualties. Inclusion criteria include age 18 years to 80 years, transferred from Level IV to Level I trauma center, or expired en route.

Results.—A total of 543 subjects (84%) met the criteria and were analyzed. Averages and confidence intervals were as follows: age of 40 years (38–41 years), males at 81%, ISS of 10 (10–11), intensive care unit stay of 2 days (1–3 days), and hospital stay of 5 days (4–6 days).

Mechanisms of injury were as follows: penetrating (15%), blunt weapon (19%), stabs (9%), burns (5%), and gunshots (5%). Eight percent received blood within the first 24 hours. Survival was at 98%. Time intervals (95% confidence interval) were as follows: prehospital at 1:43 (1:29–1:58), Level IV dwell time at 3:17 (3:06–3:28), interfacility transfer at 1:43 (1:36–1:49), and total at 6:39 (6:20–6:58). RemTORN cases were older, spent longer time en route to Level I, and had ISS similar to combat casualties. Rates of blood transfusion in the first 24 hours and survival were similar in order of magnitude.

Conclusion.—The RemTORN platform is operational. Demographic, epidemiologic, and temporal characteristics as observed will support clinical investigations of traumatic coagulopathy, shock, and potential interventions before Level I arrival. Results of such investigations will likely be applicable to the contemporary and future battlefield.

▶ The RemTORN model described in this selection represents a currently functioning military-civilian prehospital research model. The RemTORN model has many features that have the potential to mitigate bias and confounding variables to support the study of prehospital interventions and processes. Also, this model provides unique and important insight into the interplay of prehospital circumstance and intervention. If this model is allowed to mature to its potential, it stands to improve the military's ability to develop the next generation of lifesaving interventions for combatants and domestic patients of trauma. This study characterizes injury patterns, severity of injury, and medical evacuation times in a large civilian trauma system interfacing with the US Department of Defense's only Level 1 trauma center. Although not completely alike, similarities do exist between observations within this civilian prehospital trauma network and casualties cared for by the military today. Findings from this study demonstrate the feasibility of a stateside, civilian-military collaboration in prehospital research. With this model, the military has the ability to perform prehospital research pertaining to casualty data collection, casualty monitoring, and casualty resuscitation between military conflicts.

D. W. Mozingo, MD

Influencing Medical Student Education Via a Voluntary Shadowing Program for Trauma and Acute Care Surgery

Stroh DA, Ray-Mazumder N, Norman JA, et al (The Johns Hopkins Univ School of Medicine, Baltimore, MD)

JAMA Surg 148:968-970, 2013

Decreasing application into trauma surgery may be attributed to decreased exposure during medical school. We instituted a voluntary trauma call program for students to provide exposure to the field. After 3 years, participants completed a survey to gauge their experience. Of 126 students who participated, 68 completed the survey (54%). Interest in trauma surgery among students not previously planning on a career in surgery (n = 48) improved after the experience (4.4-5.3 of 10 points; $P < .005$). Operative experience, exposure to a higher number of trauma cases, and time with residents were associated with increased interest in trauma surgery. Witnessing patient death for the first time was associated with decreased interest in trauma surgery. A voluntary overnight shadowing program improves medical students' perceptions of trauma surgery and increases their reported likelihood to apply into a surgical residency.

▶ Attempts to direct medical students into careers in general and trauma surgery have been met with various degrees of success. Although some suggest the key time to encourage entry into a surgical field is the required third-year clerkship, recent data have shown that by then it is too late. Role models are one of the most important factors in career choice, and most surgical residents have decided their careers by the first year. Student shadowing programs have been shown to increase interest in emergency medicine and cardiothoracic surgery. Because trauma and acute care surgery are not mandatory in most medical school curricula, most medical students complete training without exposure to the field. The purpose of this study was to investigate whether a voluntary, student-initiated trauma shadowing program could improve student perceptions of general and trauma surgery. Interest in both surgery in general and trauma in particular improved significantly among medical students after a single overnight shadowing experience. Although most students were only slightly influenced toward a career in trauma surgery, a select few had dramatic increases in their interest. Notably, these students shadowed on active nights, observed a substantial amount of trauma patient care, and were actively engaged. This paradigm for early exposure may serve as a catalyst to drive interest in surgery for young clinicians in training and could be implemented at other academic institutions by engaging the interested students.

D. W. Mozingo, MD

Prospective Evaluation of the Role of Computed Tomography in the Assessment of Abdominal Stab Wounds

Inaba K, Okoye OT, Rosenheck R, et al (Univ of Southern California, Los Angeles; et al)

JAMA Surg 148:810-816, 2013

Importance.—An important adjunct in the management of abdominal gunshot wounds, the role of computed tomography (CT) in the diagnostic workup of abdominal stab wounds remains controversial.

Objective.—To prospectively compare CT against serial physical examination in the evaluation of patients who have sustained a stab wound to the abdomen.

Design, Setting, and Patients.—Prospective single-center observational study of all patients sustaining abdominal stab wounds from March 1, 2009, through March 31, 2011. Patients who were hemodynamically unstable, unevaluable, peritonitic, or eviscerated proceeded directly to laparotomy (n = 249). The remainder underwent CT evaluation. The impact of CT findings and physical examination on the decision to operate was analyzed.

Main Outcomes and Measures.—Diagnostic accuracy of CT vs physical examination in determining the need for therapeutic laparotomy.

Results.—A total of 249 patients were enrolled (94% male; mean [SD]: age, 30.8 [12.9] years [range, 16-87 years]; systolic blood pressure, 128 [28] mm Hg; Glasgow Coma Scale score, 14 [2]; Injury Severity Score, 6.8 [6.5]). Forty-five patients (18.1%) underwent immediate laparotomy, 27 (10.8%) had superficial injuries allowing immediate discharge, and the remaining 177 (71.1%) underwent CT. Of these, 154 (87.0%) were successfully observed, with 20 (11.3%) requiring laparotomy, 2 (1.1%) thoracotomy, and 1 (0.6%) sternotomy. Of the 20 laparotomies, 16 (80.0%) were therapeutic. All patients who underwent therapeutic laparotomy did so based on their physical examination. The most common finding leading to laparotomy was the development of peritonitis in 70%. The CT scan findings did not alter clinical decision making. The sensitivity and specificity of physical examination were 100.0% and 98.7%, respectively, while those of CT were 31.3% and 84.2%, respectively.

Conclusions and Relevance.—In this prospective evaluation of abdominal stab wound management, serial physical examination was able to discriminate between patients requiring a therapeutic laparotomy and those who could be safely observed. A physical examination-based diagnostic algorithm was effective and decreased radiation burden in the management of abdominal stab wounds.

► For patients sustaining a penetrating injury to the abdomen, nonoperative management remains a safe treatment option. Unevaluable patients, or those presenting with hemodynamic instability, peritonitis, or evisceration, are not candidates for observation or additional imaging. For the remainder, imaging is often used as a diagnostic adjunct. If the injury results from an abdominal gunshot wound, computed tomography (CT) can delineate patients into those who have an injury requiring laparotomy, those with trajectories that are clear of any intra-abdominal contents, and those with questionable injuries requiring further clinical observation. In the case of stab wounds, the optimal management plan and, in particular, the role of CT are unclear. With increased awareness of radiation burden and the ever-increasing accessibility and use of CT, the value of this extra imaging in the diagnostic workup of abdominal stab wounds remains a practical unanswered question. The authors of this selection sought to evaluate the diagnostic contribution made by CT in patients who have sustained an abdominal stab wound and to compare this with the physical examination. Their hypothesis was that, compared with a carefully performed physical examination, CT would not impact clinical management. In this prospective evaluation of abdominal stab wound management, serial physical examination was able to discriminate between patients requiring a therapeutic laparotomy and those who could be safely observed. A physical examination—based diagnostic algorithm (Fig 1 in the original article) was effective and decreased radiation burden in the management of abdominal stab wounds.

D. W. Mozingo, MD

Fibrinolysis greater than 3% is the critical value for initiation of antifibrinolytic therapy

Chapman MP, Moore EE, Ramos CR, et al (Univ of Colorado-Denver; Denver Health Med Ctr, CO; et al)

J Trauma Acute Care Surg 75:961-967, 2013

Background.—The acute coagulopathy of trauma is present in up to one third of patients by the time of admission, and the recent CRASH-2 and MATTERs trials have focused worldwide attention on hyperfibrinolysis as a component of acute coagulopathy of trauma. Thromboelastography (TEG) is a powerful tool for analyzing fibrinolyis, but a clinically relevant threshold for defining hyperfibrinolysis has yet to be determined. Recent data suggest that the accepted normal upper bound of 7.5% for 30-minute fibrinolysis (LY30) by TEG is inappropriate in severe trauma, as the risk of death rises at much lower levels of clot lysis. We wished to determine the validity of this hypothesis and establish a threshold value to treat fibrinolysis, based on prediction of massive transfusion requirement and risk of mortality.

Methods.—Patients with uncontrolled hemorrhage, meeting the massive transfusion protocol (MTP) criteria at admission (n = 73), represent the most severely injured trauma population at our center (median Injury Severity Score [ISS], 30; interquartile range, 20–38). Citrated kaolin TEG was performed at admission blood samples from this population, stratified by LY30, and evaluated for transfusion requirement and 28-day mortality. The same analysis was conducted on available field blood samples from all non-MTP trauma patients (n = 216) in the same period. These represent the general trauma population.

Results.—Within the MTP-activating population, the cohort of patients with LY30 of 3% or greater was shown to be at much higher risk for requiring a massive transfusion (90.9% vs. 30.5%, $p = 0.0008$) and dying of hemorrhage (45.5% vs. 4.8%, $p = 0.0014$) than those with LY30 less than 3%. Similar trends were seen in the general trauma population.

Conclusion.—LY30 of 3% or greater defines clinically relevant hyperfibrinolysis and strongly predicts the requirement for massive transfusion and an increased risk of mortality in trauma patients presenting with uncontrolled hemorrhage. This threshold value for LY30 represents a critical indication for the treatment of fibrinolysis.

Level of Evidence.—Prognostic study, level III (Fig 4).

▶ The acute coagulopathy of trauma is established in up to one-third of patients by the time they reach the hospital. Two-thirds of patients who die of hemorrhage will do so within the first 6 hours after injury, and up to 80% of the

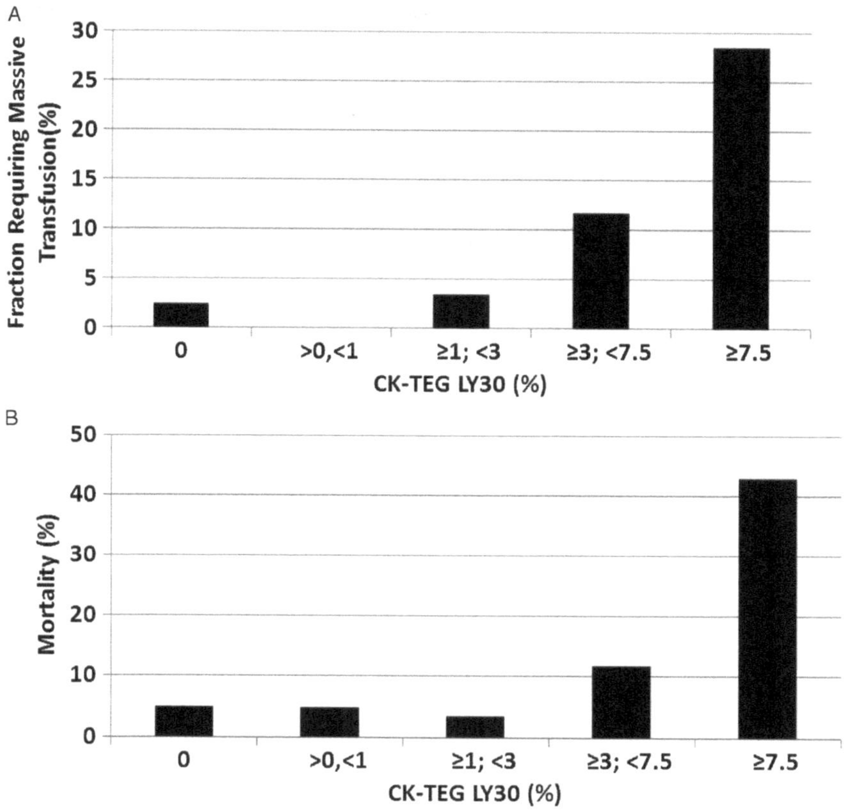

FIGURE 4.—Outcomes versus LY30 in the GT population. *A*, Plot of massive transfusion risk versus LY30 shows trend of increasing risk with increasing LY30. *B*, Plot of all-cause 28-day mortality versus LY30 demonstrates trend of increasing mortality with increasing LY30. Both of these outcomes display the same pattern of a sharp increase in risk at the threshold of LY30 of 3% or greater as in the MTP-activating population; however, the effect is much more marked at the 7.5% threshold, reflecting the lower pretest probability of massive transfusion or death in the highly heterogeneous GT population. (Reprinted from Chapman MP, Moore EE, Ramos CR, et al. Fibrinolysis greater than 3% is the critical value for initiation of antifibrinolytic therapy. *J Trauma Acute Care Surg*. 2013;75:961-967, with permission from Lippincott Williams & Wilkins.)

blood products transfused will be given within these first 6 hours. Therefore, a need exists for the rapid diagnosis and treatment of acute coagulopathy of trauma. The development and widespread adoption of point-of-care viscoelastic coagulation assays, for example, thromboelastography (TEG), have been found to be very useful scientifically and clinically for the study of the acute coagulopathy of trauma. In this prospective study of severely injured trauma patients, the authors found that an admission CK-TEG LY30 value of 3% or greater was a powerful predictor of requiring a massive transfusion within 6 hours of injury with a positive predictive value of 91%. This reflects a high specificity of 98% for predicting massive transfusion requirement as well as a moderately high probability (44%) of requiring a massive transfusion in this population. Fig 4 is included, showing these findings and the associated mortality risk. These patients were all deemed likely enough to require a massive transfusion to activate the massive transfusion protocol, but a positive test finding for LY30 of 3% or greater is a vastly superior predictor to clinical judgment alone. The sensitivity of the test is poor, however. This is not surprising because acute coagulopathy of trauma is a multifactorial entity, and not all occurrences of coagulopathy necessarily manifest hyperfibrinolysis. Also, not all massive traumatic bleeding is necessarily caused by coagulopathy.

D. W. Mozingo, MD

Regional collaboration across hospital systems to develop and implement trauma protocols saves lives within 2 years

Claridge JA, Allen D, Patterson B, et al (Case Western Reserve Univ School of Medicine, Cleveland, OH)
Surgery 154:875-884, 2013

Background.—The Northern Ohio Trauma System (NOTS) was created with the expressed goal of improving trauma care through collaboration, system-wide protocol implementation, and evidence-based process improvement. The primary goal of this study was to evaluate the mortality of trauma patients seen across the region after 2 years of beginning NOTS.

Methods.—Regional data was compared with the 2 years pre-NOTS (2008 and 2009) to the 2 years post-NOTS (2010 and 2011). The regional system consisted of two large hospital systems, initially including one level 1 center, four level 2 centers, seven nontrauma hospitals, and local emergency medical services groups. Two level 2 trauma centers closed during the study period. Mortality was the primary outcome for this study. Multivariate logistic regression also was performed to evaluate for independent predictors of mortality. An odds ratio (OR) and 95% confidence interval (CI) of survival were determined after we adjusted for other factors associated with mortality.

Result.—During the 4-year period 29,890 trauma patients were seen throughout NOTS. The mean age was 44 with a mean Injury Severity Score (ISS) of 8; 65% of the patients were male. Racial breakdown demonstrated that 64.0% were white, 31.9% were black, and 4.1% were other races. The hospital stay (mean ± SD) was 3.0 ± 5.2 days, and overall mortality was 3.4%. A separate analysis in which we used multivariate logistic regression demonstrated that patients treated in the post-NOTS period was an independent predictor for survival when we controlled for age, sex, ethnicity, mechanism, and ISS. The OR of survival of post NOTS was 0.81 (95% CI 0.70–0.94) when we evaluated all patients. The OR for admitted patients was 0.79 (95% CI 0.67–0.94) and 0.76 (0.62–0.95) in patients with ISS >24. There was an increase in the percentage of patients seen at the level 1 center in the post-NOTS period, which was especially demonstrated in patients with greater ISS.

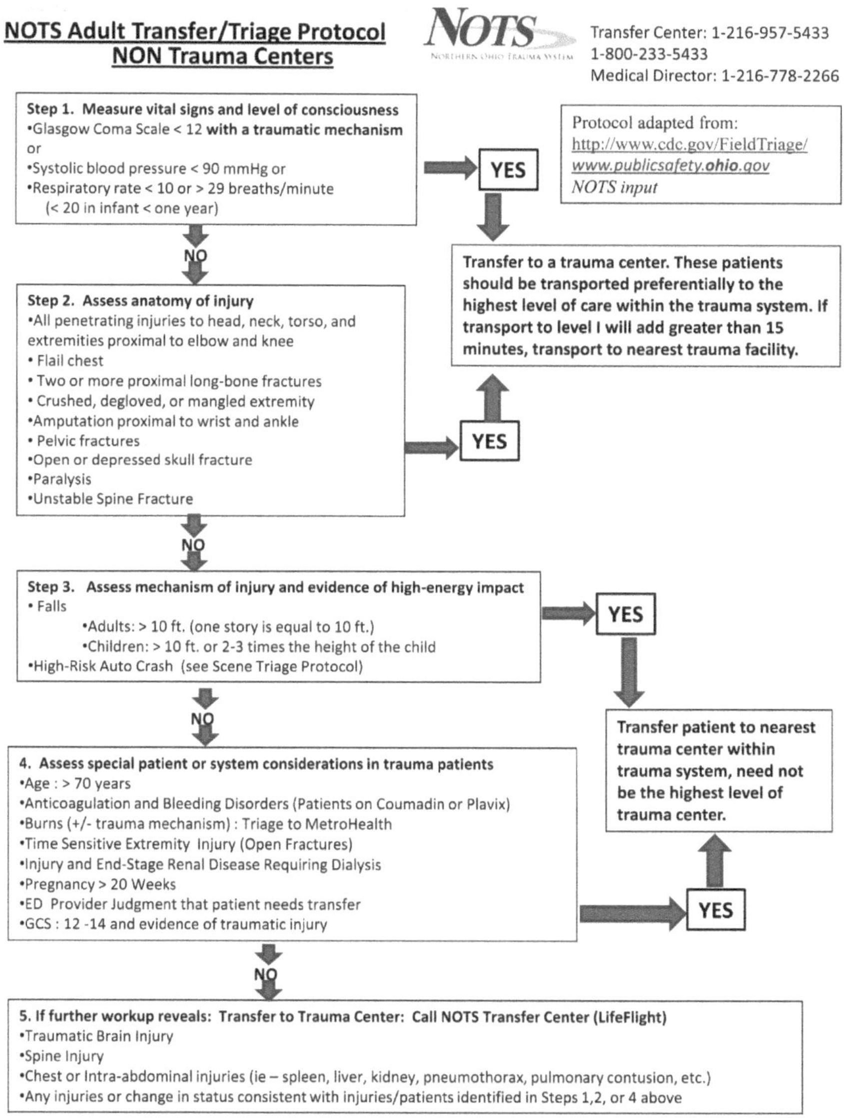

FIGURE.—NOTS nontrauma hospital transfer protocol. (Color version of figure is available online.) (Reprinted from Claridge JA, Allen D, Patterson B, et al. Regional collaboration across hospital systems to develop and implement trauma protocols saves lives within 2 years. *Surgery.* 2013;154:875-884, Copyright 2013, with permission from Elsevier.)

Conclusion.—NOTS appears to have contributed to the saving of lives within 2 years of its formation. Regionalized protocols, collaboration, and consolidation resulted in an improvement in mortality (Fig).

▶ There is evidence that a regional approach to trauma care saves resources and improves outcomes. Much of this evidence has been shown in other countries. Despite this evidence, there is a paucity of recent data in the United States showing that there is regionalization and collaboration between hospital systems to care for trauma patients. The implementation of trauma systems has evolved during the last several decades. Trauma systems have been implemented on the national, state, and regional levels with some success. The Northern Ohio Trauma System described in this selection has found that collaboration can improve outcomes dramatically, even with the closure of trauma centers. The referral algorithm for nontrauma center hospitals is included as Fig. The consolidation of resources and collaboration helped reduce mortality within 2 years by as much as 41%. The data from this study are critical to help guide the development of future trauma systems. Often, the first thought by individuals is that more trauma centers are needed. These data show that collaboration, protocol development, and consolidation of resources can lead to substantial improvements. Nearly 300 lives have been saved potentially since the implementation of this collaborative system.

D. W. Mozingo, MD

The injured elderly: A rising tide

Ciesla DJ, Pracht EE, Tepas JJ III, et al (Univ of South Florida Colleges of Medicine, Tampa, FL; Univ of South Florida College of Public Health, Tampa, FL; Univ of Florida College of Medicine, Jacksonville; et al)
Surgery 154:291-298, 2013

Background.—Injury remains a public health challenge despite advances in trauma care. Periodic survey of injury epidemiology is essential to the trauma system's continuous performance improvement. We undertook this study to characterize the changes in Florida injury rates during the past 15 years.

Methods.—Injured patients were identified with the use of a statewide database over 15 years ending in 2010. Population data were obtained from the U.S. Census. Severe injury was defined by International Classification Injury Severity Scores less than 0.85. Injury rates were expressed in discharges per 100,000 residents. Trends were analyzed by linear regression.

Results.—The 1.5 million patient discharges consisted of 5.2% children, 39.7% adults, and 55.1% elderly. The overall injury rate decreased in children by 18% but increased in adults by 2% and in the elderly by 17% during the study period. The proportion of severe injuries decreased in children and the elderly but did not change in adults. Injury patterns changed in all age groups.

Conclusion.—Injury in the elderly is increasing at a rate seven times that of adults. In 2010, the elderly accounted for only 17% of the population

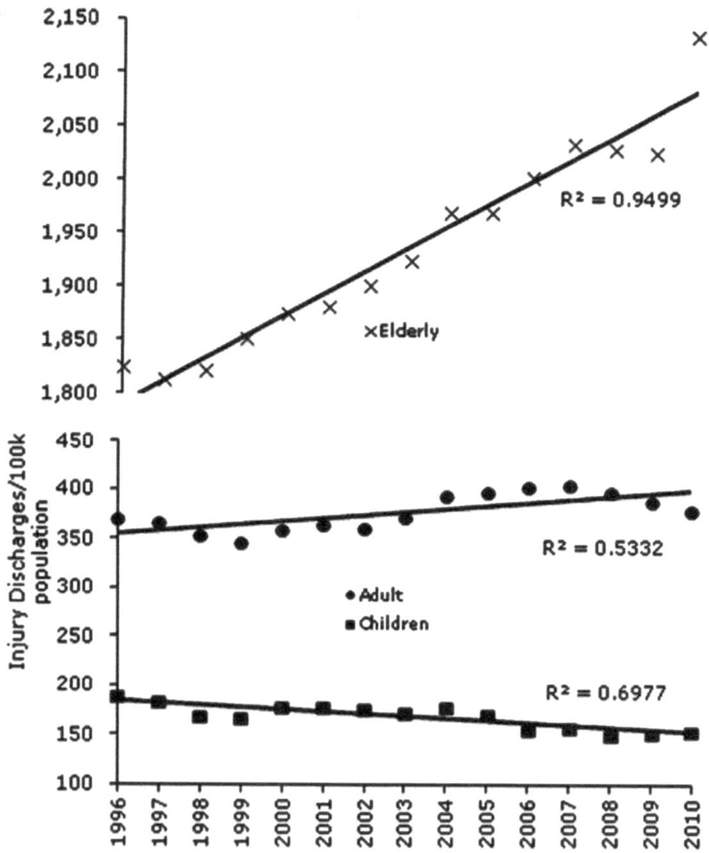

FIGURE 2.—Annual injured patient discharges per 100,000 population: elderly (age 65+), adults (age 15–64), and children (age 0–14). R2 = linear model R2 value. (Reprinted from Ciesla DJ, Pracht EE, Tepas JJ III, et al. The injured elderly: a rising tide. *Surgery*. 2013;154:291-298, Copyright 2013, with permission from Elsevier.)

but 55% of injury-related discharges. These trends have dramatic implications for the design of future trauma systems and health care resource use (Fig 2).

▶ Periodic surveys of injury epidemiology and burden of disease are essential to the continuous performance assessment and improvement of trauma systems. This study has several important implications. First, common conceptions that injury is a disease of the young may not be accurate today. Although trauma may be the leading cause of years of lost life, the elderly account for most of the burden of disease. Second, overall and specific injury rates are not static and in some cases changes drastically in the span of less than two decades. Fig 2 shows this point. This observation suggests that reliance on historic injury rates for planning trauma systems may lead to a mismatch of need and resources. Third, the changing injured demographic calls for concurrent performance and outcome assessment of the trauma system. Assumptions regarding the benefits of improved outcome in trauma centers based on a young patient population may not be accurate in the aging patient. The fraction of the population older than 65 years is predicted to continue to increase until 2020. Preparing for this surge in the elderly trauma population will be paramount.

D. W. Mozingo, MD

Flow disruptions in trauma care handoffs

Catchpole KR, Gangi A, Blocker RC, et al (Cedars-Sinai Med Ctr, Los Angeles, CA; et al)

J Surg Res 184:586-591, 2013

Background.—Effective handoffs of care are critical for maintaining patient safety and avoiding communication problems. Using the flow disruption observation technique, we examined transitions of care along the trauma pathway. We hypothesized that more transitions would lead to more disruptions, and that different pathways would have different numbers of disruptions.

Methods.—We trained observers to identify flow disruptions, and then followed 181 patients from arrival in the emergency department (ED) to the completion of care using a specially formatted PC tablet. We mapped each patient's journey and recorded and classified flow disruptions during transition periods into seven categories.

Results.—Mapping the transitions of care shows that approximately four of five patients were assessed in the ED, transferred to imaging for further diagnostics, and then returned to the ED. There was a mean of 2.2 ± 0.09 transitions per patient, a mean of 0.66 ± 0.15 flow disruptions per patient, and 0.31 ± 0.07 flow disruptions per transition. Most of these (53%) were related to coordination problems. Although disruptions did not rise with more transitions, patients who went directly to the operating room or needed direct admission to intensive care unit were significantly more likely ($P = 0.0028$) to experience flow disruptions than those who took other, less expedited pathways.

Conclusions.—Transitions in trauma care are vulnerable to systems problems and human errors. Coordination problems predominate as the cause. Sicker, time-pressured, and more at-risk patients are more likely to experience problems. Safety practices used in motor racing and other industries might be applied to address these problems (Fig 4).

▶ The authors of this selection aimed to analyze flow disruptions during the care transitions that patients experience during trauma care. They hypothesized that more transitions would lead to more disruptions and that different pathways would have different disruptions. Most disruptions during trauma transitions derive from coordination issues. Second, successive handoffs do not necessarily increase the number of transition flow disruptions, and some patient pathways are at a demonstrably higher risk of transition flow disruptions. This is

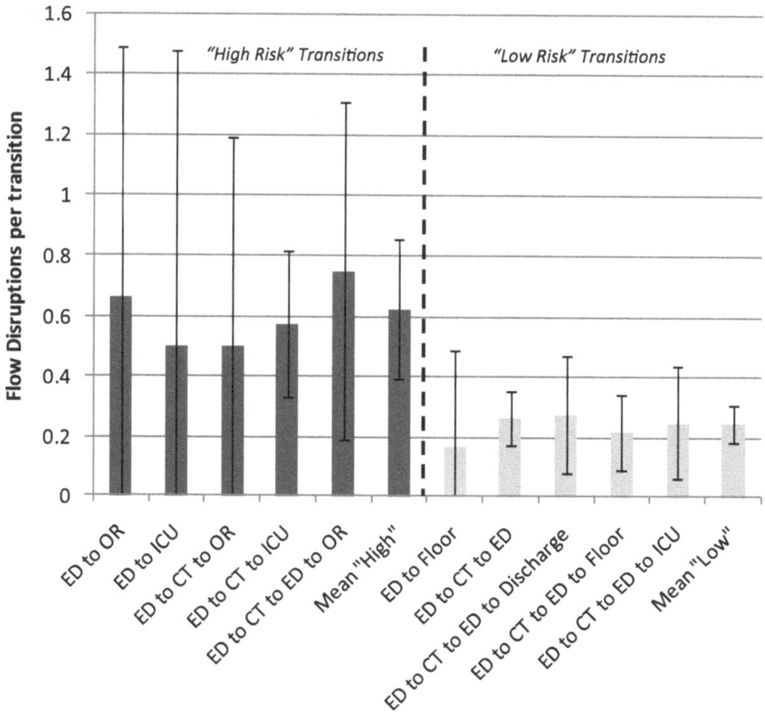

FIGURE 4.—High-risk and low-risk transitions. (Reprinted from The Journal of Surgical Research. Catchpole KR, Gangi A, Blocker RC, et al. Flow disruptions in trauma care handoffs. *J Surg Res.* 2013;184:586-591, Copyright 2013, with permission from Elsevier.)

depicted in Fig 4 included in this review. Patients taken directly to the operating room or who need immediate intensive care unit care are far more likely to experience multiple disruptions during care transitions than those who follow a more standard and less time-pressured pathway. The sickest patients who need the most rapid and specialized treatment are most at risk from coordination and other problems during their transitions to different care teams and locations. About one-half of the high-risk transitions experience a flow disruption, compared with about 1 in every 5 low-risk transitions.

D. W. Mozingo, MD

A comparison of health outcomes for combat amputee and limb salvage patients injured in Iraq and Afghanistan wars

Melcer T, Sechriest VF, Walker J, et al (Naval Health Res Ctr, San Diego, CA)
J Trauma Acute Care Surg 75:S247-S254, 2013

Background.—Treatment of military combatants who sustain leg-threatening injuries remains one of the leading challenges for military providers. The present study provides systematic health outcome data to inform decisions on the definitive surgical treatment, namely amputation versus limb salvage, for the most serious leg injuries.

Methods.—This was a retrospective analysis of health records for patients who sustained serious lower-extremity injuries in the Iraq and Afghanistan conflicts, 2001 to 2008. Patients had (1) amputation during the first 90 days after injury (early amputees, n = 587), (2) amputation more than 90 days after injury (late amputees, n = 84), or (3) leg-threatening injuries without amputation (limb salvage [LS], n = 117). Injury data and health outcomes were followed up to 24 months.

Results.—After adjusting for group differences, early amputees and LS patients had similar rates for most physical complications. Early amputees had significantly reduced rates of psychological diagnoses (posttraumatic stress disorder, substance abuse) and received more outpatient care, particularly psychological, compared with LS patients. Late amputees had significantly higher rates of many mental and physical health diagnoses, including prolonged infections and pain issues, compared with early amputees or LS patients.

Conclusion.—Early amputation was associated with reduced rates of adverse health outcomes relative to late amputation or LS in the short term. Most evident was that late amputees had the poorest physical and psychological outcomes. These findings can inform health care providers

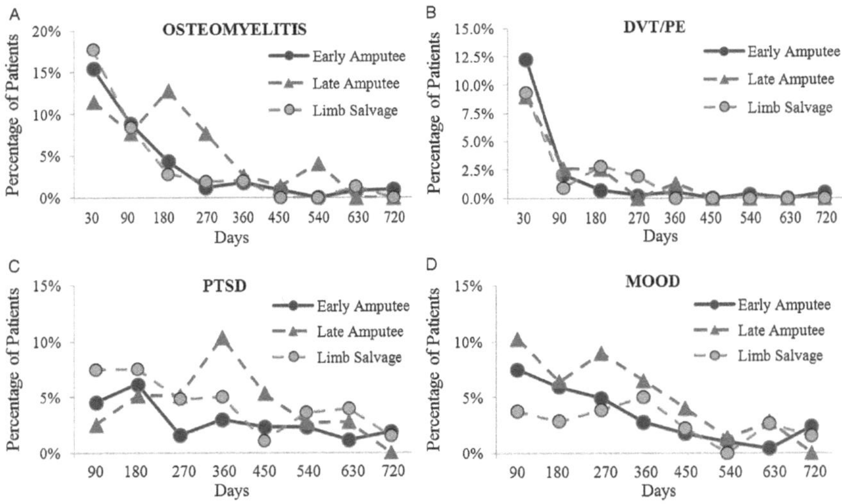

FIGURE 1.—Incidence rates of selected health outcomes during consecutive 30-day or 90-day intervals after injury for unilateral injury groups. Data are the first or onset diagnosis for each patient (e.g., Day 90 includes 0–90 days, Day 180 includes 91–180 days, Day 270 includes 181–270 days). Statistical significance during postinjury intervals through Day 360 only (χ^2 or Fisher's exact test as appropriate). Osteomyelitis: at 180 and 270 days, EA < LA, *p*'s < 0.01. DVT/PE: at 180 days, EA < LA and LS, $p < 0.05$. PTSD: at 270 days after injury, EA < LA and LS, *p*'s < 0.06; 360 days after injury, EA < LA, $p < 0.01$. Mood: combined data through 360 days, EA < LA, $p < 0.05$. (Reprinted from Melcer T, Sechriest VF, Walker J, et al. A comparison of health outcomes for combat amputee and limb salvage patients injured in Iraq and Afghanistan wars. *J Trauma Acute Care Surg.* 2013;75:S247-S254, with permission from Lippincott Williams & Wilkins.)

of the differing clinical consequences of early amputation and LS. These results indicate the need for separate health care pathways for early and late amputees and LS patients (Fig 1).

▶ During the Iraq and Afghanistan conflicts, thousands of US military personnel sustained lower-extremity injuries, many caused by high-energy trauma from powerful blast injuries. The most severe of these injuries have been limb-threatening, with complex fracture patterns, extensive soft tissue damage, and vascular and neurologic compromise. For all health care providers, one of the most challenging clinical decisions remains whether to treat such injuries with early amputation or to attempt limb salvage through reconstructive surgeries. The clinical outcome research published from the clinical data collected in the Iraq and Afghanistan conflicts has been outstanding, and this is yet another example. This is one of the first studies to quantify and compare early adverse physical and psychological outcomes for patients treated with amputation or limb salvage following combat injuries in these recent conflicts. After adjusting for covariates, the type and timing of definitive surgical treatment was significantly associated with specific health outcomes and outpatient health care use. Early amputation was associated with similar or fewer adverse health outcomes relative to patients treated with limb salvage or late amputation. Most evident was that patients treated with late amputation had relatively high rates of adverse physical and psychological outcomes. Fig 1 is included to demonstrate these findings. The present study provides treatment-specific outcomes during the first 24 months after injury, indicating apparent benefits of early amputation. For patients who sustain leg-threatening injuries that may be treated with either amputation or limb salvage, the authors of this selection currently recommend a substantial period of reflection, including clinical and family consultation before deciding on amputation or salvage. Based on these findings, providers may consider the apparent benefits of early amputation versus late amputation or limb salvage in this complex clinical decision.

D. W. Mozingo, MD

Outcomes after colon trauma in the 21st century: An analysis of the U.S. National Trauma Data Bank

Hatch Q, Causey M, Martin M, et al (Madigan Army Med Ctr, Tacoma, WA; et al)

Surgery 154:397-403, 2013

Introduction.—Most colon trauma data arise from institutional series that provide descriptive analysis. We investigated the outcome of these patients by analyzing a nationwide database.

Methods.—We queried the U.S. National Trauma Data Bank (2007–2009) using primary International Classification of Diseases, 9th edition, Clinical Modification codes to identify colon injuries. Outcomes were stratified by injury mechanism (blunt versus penetrating), segment of colon injured, and management strategy (diversion versus in continuity).

TABLE 4.—Multivariate Logistic Regression for Overall Morbidity and Mortality in 6,381 Colon Injured Patients (Controlled for Admission Vitals, Admission GCS, and Patient Comorbidity)

	OR	95% CI	*P* Value
Overall morbidity			
Age	1.03	1.02–1.04	<.001
Female gender	4.6	2.6–8.0	<.001
Blunt mechanism	0.7	0.5–1.1	.1
ISS	1.04	1.02–1.05	<.001
Fecal diversion	1.0	0.5–1.9	.9
Mortality			
Age	1.08	1.06–1.1	<.001
Female gender	1.2	0.6–1.6	.6
Blunt mechanism	0.5	0.3–1.001	.051
ISS	1.02	0.99–1.0	.1
Fecal diversion	0.7	0.2–2.5	.6

ISS, Injury Severity Score.

Results.—There were 6,817 patients who suffered primary colon injuries; 82% were male and 48% experienced blunt injuries. Blunt colon trauma patients were older, had lengthier intensive care stays, and greater rates of morbidity and mortality than those with penetrating injuries (all $P < .05$). Nonspecified injuries were the most common (36%), followed by transverse colon injuries (24%). The overall fecal diversion rate was 9%, with the highest rates seen in patients with sigmoid colon injuries (15%). Diverted patients were older, had higher injury severity scores, and increased mortality (22% vs 12%; $P < .001$). Multivariate analysis found that neither mechanism nor fecal diversion were independently associated with increased morbidity or mortality.

Conclusion.—Sigmoid colon injuries seem to be managed with fecal diversion more often than other segmental injuries. Neither blunt mechanism nor fecal diversion were independently associated with adverse outcomes in colon trauma (Table 4).

▶ The management of colon trauma has generated a considerable amount of disagreement over the years. The controversy exists, in large part, because of the devastating impact of suture-line breakdown after colon repair. The authors of this selection queried the National Trauma Data Bank to explore the national trends in operative management of colon injury and subsequent outcomes. They identified a number of other variables independently associated with adverse outcomes in colon trauma. Age, female gender, and Injury Severity Scores were all predictive of increased overall morbidity in colon trauma, whereas age was the only independent association with increased mortality. Table 4, demonstrating these findings, is included here. These variables have all been previously associated with poor outcomes in colorectal trauma. Fecal diversion was most prevalent in the management of distal colon injuries. Diversion versus in-continuity management and mechanism of injury were not independently associated with adverse outcomes on multivariate analysis. Although these results must be interpreted in light of the limitations of retrospective database studies, they do provide large-scale, population-based data regarding outcomes of colon trauma in the current clinical setting.

D. W. Mozingo, MD

Bilateral lower-extremity amputation wounds are associated with distinct local and systemic cytokine response

Lisboa FA, Forsberg JA, Brown TS, et al (Naval Med Res Ctr, Silver Spring, MD)

Surgery 154:282-290, 2013

Background.—Approximately 25% of U.S. military members sustaining extremity amputations in recent military conflicts have bilateral lower-extremity amputations (BLA). We investigated among combat-related extremity wounds whether BLA exhibit different bacterial burden, inflammatory response, and local complications.

Methods.—A total of 75 patients with combat-related extremity wounds (19 BLA) were evaluated for age, tobacco use, body mass index, Injury Severity Score, Acute Physiology and Chronic Health Evaluation II, and delayed primary closure time. Blood, wound exudates, and muscle biopsies were obtained and analyzed for cytokine and quantitative bacteriology, excluding patients using nonsteroidal anti-inflammatory medications and corticosteroids, due to potential effects on their inflammatory profile.

Results.—BLA was not associated with differences in age, tobacco use, body mass index, and delayed primary closure time, but these patients had increased Injury Severity Score, Acute Physiology and Chronic Health Evaluation II, and rates of critical colonization. Proinflammatory cytokines including tumor necrosis factor-α (exudate), interleukin (IL)-1 (exudate) and IL-6 (serum) were increased in BLA patients. They also had serum and exudate increased IL-8 and decreased IL-13 and granulocyte-macrophage colony-stimulating factor. Both wound dehiscence (WD) and heterotopic ossification (HO) were more common in BLA patients.

Conclusion.—BLA patients were more likely to exhibit critical bacterial colonization, a distinct inflammatory response, and develop WD and HO. Modulating this response represents an attractive target in an effort to prevent complications such as WD and HO (Fig 6).

► The authors of this selection state that, according to the Armed Forces Amputee Patient Care Database, 1506 US uniformed service members have sustained major limb amputations from the beginning of combat operations in Iraq and Afghanistan through July 2012, including 378 with bilateral lower-extremity amputations. They have investigated whether patients presenting with bilateral lower-extremity amputations exhibit differences in injury severity, physiologic and inflammatory response, bacterial burden, and wound-specific complications compared with patients with other combat-related extremity wounds. In this study, patients with bilateral lower extremity amputations were more severely

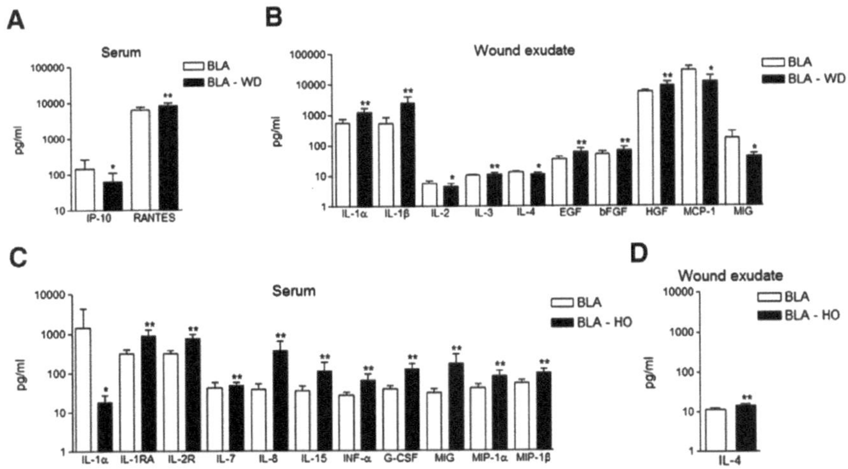

FIGURE 6.—Systemic and local cytokine levels of patients with BLA who developed wound dehiscence (WD) and/or heterotopic ossification (HO). 95% confidence intervals are depicted with a bar. (A) Serum cytokines that are different between BLA patients with and without WD. (B) Wound exudate cytokines that are different between BLA patients with and without WD. (C) Serum cytokines that are different between BLA patients with and without HO. (D) Wound exudate cytokine that was different between BLA patients with and without HO. **Statistical increase ($P < .05$) and *statistical decrease ($P < .05$). (Reprinted from Lisboa FA, Forsberg JA, Brown TS, et al. Bilateral lower-extremity amputation wounds are associated with distinct local and systemic cytokine response. *Surgery.* 2013;154:282-290, Copyright 2013, with permission from Elsevier.)

injured, more likely to be critically colonized, and exhibited distinct local and systemic inflammatory responses that differed from patients with other types of combat-related extremity wounds. Wound dehiscence and heterotopic ossification were associated with local and systemic inflammatory responses, respectively. Fig 6 demonstrates these associations. These findings provide prognostic and diagnostic insight and help justify modulation of the immune response in favor of avoiding complications such as wound dehiscence and heterotopic ossification in an effort to promote uncomplicated wound healing in these patients.

D. W. Mozingo, MD

Mechanism of injury alone is not justified as the sole indication for computed tomographic imaging in blunt pediatric trauma

Moore HB, Faulk LW, Moore EE, et al (Univ of Colorado, Denver)
J Trauma Acute Care Surg 75:995-1001, 2013

Background.—The liberal use of computed tomographic (CT) scanning during the evaluation of injured children has increased their exposure to the risks of ionizing radiation. We hypothesized that CT imaging performed for mechanism of injury alone is unnecessary and that serious or life-threatening injury is rarely identified.

TABLE 1.—Patient Demographics, CT Imaging, Radiation Dose

	Group I: Normal GCS Score/VS/PE Findings ("Mechanism")	Group II: Abnormal GCS Score	Group III: Abnormal VS/PE Findings	Group IV: Abnormal GCS Score/VS/PE Findings
Age, mean (SD), y	7 (4)	7 (5)	8 (5)	6 (5)
ISS, mean (SD)	7 (6)	17 (13)	9 (8)	16 (10)
Mortality, %	0	12	0	15
Imaged by CT	82% (54/66)	100% (25/25)	86% (49/57)	96% (25/26)
Radiation dose, mean (SD) per child, mSv	17 (14)	29 (13)	20 (16)	27 (17)
No. scans per patient	1.68	3.08	1.95	2.77
Serious injury on CT imaging	0% (0/111)	22% (17/77)	23% (25/109)	25% (18/72)
(Head/neck/chest/abdomen/pelvis)	0/0/0/0	13/2/0/2	4/3/0/18	13/2/0/3

Methods.—All pediatric blunt trauma team evaluations (age < 15 years) at a pediatric Level 2 trauma center over 72 months were reviewed. CT findings in patients with normal Glasgow Coma Scale (GCS) score, vital signs (VS), and physical examination (PE) (Group I) were compared with Group II (GCS score < 15), Group III (abnormal VS/PE), and Group IV (abnormal GCS score, VS/PE). Variables associated with any positive finding were entered into a multiple logistic regression model to assess for independent contributions. Each patient's total effective radiation dose from CT scans in millisieverts was calculated using an age-adjusted scale.

Results.—A total 174 children met trauma team activation criteria (mean [SD] age, 7 [5] years; 63% male; mean [SD] Injury Severity Score [ISS], 10 [10]). A total of 153 (88%) were imaged by CT (I, 54 of 66; II, 25 of 25; III, 49 of 57; IV, 25 of 26). No patient in Group I had a serious finding on CT compared with Group II (17 of 77), III (25 of 111), and IV (18 of 72). Mortality was 4%. Radiation dose (mSv) from CT was not different among the groups (I, 17 [14]; II, 29 [13]; III, 21 [16]; IV, 27 [17]). By univariate analysis, GCS score of less than 15 ($p < 0.01$) and respiratory rate of greater than 30 ($p = 0.09$) were associated with a positive CT finding. By logistic regression analysis, GCS score of less than 15 remained the only variable associated significantly with a positive finding (odds ratio, 6.7; 95% confidence interval, 3–14; $p < 0.01$).

Conclusion.—In children imaged based only on mechanism, no patient had a serious positive finding but was subjected to radiation doses associated with an increased risk of future malignancy. The use of CT imaging in injured children in the absence of a physiologic or anatomic abnormality does not seem to be justified.

Level of Evidence.—Care management study, level IV. (Table 1).

▶ Radiologic imaging with ionizing radiation remains the standard of care for diagnosing many injuries. However, ionizing radiation causes cancer. It is recognized that the impact of this potential oncogenic health risk can take up to

30 years before it will manifest with clinical symptoms. The authors of this selection have shown that computed tomography (CT) imaging is highly prevalent when the trauma team is activated at their level 1 trauma center. They demonstrated that normal physical examination and vital signs are superior to mechanism of injury for directing high-yield CT imaging. Table 1 summarizes these findings. Similarities exist between overtriage for trauma activation and low-yield CT imaging. Although the relative risk of cancer from this imaging modality seems almost inconsequential, the high frequency with which this modality is used to diagnose traumatic injuries in children and young adults warrants continued scrutiny. The results of this study suggest that we can improve our clinical decision making in pediatric trauma patients to reduce the amount of iatrogenic radiation these patients receive.

D. W. Mozingo, MD

Vasopressor use after initial damage control laparotomy increases risk for anastomotic disruption in the management of destructive colon injuries

Fischer PE, Nunn AM, Wormer BA, et al (F.H. "Sammy" Ross Trauma Ctr, Charlotte, NC)

Am J Surg 206:900-903, 2013

Background.—Management of destructive colon injuries during damage control (DC) laparotomy is debated. The authors reviewed a single institution's experience with destructive colon injuries to identify risk factors for anastomotic failure after colon reconstruction.

Methods.—The authors identified all trauma patients sustaining destructive colon injuries between 2002 and 2011 from their medical center's trauma registry. Anastomotic leak was defined as suture or staple line disruption or enteral fistula formation.

Results.—Of 171 identified patients, 68 had DC procedures, 41 (60%) had subsequent anastomoses performed during the same hospitalization, and 27 (40%) were diverted. The colon anastomotic leak rate in patients who underwent DC laparotomy was higher than in patients who were reconstructed at the primary operation in a non-DC setting (17% vs 6%, $P = .09$). The use of vasopressors after the initial DC operation more than quadrupled the leak rate to 50% ($P = .02$).

Conclusions.—Colonic anastomotic disruptions yield deadly consequences, and diversion rather than anastomosis should be used in patients who require vasopressor support after the initial DC procedure (Table 4).

▶ The management of traumatic colon injuries has evolved substantially over the past half century. The most conservative would argue that the safest option for the management of any colon injury is mandatory fecal diversion, whereas many others will cite the success of primary repair in most circumstances. In this study, the authors examined the safety of colonic anastomosis after destructive colon wounds after resection. Patients in the non–damage control group who underwent anastomoses had a 6% leak rate. Of concern, in the

TABLE 4.—Anastomotic Leaks in Patients Undergoing DC Procedures

Variable	Leak (n = 7)	No leak (n = 34)	*P*
Age (y)	38 (36)	29 (15)	.61
Blood transfused in the first 24 h (U)	8 (7)	3 (13)	.60
Type of anastomosis			
Ileocolonic	3 (42%)	20 (58%)	.43
Colocolonic	4 (58%)	14 (42%)	
Hand sewn	3 (42%)	16 (48%)	.78
Vasopressors	4 (57%)	4 (12%)	.02
Length of ICU stay	25 (18)	7 (15)	.01
Length of hospital stay	38 (26)	17 (19)	.07
Mortality	2 (29%)	1 (3%)	.02

Continuous variables are expressed as median (interquartile range), and categorical variables are expressed as number (percentage).
DC = damage control; ICU = intensive care unit.

damage control setting, the anastomotic leak rate rose to 17%. A comparison of these groups is included in Table 4. Although this represents a clinically significant increase in the rate of anastomotic disruption, the groups are difficult to compare. The damage control group, by the nature of the damage control procedure, represents a population that experienced more profound shock and often has more associated injuries. These factors alone would be expected to raise the complication rate.

D. W. Mozingo, MD

A Paradigm Shift in Trauma Resuscitation: Evaluation of Evolving Massive Transfusion Practices

Kutcher ME, Kornblith LZ, Narayan R, et al (Univ of California, San Francisco)
JAMA Surg 148:834-840, 2013

Importance.—The evolution of damage control strategies has led to significant changes in the use of resuscitation after traumatic injury.

Objective.—To evaluate changes in the administration of fluids and blood products, hypothesizing that a reduction in crystalloid volume and a reduced red blood cell (RBC) to fresh frozen plasma (FFP) ratio over the last 7 years would correlate with better resuscitation outcomes.

Design.—Observational prospective cohort study.

Setting.—Urban level I trauma center.

Participants.—A total of 174 trauma patients receiving a massive transfusion (>10 units of RBCs in 24 hours) or requiring the activation of the institutional massive transfusion protocol from February 2005 to June 2011.

Exposure.—Patients had to either receive a massive transfusion or require the activation of the institutional massive transfusion protocol.

Main Outcomes and Measures.—In-hospital mortality.

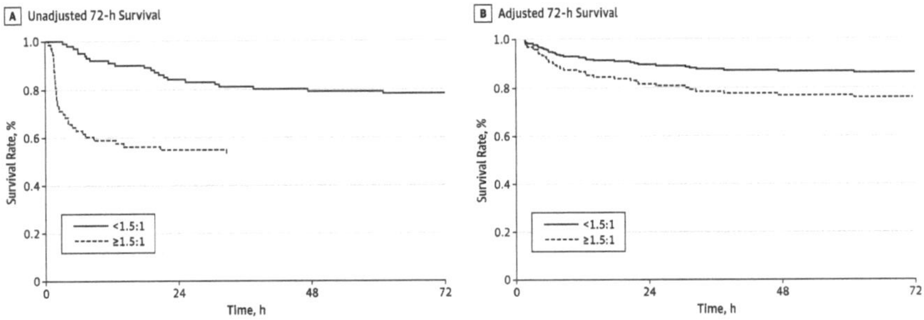

FIGURE 2.—Unadjusted and Adjusted Survival Plots. Kaplan-Meier 72-hour survival plots based on the red blood cell (RBC) to fresh frozen plasma (FFP) ratio transfused within 24 hours of admission are shown for unadjusted survival ($P < .001$ determined by log-rank test) (A) and adjusted for age, Injury Severity Score, Glasgow Coma Scale score, and base deficit at admission using Cox proportional hazards regression (B). The Harrell C index was 0.808 for the adjustment model. By convention, the solid line indicates a plasma-based ratio (RBC:FFP ratio < 1.5:1), and the dashed line indicates an erythrocyte-based ratio (RBC:FFP ratio ≥ 1.5:1). (Reprinted from Kutcher ME, Kornblith LZ, Narayan R, et al. A paradigm shift in trauma resuscitation: evaluation of evolving massive transfusion practices. *JAMA Surg*. 2013;148:834-840.)

Results.—The mean (SD) Injury Severity Score was 28.4 (16.2), the mean (SD) base deficit was -9.8 (6.3), and median international normalized ratio was 1.3 (interquartile range, 1.2-1.6); the mortality rate was 40.8%. Patients received a median of 6.1 L of crystalloid, 13 units of RBCs, 10 units of FFP, and 1 unit of platelets over 24 hours, with a mean RBC:FFP ratio of 1.58:1. The mean 24-hour crystalloid infusion volume and number of the total blood product units given in the first 24 hours decreased significantly over the study period ($P < .05$). The RBC:FFP ratio decreased from a peak of 1.84:1 in 2007 to 1.55:1 in 2011 ($P = .20$). Injury severity and mortality remained stable over the study period. When adjusted for age and injury characteristics using Cox regression, each decrease of 0.1 achieved in the massive transfusion protocol's RBC:FFP ratio was associated with a 5.6% reduction in mortality ($P = .005$).

Conclusions and Relevance.—There has been a shift toward a reduced crystalloid volume and the recreation of whole blood from component products in resuscitation. These changes are associated with markedly improved outcomes and a new paradigm in the resuscitation of severely injured patients (Fig 2).

▶ In the past 10 years, a paradigm shift has occurred in the resuscitation of critically injured patients. Early in this era, iatrogenic and resuscitation-associated causes of coagulopathic bleeding after traumatic injury were identified, and hypothermia, metabolic acidosis, and dilutional coagulopathy were recognized as the primary causes of this problem. In response to these observations, rewarming efforts, early correction of acidosis, and the limitation of crystalloid became the new goals of trauma resuscitation. This focus on early correction of physiological abnormalities, as opposed to definitive surgical repair, defined the beginning of damage-control surgery. Concurrently, large retrospective military and civilian series suggested a survival benefit with transfusion strategies using earlier and more frequent use of plasma, particularly in patients receiving massive transfusion. In this selection, the authors described their alterations in massive transfusion practices during a changing era of trauma resuscitation. They further identified univariate and multivariate associations of the effect of these trends on in-hospital mortality. They observed trends toward reduced overall transfusion practices, earlier empirical plasma transfusion, and more plasma-based red blood cell (RBC) to fresh frozen plasma (RBC:FFP) transfusion ratios, in parallel with countrywide trends in massive transfusion. They further investigated the association of these trends with improved survival, finding a clinically and statistically significant association of lower RBC:FFP transfusion ratios with reductions in both unadjusted and injury-adjusted in-hospital mortality. These trends are depicted in Fig 2, included with this selection. The authors point out the dearth of randomized or multicenter trials in this area; however, it appears that clinicians who care for injured patients are forging ahead, regardless of the controversies in clinical evidence, by adopting crystalloid-restricted, more plasma-based massive transfusion practices.

D. W. Mozingo, MD

Excessively Long Hospital Stays After Trauma Are Not Related to the Severity of Illness: Let's Aim to the Right Target!

Hwabejire JO, Kaafarani HMA, Imam AM, et al (Massachusetts General Hosp and Harvard Med School, Boston)

JAMA Surg 148:956-961, 2013

Importance.—Reduction in length of hospital stay is a veritable target in reducing the overall costs of health care. However, many existing approaches are flawed because the assumptions of what cause excessive length of stay are incorrect; we methodically identified the right targets in this study.

Objective.—To identify the causes of excessively prolonged hospitalization (ExProH) in trauma patients.

Design.—The trauma registry, billing databases, and medical records of trauma admissions were reviewed. Excessively prolonged hospitalization was defined by the standard method used by insurers, which is a hospital stay that exceeds the Diagnosis Related Group-based trim point. The causes of ExProH were explored in a unique potentially avoidable days database, used by our hospital's case managers to track discharge delays.

Setting.—Level I academic trauma center.

Participants.—Adult trauma patients admitted between January 1, 2006, and December 31, 2010.

Main Outcomes and Measures.—Excessively prolonged hospitalization and hospital cost.

Results.—Of 3237 patients, 155 (5%) had ExProH. The patients with ExProH compared with non-ExProH patients were older (mean [SD] age, 53 [21] vs 47 [22] years, respectively; $P = .001$), were more likely to have blunt trauma (92% vs 84%, respectively; $P = .03$), were more likely to be self-payers (16% vs 11%, respectively; $P = .02$) or covered by Medicare/Medicaid (41% vs 30%, respectively; $P = .002$), were more likely to be discharged to post-acute care facilities than home (65% vs 35%, respectively; $P < .001$), and had higher hospitalization cost (mean, \$54 646 vs \$18 444, respectively; $P < .001$). Both groups had similar Injury Severity Scores, Revised Trauma Scores, baseline comorbidities, and in-hospital complication rates. Independent predictors of mortality were discharge to a rehabilitation facility (odds ratio = 4.66; 95% CI, 2.71-8.00; $P < .001$) or other post-acute care facility (odds ratio = 5.04; 95% CI, 2.52-10.05; $P < .001$) as well as insurance type that was Medicare/Medicaid (odds ratio = 1.70; 95% CI, 1.06-2.72; $P = .03$) or self-pay (odds ratio = 2.43; 95% CI, 1.35-4.37; $P = .003$). The reasons for discharge delays were clinical in only 20% of the cases. The remaining discharges were excessively delayed because of difficulties in rehabilitation facility placement (47%), in-hospital operational delays (26%), or payer-related issues (7%).

Conclusions and Relevance.—System-related issues, not severity of illness, prolong hospital stay excessively. Cost-reduction efforts should target operational bottlenecks between acute and postacute care.

► Excessively prolonged hospitalization (ExProH) is associated with significant clinical risks and increased cost. These clinical risks may include nosocomial infections, deep venous thrombosis, adverse drug reactions, medication errors, and multiple other adverse events. The authors of this selection sought to determine the primary reasons for ExProH in their trauma patient population. The primary outcome was ExProH. The Diagnosis Related Group (DRG) of each patient was reviewed, and the trim point for length of stay (LOS) for that DRG was determined. The trim point for LOS is defined as 2 standard deviations above the mean LOS for cases within a DRG. Insurers also use this trim point to determine prolonged hospitalization, and the authors used the same value to define ExProH. In surgical care, there is a prevailing belief that the patient's physiologic condition, mainly determined by preexisting comorbidities and the occurrence of postoperative complications, is the major determinant of ExProH. A logical conclusion would then be that ExProH can be reduced by better medical care to optimize patients for surgery and avoid subsequent complications. The results of this study show that this is not the case at all. This study shows that delays in discharge are typically not caused by medical factors. In most cases, ExProH was related to administrative issues, predominantly the inability to place a patient in an appropriate rehabilitation facility, and to operational and insurance issues. The financial burden of such unnecessary hospitalization is significant. Although physicians should always participate in all aspects of patient care, there is little they can do to improve these specific issues. Health care policy makers should shift the focus toward the right target to reduce excessive hospital stays and cost in trauma patients.

D. W. Mozingo, MD

Blunt cerebrovascular injury in children: Underreported or underrecognized?: A multicenter ATOMAC study

Azarakhsh N, Grimes S, Notrica DM, et al (Univ of Tennessee Health Science Ctr, Memphis; Lebonheur Children's Hosp, Memphis, TN; Univ of Arizona, Phoenix; et al)

J Trauma Acute Care Surg 75:1006-1012, 2013

Background.—Blunt cerebrovascular injury (BCVI) has been well described in the adult trauma literature. The risk factors, proper screening, and treatment options are well known. In pediatric trauma, there has been very little research performed regarding this injury. We hypothesize that the incidence of BCVI in children is lower than the 1% reported incidence in adult studies and that many children at risk are not being screened properly.

Methods.—This is a multi-institutional retrospective cohort study of pediatric patients (<15 years) admitted with blunt trauma to six American College of Surgeons—verified Level 1 pediatric trauma centers between October 2009 and June 2011. All patients with head, neck, or face injuries who were high risk for BCVI based on Memphis criteria were analyzed.

Results.—Of 5,829 blunt trauma admissions, 538 patients had at least one of the Memphis criteria. Only 89 (16.5%) of these patients were screened (16 patients had more than one test) by angiography (64 by computed tomography angiography, 39 by magnetic resonance angiography, and 2 by conventional angiography), while 459 (83.5%) were not screened. Screened patients differed from unscreened patients in Injury Severity Score (ISS) (22.6 ± 13.3 vs. 13.3 ± 9.9, $p < 0.0001$) and head and neck Abbreviated Injury Scale (AIS) score (3.7 ± 1.2 vs. 2.8 ± 1.2, $p < 0.0001$). The incidence of BCVI in our total population was 0.4% (23 patients). Of the 23 patients with BCVI, 3 (13%) had no risk factors for the injury. The odds of having sustained BCVI in a patient with one or more of the risk factors was 4.0 (95% confidence interval, 1.1–14.2).

Conclusion.—BCVI in Level 1 pediatric trauma centers is diagnosed less frequently than in adult centers. However, screening was performed in a minority of high-risk patients who may explain the reported lower incidence of BCVI in children. Pediatric surgeons need to become more vigilant about screening pediatric patients with high-risk criteria for BCVI.

Level of Evidence.—Prognostic/epidemiologic study, level III; therapeutic study, level IV (Table 2).

▶ Blunt cerebrovascular injury (BCVI) has been studied extensively in adults during the last 2 decades, and there are screening criteria for BCVI in the adult population. None of the recommended guidelines or screening criteria, however, has approached detecting all BCVI patients. In fact, 15% to 20% of patients are still missed despite current adult screening criteria. In addition, controversy still exists regarding whether digital subtraction angiography or computed tomography angiography is the best approach to detect BCVI in high-risk patients. The controversies surrounding BCVI have kept it in the forefront among adult trauma

TABLE 2.—High-Risk Patients Based on Memphis Criteria: Imaging and BCVI Diagnosis

Risk Factor	Total	Patients Screened*	+BCVI**
Cervical spine fracture	40	8 (19.5)	1 (12.5)
Skull base fracture	283	26 (8)	7 (27)
Le Fort II/III fracture	40	4 (10)	0 (0)
Neck soft tissue injury	93	24 (26)	4 (17)
Anisocoria	1	0 (0)	0 (0)
Neurologic examination not explained by brain imaging	18	3 (17)	0 (0)
Combination of ≥2	63	24 (36)	8 (33)
Total	538	89 (16)	20 (22.4)

*Number of the patients with this injury who were screened (percentage of the total).
**Number of the patients with this injury who were diagnosed with BCVI (percentage of those who had been screened).

surgeons. Pediatric surgeons, however, seem to have had less exposure to this debate, which may have blunted the index of suspicion for BCVI in seriously injured children. This study represents the largest multi-institutional study to date investigating the incidence of BCVI in children admitted to the hospital with blunt injuries. The authors hypothesized that the incidence of BCVI was lower than the 1% reported in the adult literature. However, it was also of concern that well-accepted criteria for BCVI screening, like the Memphis criteria, may not be familiar to pediatric surgeons who function in free-standing children's hospitals. The Memphis screening criteria applied to the study population is included as Table 2. Adoption of the adult guidelines, while increasing the exposure to ionizing radiation, will be necessary to determine the true incidence of this injury in the pediatric trauma patient population. Considering the established correlation between the risk factors and BCVI, an incidence of 0.4% among injured children, and the demonstration that treatment seems to lower the risk of subsequent stroke, pediatric screening of patients at high risk for BCVI is warranted. With the current low rates of angiographic imaging of pediatric patients in the high-risk group, an opportunity to improve care at pediatric trauma centers exists with further study of this at-risk population.

D. W. Mozingo, MD

3 Burns

A Protocol of Early Aggressive Acceleration of Tube Feeding Increases Ileus Without Perceptible Benefit in Severely Burned Patients

Kesey J, Dissanaike S (Univ Med Ctr, Lubbock, TX; Tech Univ Health Sciences Ctr, Lubbock, TX)

J Burn Care Res 34:515-520, 2013

Optimal nutrition is essential to the recovery of burned patients. The authors evaluated the efficacy of an aggressive nutrition delivery protocol. The following protocol was implemented: initiation of tube feeds within 4 hours, acceleration to goal rate within 8 hours, and tolerance of gastric residual volumes of 400 ml. Patients on the protocol formed the study group whereas patients admitted immediately before implementation served as controls for a study period of 7 days after admission. Outcome variables included ileus, prokinetic medication use, intensive care unit and overall length of stay, ventilator days and mortality. Variables were compared using bivariate analysis. The 42 study subjects and 34 controls were similar at baseline. Time to initiation was similar (6.8 vs 9.4 hours; $P = .226$), however, goal rate was achieved much sooner in the study group (11.2 vs 20.9 hours; $P < .001$). Number of hours spent at goal was different on days 1 and 2 (6.62 vs 2.74, $P = .003$ and 17.24 vs 13.18, $P = .032$) with no difference thereafter. Residual volumes in the study group were higher from day 2 onward, and remained increased throughout the study period (401 vs 234ml average; $P = .449$). Clinical ileus was much more common in the study group (8 cases vs 1, $P = .037$). There was no difference in length of stay or mortality. The protocol was successfully implemented and resulted in early achievement of goal tube feed rates. However, this resulted in tube feed intolerance as manifested by more cases of clinical ileus.

► Burn-injured patients have among the highest metabolic demands of all critically ill or injured patients. Burn injury results in an increase in the hypothalamic set-point for the production of endogenous catecholamines, cortisol, and glucocorticoids resulting in hypermetabolism. Delivering early nutrition therapy can reduce disease severity, reduce complications, decrease length of stay, and improve outcomes. Enteral nutrition is preferred over parenteral nutrition whenever possible. Early nutrition is typically defined as initiation of feedings within the first 24 hours of burn injury. Patients with extensive burn or those requiring mechanical ventilation often require supplemental enteral feeding to meet their high caloric and protein requirements. The goal of nutrition supplementation is to promote wound healing, prevent infection, and attenuate the loss of lean body mass, often associated with increased mortality and poorer long-term outcomes. On the basis of these findings, the authors of this selection created an aggressive protocol for nutrition support in severely burned patients. This protocol involved reducing the time to initiation of enteral feeding, faster acceleration of rate of delivery, tolerating higher gastric residual volumes, and continuing tube feeding during operations and procedures. They hypothesized that this aggressive enteral nutrition protocol would result in improved clinical outcomes in critically ill burn patients. Their findings were not as expected. Initiation of this feeding regimen resulted in an increase in the incidence of clinical ileus manifested in 8 cases in the study group and only one in the control ($P = .037$) group.. Gastric residual volumes were significantly higher in the study group. Overall provision of nutrition was not different between groups throughout the hospital stay. I guess that more is not always better.

D. W. Mozingo, MD

Time to Rehabilitation in the Burn Population: Incidence of Zero Onset Days in the UDSMR National Dataset

Schneider JC, Tan W-H, Goldstein R, et al (Spaulding Rehabilitation Hosp, Boston, MA; et al)

J Burn Care Res 34:666-673, 2013

A preliminary investigation of the burn rehabilitation population found a large variability of zero onset day frequency between facilities. Onset days is defined as the time from injury to inpatient rehabilitation admission; this variable has not been investigated in burn patients previously. This study explored if this finding was a facility-based phenomena or characteristic of burn inpatient rehabilitation patients. This study was a secondary analysis of Uniform Data System for Medical Rehabilitation (UDSMR®) data from 2002 to 2007 examining inpatient rehabilitation characteristics among patients with burn injuries. Exclusion criteria were age less than 18 years and discharge against medical advice. Comparisons of demographic, medical and functional data were made between facilities with a high frequency of zero onset days versus facilities with a low frequency of zero onset days. A total of 4738 patients from 455 inpatient rehabilitation facilities were included. Twenty-three percent of the population exhibited zero onset days ($n = 1103$). Sixteen facilities contained zero onset patients; two facilities accounted for 97% of the zero onset subgroup. Facilities with a high frequency of zero onset day patients demonstrated significant differences in demographic, medical, and functional variables compared to the remainder of the study population. There were significantly more zero onset day admissions among burn patients (23%) than other diagnostic groups (0.5–3.6%) in the Uniform Data System for Medical Rehabilitation database, but the majority (97%) came from two inpatient rehabilitation facilities. It is unexpected for patients with significant burn injury to be admitted to a rehabilitation facility on the day of injury. Future studies investigating burn rehabilitation outcomes using the Uniform Data System for Medical Rehabilitation database should exclude facilities with a high percentage of zero onset days, which are not representative of the burn inpatient rehabilitation population.

▶ In this selection, the authors found that there were significantly more zero-onset day admissions among burn patients than other diagnostic groups in the Uniform Data System for Medical Rehabilitation (UDSMR®) database, but most came from 2 inpatient rehabilitation facilities. It is unexpected for patients with significant burn injury to be admitted to a rehabilitation facility on the day of injury. They concluded that studies examining burn rehabilitation using the UDSMR database should exclude zero-onset facilities, as these facilities are not representative of the burn rehabilitation population as shown by their statistically significant differences in demographic, medical, and rehabilitation characteristics. All other facilities with typical frequencies of zero-onset day patients represent the largest national burn rehabilitation dataset and a rich potential source for further study of this population. Future studies examining burn rehabilitation outcomes using multifacility data should look for facility-specific effects as sources of findings that appear irreconcilable with clinical circumstances.

D. W. Mozingo, MD

Treatment of Patients With Severe Burns—Costs and Health-Related Quality of Life Outcome

Koljonen V, Laitila M, Rissanen AM, et al (Helsinki Univ Central Hosp, Finland; Helsinki and Uusimaa Hosp District, Finland; et al)

J Burn Care Res 34:e318-e325, 2013

To study the effectiveness of the treatment of patients with severe burns, the authors collected health-related quality of life (HRQoL) data with the 15D instrument, 17 to 29 months after treatment had commenced at the national burns unit. The costs of each patient's secondary care treatment were followed for a mean of 66 months. During the 1-year study period, 107 patients were treated at the burns unit, eight for scar surgery, the remainder for primary treatment of a burn injury; 19 had died or could not be located during the time of the HRQoL survey. Of the remaining 88 patients, 43 (49%; mean [SD] age 45.7 [14.8] years; 70% men) returned the questionnaire. Their mean (SD) HRQoL score (0.909[0.113]) was only slightly, and not significantly, lower than that of the age- and sex-standardized general population (0.928[0.080]). The mean (SD) secondary care cost of burn treatment of for all the 107 patients, over the 60- to 72-month observation time, was 42,838 USD (73,569 USD; range 1319–34,8741 USD). The largest portion of the total cost was because of inpatient treatment (61%) followed by operations (22%), and outpatient visits. In addition to the costs of burns treatment, the patients consumed other secondary care services to a value of nearly 12,229 USD.

The HRQoL in patients treated for severe burns is good, thus the observed high-treatment costs can be considered acceptable.

▶ The major strength of this study is that it reports the outcome and costs of treatment of patients with severe burns under everyday conditions in a real-world setting. The study setting includes all patients treated as inpatients in a burn center for 1 year. The findings are based on an unselected population and reflect normal practice as closely as possible. Furthermore, the fact that they are analyzing patient-reported outcome is a strength. A limitation of this study is that the costs were estimated from the health care provider's perspective only, as only direct hospital costs covering both in-hospital and outpatient care were included. Data on productivity costs would broaden the perspective of the cost analysis. Another limitation is the relatively low response rate of 49%. However, among severely burned individuals with a median percentage of total burn surface area of 87.5, the response rate was only 27%. The authors chose not to contact the patients directly but rather mailed them the questionnaire so that they could freely decide whether they wanted to participate. It might be supposed that individuals who respond are those who are satisfied with the outcome, and those unsatisfied are unlikely to return the surveys.

D. W. Mozingo, MD

Doxycycline attenuates burn-induced microvascular hyperpermeability

Stagg HW, Whaley JG, Tharakan B, et al (Texas A&M Health Science Ctr College of Medicine and Scott & White Healthcare, Temple; et al)

J Trauma Acute Care Surg 75:1040-1046, 2013

Background.—Burns induce systemic microvascular hyperpermeability resulting in shock, and if untreated, cardiovascular collapse. Damage to the endothelial cell adherens junctional complex plays an integral role in the pathophysiology of microvascular hyperpermeability. We hypothesized that doxycycline, a known inhibitor of matrix metalloproteinases (MMPs), could attenuate burn-induced adherens junction damage and microvascular hyperpermeability.

Methods.—Male Sprague-Dawley rats were divided into sham, burn, and burn + doxycycline (n = 5). The experimental groups underwent a 30% total body surface area full-thickness burn. Fluorescein isothiocyanate-albumin was administered intravenously. Mesenteric postcapillary venules were examined with intravital microscopy to determine flux of albumin from the intravascular space to the interstitium. Fluorescence intensity was compared between the intravascular space to the interstitium at 30, 60, 80, 100, 120, 140, 160, and 180 minutes after burn. Parallel experiments were performed in which rat lung microvascular endothelial cells were treated with sera from sham or burn animals as well as separate groups pretreated with either doxycycline or a specific inhibitor of MMP-9. Monolayer permeability was determined by fluorescein isothiocyanate albumin-flux across Transwell plates and immunofluorescense staining for the

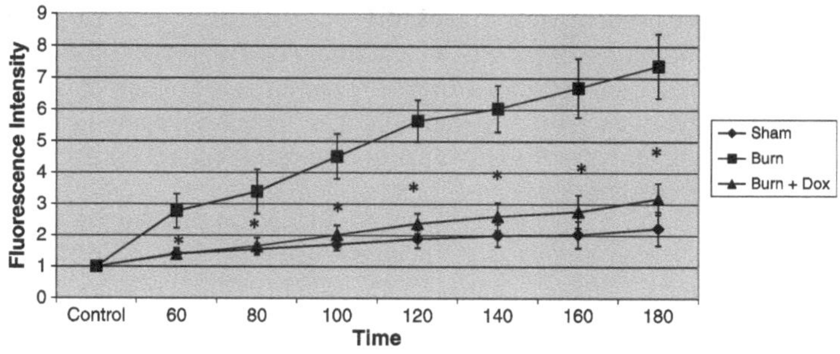

FIGURE 5.—Graphical representation of the changes in microvascular permeability in mesenteric postcapillary venules of sham, burn, and doxycycline treatment before burn. Burn trauma group shows significant increase in vascular permeability evidenced by significant extravasation of the FITC-albumin compared with the sham-control rats ($p < 0.05$). Doxycycline pretreatment decreases burn-induced hyperpermeability significantly ($p < 0.05$). (Reprinted from Stagg HW, Whaley JG, Tharakan B, et al. Doxycycline attenuates burn-Induced microvascular hyperpermeability. *J Trauma Acute Care Surg.* 2013;75:1040-1046, with permission from Lippincott Williams & Wilkins.)

adherens junction protein β-catenin was performed. Western blot and gelatin zymography were performed to assess MMP-9 level and activity.

Results.—MMP-9 levels were increased after burn. Monolayer permeability was significantly increased with burn serum treatment; this was attenuated with doxycycline as well as the specific MMP-9 inhibitor ($p < 0.05$). Damage of the endothelial cell adherens junction complex was induced by serum from burned rats, and doxycycline restored the integrity of the adherens junction similar to the MMP-9 inhibitor. Intravital microscopy revealed microvascular hyperpermeability after burn; this was attenuated with doxycycline ($p < 0.05$).

Conclusion.—Burns induce microvascular hyperpermeability via endothelial adherens junction disruption associated with MMP-9, and this is attenuated with doxycycline (Fig 5).

▶ The cause of microvascular hyperpermeability after burn is multifactorial. Oxidant injury plays a vital role in this process, mainly through initiating the apoptotic cascade. Inflammatory biochemical factors such as cytokines, kinins, prostaglandins, and histamines also contribute to the induction of hyperpermeability. The release of these factors results in damage to the adherens junctional complex. Matrix metalloproteinases (MMPs) are a family of zinc endopeptidases involved in a number of processes, both physiologic and pathologic. MMP-9 has been found to be involved in microvascular hyperpermeability, possibly as a downstream effector of many proinflammatory cytokines such as tumor necrosis factor, interleukin 6, interleukin 8, transforming growth factor alpha, and vascular endothelial growth. MMP-9 is a potential therapeutic target in the treatment of microvascular hyperpermeability associated with burn shock. The beneficial effect of doxycycline administration on the reduction of vascular permeability is evident as shown in Fig 5. The major drawback of this study is that animals were pretreated with doxycycline instead of given the dose after the injury in a more clinically relevant scenario. Prevention of postburn microvascular hyperpermeability and maintenance of the endothelial cell barrier could significantly decrease the morbid consequences of burn edema. MMP-9 is an effector of burn-associated microvascular hyperpermeability; its effects can be significantly attenuated with the common drug doxycycline, and this could represent a valuable adjunct in the treatment of burn shock.

D. W. Mozingo, MD

Burn-Induced Cardiac Dysfunction Increases Length of Stay in Pediatric Burn Patients

Howard TS, Hermann DG, McQuitty AL, et al (Univ of Texas Med Branch, Galveston)
J Burn Care Res 34:413-419, 2013

The aim of this study was to evaluate cardiac function and clinical outcomes in perioperative pediatric burn patients. Transesophageal echocardiography data were collected on 40 patients from 2004 to 2007. Of the 40 patients who received exams, a complete set of cardiac parameters and outcome variables was obtained in 26 patients. The mean age of the patients was 9.7 ± 0.9 years, and the mean TBSA burn size was 64 ± 3%. Patients were divided into two groups based on systolic function. One group represented patients with ejection fractions of >50% and the other ≤50%. Clinical variables were then compared among the groups. In our cohort, systolic dysfunction was observed in 62% of patients (EF ≤ 50%). Systolic dysfunction was associated with a statistically significant increase in number of surgeries, ventilator days, and length of stay in the intensive care unit. The length of stay in patients with preserved systolic function and those with systolic dysfunction was 34.3 ± 3.3 days and 67.2 ± 4.0 days, respectively. Diastolic function measurements were obtained in 65%, and 88% had evidence of diastolic dysfunction. Diastolic dysfunction was not associated with any statistically significant correlations. This study lends evidence to the well-supported basic science models showing cardiac dysfunction after burns. Additionally, it shows that cardiac dysfunction can have clinical consequences. To our knowledge, this is the first study that shows the clinical sequelae of systolic dysfunction in the perioperative pediatric burn population (Fig 2).

▶ Mechanisms for cardiac dysfunction after burn injury have been extensively reported. It has been found that thermal injury produces myocardial depression. It is known that circulating inflammatory cytokines are systemically released after burn injury and contribute to myocardial depression. In this selection, the authors examined a cohort of 26 burned children for which transesophageal echocardiography (TEE) data on systolic function were compared with outcome variables during their perioperative intensive care unit (ICU) stay. This is the first study to evaluate the clinical sequelae of cardiac dysfunction in burned children during the perioperative period. TEE was performed in the operating room,

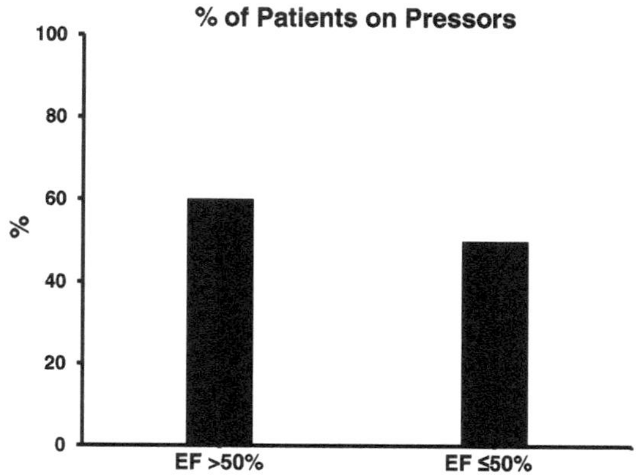

FIGURE 2.—Systolic function and pressor support during echocardiography of children with ≥35% TBSA. Use of cardiovascular supportive agents was independent of systolic function for both preserved (EF > 50%) and dysfunctional (EF ≤ 50%) systolic function groups. (Reprinted from Howard TS, Hermann DG, McQuitty AL, et al. Burn-induced cardiac dysfunction increases length of stay in pediatric burn patients. *J Burn Care Res.* 2013;34:413-419, with permission from the American Burn Association.)

before surgical incision, or in the patient's ICU room. The authors discovered that a significant number of children with large total body surface area burns had reduced systolic function, defined as an ejection fraction ≤50%. Additionally, systolic dysfunction was associated with approximately a 2-fold increase in ICU stay, increased number of days on ventilation support, increased creatinine, and number of surgeries. Fig 2 shows the effect of systolic dysfunction on ICU length of stay. Diastolic dysfunction was not significantly associated with length of stay or any of the other clinical parameters.

D. W. Mozingo, MD

Admission Temperature and Survival in Patients Admitted to Burn Centers

Hostler D, Weaver MD, Ziembicki JA, et al (Univ of Pittsburgh, PA; UPMC Mercy Trauma and Burn Ctr, PA)

J Burn Care Res 34:498-506, 2013

It is commonly believed that hypothermia occurring during burn resuscitation is associated with poor outcome, but there is little direct supporting evidence. The authors conducted an analysis of a statewide trauma registry to determine whether hypothermia (T ≤36.5 C) was associated with mortality when controlling for clinical confounders. They included all patients treated at an accredited burn center from 2000 to 2011 where the trauma registrar recorded the primary injury type as a burn. They excluded records with missing data and nonphysiologic temperature (<26° C or >42° C). The primary exposure of interest was hypothermia. The authors constructed a hierarchical, multivariable logistic regression model to examine the effect of hypothermia on survival, controlling for potentially confounding variables. Predictors of mortality are presented as odds ratio (95% confidence

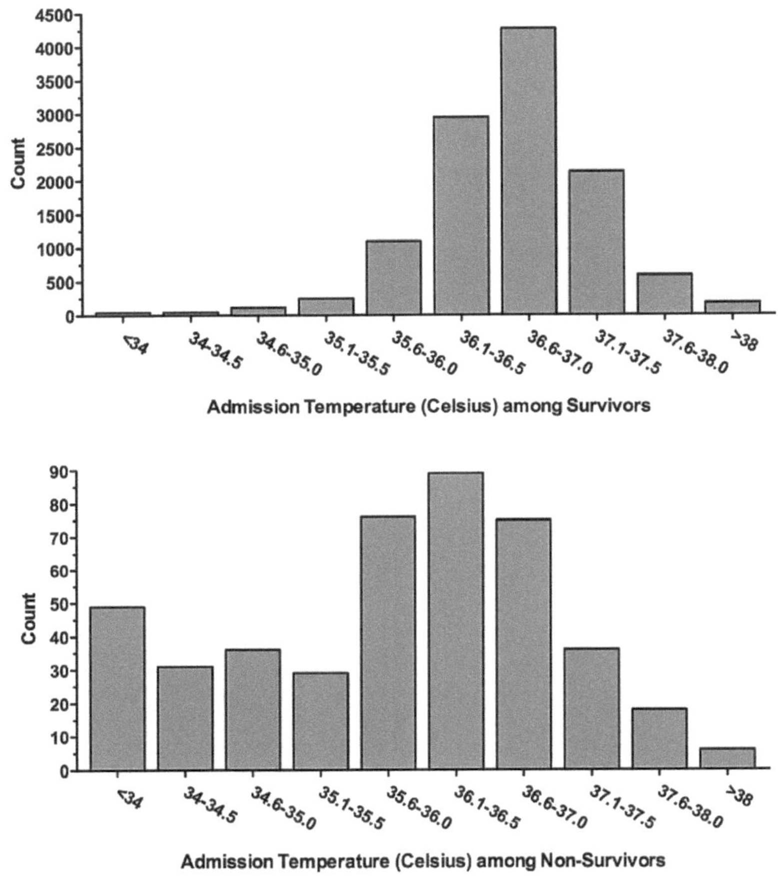

FIGURE 3.—Frequency distribution of admission temperature for survivors and nonsurvivors. (Reprinted from Hostler D, Weaver MD, Ziembicki JA, et al. Admission temperature and survival in patients admitted to burn centers. *J Burn Care Res*. 2013;34:498-506, with permission from the American Burn Association.)

interval). Primary burn injury was coded 17,098 times during the study period. Of these, 3809 were not treated at a burn center and 1192 were excluded for missing data. Admission hypothermia was independently associated with mortality (1.91 [1.58–2.29]) when adjusting for age, sex, total second- and third-degree burn surface area (TBSA), comorbid conditions, injury severity score, direct transport vs referral, method of temperature measurement, year, and the hospital providing care. Increasing age, female sex, TBSA > 40%, presence of multiple comorbid conditions, and increasing injury severity score were associated with mortality. Other variables in the model were not independently associated with outcome. There was a weak correlation between TBSA and admission temperature ($r = .18$). Hypothermia at hospital admission is independently associated with mortality in burn patients when controlling for clinical confounders.

Future studies should address potential causes underlying this observation (Fig 3).

▶ Similar to previous studies of trauma patients, the authors of this selection have shown that hypothermia at hospital admission is independently associated with death in a large, multiyear cohort of burn patients collected from a statewide trauma registry. However, given the weak correlation between burn size and admission temperature in this study, it is possible that this hypothermia is not simply a function of burn size and severity. Fig 3 demonstrates the difference in admission temperature for survivors and nonsurvivors. Although it is impossible to determine causality with this data set, the authors noted that burn patients arriving with temperatures < 36.5°C were more likely to be severely burned, severely injured, and receive large volumes of prehospital fluids. Therefore, it is unclear whether hypothermia was the result of the injury, treatment, or simply the lack of prevention of the loss of body heat. The authors have shown that nearly 40% of burn patients in a large trauma registry present to the burn center as mildly or moderately hypothermic and that core body temperature is only weakly correlated with burn size. After adjusting for related risk factors, hypothermia, age > 50 years, and female sex remain independent predictors of mortality.

D. W. Mozingo, MD

Acute burn induced coagulopathy

Sherren PB, Hussey J, Martin R, et al (Greater Sydney Area Helicopter Emergency Med Service (GSA-HEMS), New South Wales, Australia; St. Andrew's Burn Centre, UK; et al)

Burns 39:1157-1161, 2013

Background.—Acute traumatic coagulopathy is well described in the trauma population. Major burns are characterised by a similar endothelial injury and cellular hypoperfusion. These features could be a driver for an acute burn induced coagulopathy (ABIC).

Methods.—Patients admitted to a regional burn centre over a 71 months period with a total body surface area burn of 30% or more were identified. The metavision electronic patient database was scrutinised for a predetermined list of demographics, interventions and admission investigations to identify any clinically significant ABIC.

Results.—On admission 39.3% of the 117 patients analysed met our criteria for a coagulopathy. Of the patients with a coagulopathy, 71.7% had an elevated Prothrombin Time (PT), 2.2% had an elevated Activated Partial Thromboplastin time (APPT) and 26.1% had an elevation of both. Patients with a coagulopathy received a similar volume of fluid ($p = 0.08$). There was a statistically significant correlation between the PT and the abbreviated burn severity index ($p = 0.0013$, $r = 0.292$) and serum lactate ($p = 0.0013$, $r = 0.292$). ABIC was an independent predictor of 28 day mortality, OR 3.42 (1.11–10.56).

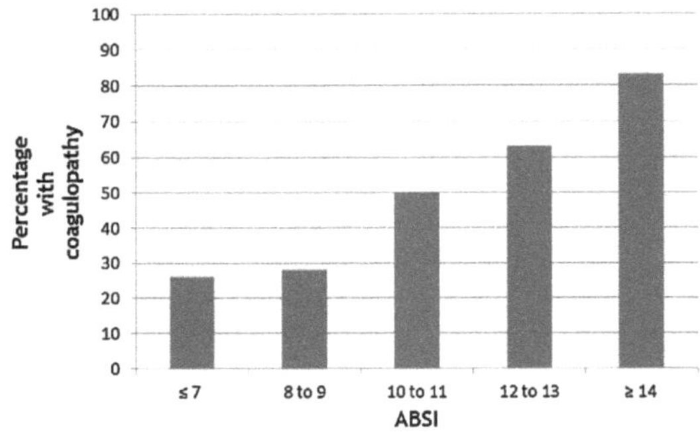

FIGURE 2.—Incidence of coagulopathy with varying abbreviated injury severity score (ABSI). (Reprinted from Sherren PB, Hussey J, Martin R, et al. Acute burn induced coagulopathy. *Burns*. 2013;39:1157-1161, Copyright 2013, with permission from International Society for Burn Injuries.)

Conclusion.—In patients with major thermal injuries a clinically significant ABIC exists. Early diagnosis and treatment of ABIC should be considered particularly in those undergoing total burn wound excision (Fig 2).

► Acute traumatic coagulopathy is a well-described phenomenon in the trauma population. It represents an impairment of hemostasis involving a complex dynamic interaction between endogenous anticoagulants and fibrinolysis that is initiated immediately after an injury. Acute traumatic coagulopathy is induced by endothelial injury and hypoperfusion, which results in increased thrombomodulin expression and activation of protein C. It is associated with an increase in transfusion requirements, injury severity scores, organ dysfunction, and mortality. Major burn injury also causes a similar direct endothelial injury and acute phase response with release of pro-inflammatory cytokines. This is accompanied by hypovolemia, impaired myocardial contractility, and cellular hypoperfusion. The authors of this selection suggest that this combination of features could be a driver for an acute burn-induced coagulopathy. The investigators found that just over 40% of patients with a major thermal injury had a coagulopathy on admission. They demonstrated that the coagulopathy is unrelated to fluid resuscitation and was an independent predictor of 28-day mortality. The presence of acute burn-induced coagulopathy correlated to the severity of the burn and was associated with a significant increase in total body surface area burn, inhalational injuries, incidence of full-thickness burns, and the abbreviated burn severity index. Fig 2 was included, demonstrating this finding. Patients with a major burn and coagulopathy who require early burn wound excision may be at an increased risk of bleeding and massive transfusion. Functional whole blood coagulation tests and laboratory tests should be used to make an early diagnosis and monitor progression. These patients may benefit from early transfusion of plasma and antifibrinolytic agents. Additional trials are required to delineate any morbidity or mortality benefit to such strategies.

D. W. Mozingo, MD

Evaluation of an Enoxaparin Dosing Calculator Using Burn Size and Weight

Faraklas I, Ghanem M, Brown A, et al (Univ of Utah Health Care, Salt Lake City)

J Burn Care Res 34:621-627, 2013

Previous research has shown that inadequate antifactor Xa levels (anti-Xa) occur in burn patients and may increase the risk of venous thromboembolic events (VTE). The objective of this retrospective review was to investigate the usefulness of an enoxaparin dosing algorithm using a previously published equation. With institutional review board approval, all acute burn patients at an American Burn Association–verified regional burn center who were treated with enoxaparin for VTE prophylaxis and had at least one anti-Xa from May 1, 2011 to December 15, 2012 were included. Patients with subprophylactic anti-Xa received increased enoxaparin dose per unit protocol with the goal of obtaining a prophylactic anti-Xa (0.2–0.4 U/ml). Sixty-four patients were included in our analysis. The regression equation was used in 33 patients for initial enoxaparin dosing (Eq) whereas 31 patients received traditionally recommended prophylaxis dosing (No-Eq). Groups were comparable in sex, age, weight, inhalation injury, and burn size. Initial enoxaparin dosing in Eq was significantly more likely to reach target than in No-Eq (73 vs 32%; $P = .002$). No episodes of hemorrhage, thrombocytopenia, or heparin sensitivity were documented in either group. Median final enoxaparin dose required to reach prophylactic level was 40 mg every 12 hours (range, 30–80 mg). Twenty-one No-Eq patients ultimately reached target, and 11 of these final doses were equivalent to or greater than the predicted equation. Ten patients never reached prophylactic anti-Xa before enoxaparin was discontinued (nine from No-Eq). Two patients, one from each group, developed VTE complications despite appropriate anti-Xa for prophylaxis. A strong correlation was shown between weight, burn size, and enoxaparin dose ($r^2 = .68$; $P < .001$). Use of the enoxaparin dosing algorithm significantly increased the frequency of obtaining a target initial anti-Xa. There were no bleeding complications. Enoxaparin dosing correlates to burn size and weight, making a standard dose inappropriate because patient habitus and extent of burn injury are highly variable. This simple equation improves enoxaparin dosing for acute adult burn patients (Fig 2).

► In burn patients with additional risk factors, including advanced age, morbid obesity, extensive or lower-extremity burns, other trauma, prolonged immobility, or femoral venous catheters, routine thromboprophylaxis is recommended. Estimates of the incidence of venous thromboembolic events (VTEs) in burn patients range from as low as 0.4% when identified clinically to as high as 23% when detected by screening ultrasound. Practice guidelines published by the American Burn Association's Committee on the Organization and Delivery of Burn Care indicate that, although complications related to prophylaxis are unknown, prophylactic measures are warranted based on a suspicion that deep vein thrombosis incidence is greater than historically believed. The authors of this selection adopted a thromboembolic prophylaxis protocol using enoxaparin. Using linear

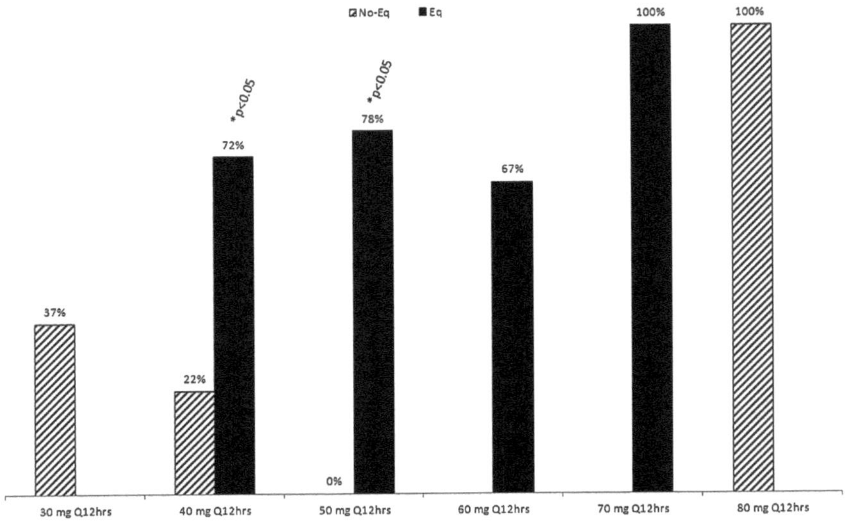

FIGURE 2.—Percentage of patients who achieve target anti-Xa levels with initial enoxaparin dose. There were no patients in the regression equation (Eq) group that initially received 30 or 80 mg every 12 hours (Q12Hrs), and correspondingly there were no patients in the not using the regression equation (No-Eq) group that received 60 or 70 mg Q12Hrs. (Reprinted from Faraklas I, Ghanem M, Brown A, et al. Evaluation of an enoxaparin dosing calculator using burn size and weight. *J Burn Care Res.* 2013;34:621-627, with permission from the American Burn Association.)

regression analysis, they identified that burn injury size (TBSA) and weight affected dose, generating the following equation for VTE prophylaxis: enoxaparin dose in milligrams every 12 hours = 22.8 + (3.3 × %TBSA/10) + (1.89 × (weight in kg)/10). The objective of the current study was to evaluate this equation by demonstrating that it enabled more patients to achieve prophylaxis with initial dosing. Fig 2 is included here, which demonstrates the beneficial effect of including weight and burn size in the enoxaparin dosing regimen.

D. W. Mozingo, MD

Noninvasive Measurement of Intestinal Inflammation After Burn Injury

Sigman M, Conrad P, Rendon JL, et al (Loyola Univ Chicago, Maywood, IL)
J Burn Care Res 34:633-638, 2013

Intestinal inflammation has been linked with multiorgan failure in patients with burn and other traumatic injuries. We hypothesized that markers of intestinal inflammation are detectible noninvasively. Fecal samples were collected from seven severely burned patients and 15 control patients for the measurement of inflammatory cytokines using a multiplex assay kit. In addition, fecal levels of myeloperoxidase (MPO) and elastase were measured using standard procedures. Compared with a control group, levels of inflammatory cytokines were significantly increased in the burn group. Interleukin (IL)-6 increased to a mean (± SEM) of

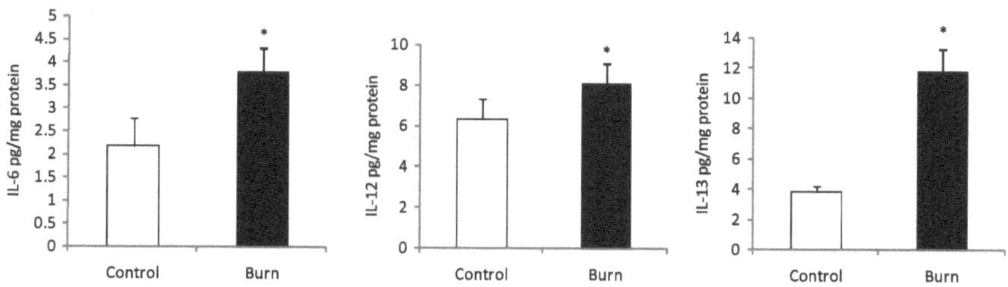

FIGURE 1.—Fecal levels of cytokines after burn injury. Feces collected from patients at various time points after burn injury was used to determine the levels of cytokines using multiplex kit. Interleukin (IL)-6 (A), IL-12(B), and IL-13 (C) are increased in the burn group compared with the control group. Data are shown as mean ± SEM. **P* < .05 compared with control group. (Reprinted from Sigman M, Conrad P, Rendon JL, et al. Noninvasive measurement of intestinal inflammation after burn injury. *J Burn Care Res.* 2013;34:633-638, with permission from the American Burn Association.)

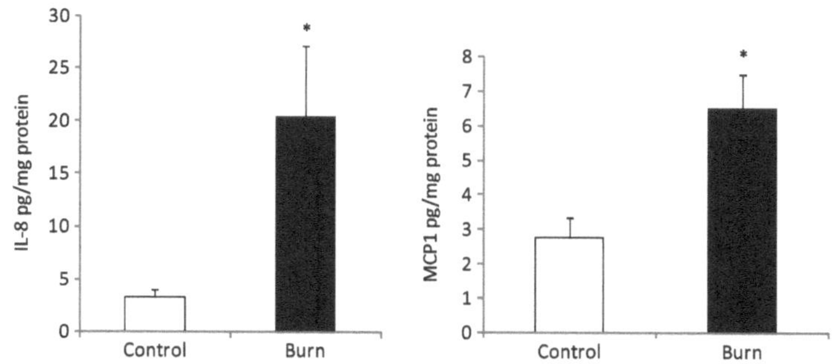

FIGURE 2.—Fecal levels of chemokines interleukin (IL)-8 (A) and monocyte chemoattractant protein (MCP)-1 (B) after burn injury. Inflammatory chemokines IL-8 and MCP-1 also were increased in the burn group compared with the control group. Data are shown as mean ± SEM. **P* < .05 compared with control group. (Reprinted from Sigman M, Conrad P, Rendon JL, et al. Noninvasive measurement of intestinal inflammation after burn injury. *J Burn Care Res.* 2013;34:633-638, with permission from the American Burn Association.)

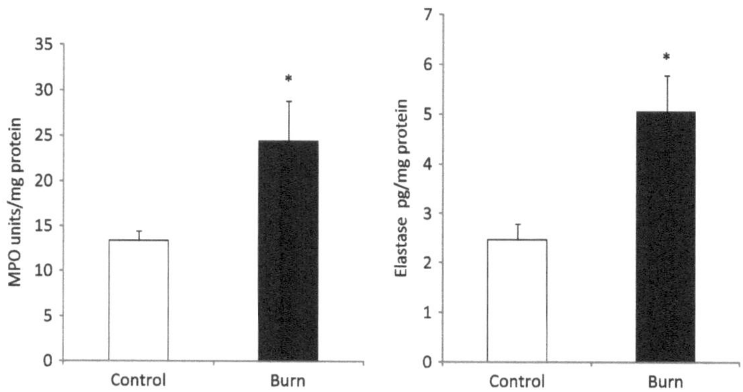

FIGURE 3.—Fecal levels of neutrophil markers myeloperoxidase (MPO) (A) and elastase (B) were increased in the burn sample compared with the control sample. Data are shown as mean ± SEM. **P* < .05 compared with control group. (Reprinted from Sigman M, Conrad P, Rendon JL, et al. Noninvasive measurement of intestinal inflammation after burn injury. *J Burn Care Res.* 2013;34:633-638, with permission from the American Burn Association.)

2.16 ± 0.61 to 3.81 ± 0.49 pg/mg ($P < .05$), as did IL-8 (3.32 ± 0.76 to 20.51 ± 6.65 pg/mg; $P < .05$), IL-12 (6.23 ± 0.98 to 8.11 ± 0.95 pg/mg; $P = 0.01$), IL-13 (3.86 ± 0.32 to 11.83 ± 1.47 pg/mg; $P < .05$), monocyte chemoattractant protein-1 (2.78 ± 2.61 to 6.5 ± 3.97 pg/mg; $P < .05$), MPO (13.41 ± 1.40 to 24.52 ± 4.31 units/mg protein; $P < .05$), and elastase (2.46 ± 0.38 to 5.08 ± 0.72 pg/mL; $P < .05$). Our results suggest that markers of intestinal inflammation are measurable by noninvasive means and are increased after burn injury compared with controls. Of note, increased IL-8 correlated with increased MPO and elastase activity, suggesting a role for neutrophil activation in burn-mediated intestinal inflammation. Thus, these inflammatory cytokine profiles may be valuable biomarkers of intestinal inflammation after burn injury (Figs 1-3).

► The human colon is the major reservoir of bacteria within the body. Under healthy conditions, it maintains an effective barrier against luminal bacteria; however, it is known that this barrier is disrupted after burn injury. This compromised barrier may play a role in the process that leads to organ and immune dysfunction after burn, but the exact role is uncertain. There is evidence that it is not the actual bacteria themselves that translocate and lead to this immune dysfunction; instead, it is the cytokine milieu induced by our immune system's interaction with these bacteria that seems to be the cause. The situation that is created by a burn injury is one in which a permeable gut loaded with intestinal bacteria sets the stage for an abnormal immune interaction, leading to the production of mediators that can fuel organ and immune dysfunction. This study demonstrates that fecal samples of burned patients show increased markers of inflammation, as depicted in Figs 1-3. Although more studies are needed to confirm this observation within a large burn-patient population, the findings suggest that fecal levels of inflammatory markers may be considered for determining gut inflammation after burn injury.

D. W. Mozingo, MD

Fluid Therapy LiDCO Controlled Trial—Optimization of Volume Resuscitation of Extensively Burned Patients through Noninvasive Continuous Real-Time Hemodynamic Monitoring LiDCO

Tokarik M, Sjöberg F, Balik M, et al (Charles Univ, Prague, Czech Republic; Linköping Univ, Sweden)

J Burn Care Res 34:537-542, 2013

This pilot trial aims at gaining support for the optimization of acute burn resuscitation through noninvasive continuous real-time hemodynamic monitoring using arterial pulse contour analysis. A group of 21 burned patients meeting preliminary criteria (age range 18–75 years with second-third- degree burns and TBSA ≥10–75%) was randomized during 2010. A hemodynamic monitoring through lithium dilution cardiac output was used in 10 randomized patients (LiDCO group), whereas those without LiDCO monitoring were defined as the control group. The modified Brooke/Parkland formula as a starting resuscitative formula, balanced

TABLE 2.—FACT Algorithm

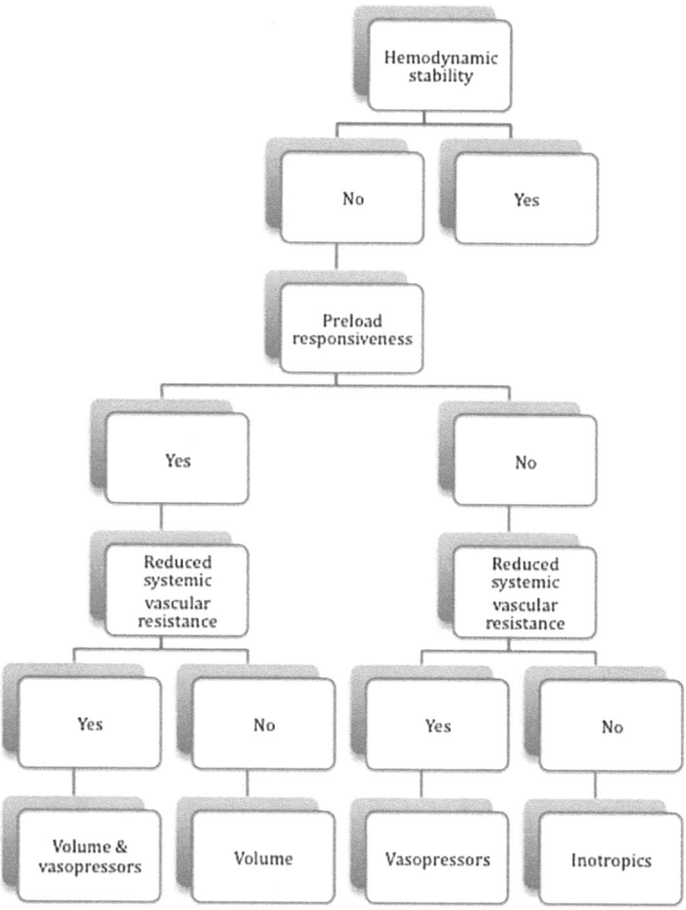

Algorithm of volume and vasopressor/inotropic (noradrenaline/dobutamine) support.
Hemodynamic instability: mean arterial pressure < 65 T and oliguria < 0.5 ml/kg/hr.
Preload responsiveness based on dynamic preload parameters (systolic pressure variation > 10 mm Hg, pulse pressure variation > 15%, stroke volume variation > 15%).
Physiological range: CI: 2.5–4.0 l/min l/min/m2, systemic vascular resistence index: 1970–2390 dynes·sec/cm5/m2.
Source: From Reference 13.
Editor's Note: Please refer to original journal article for full references.

crystalloids as the initial solutions, urine output of 0.5 ml/kg/hr as a crucial value of adequate intravascular filling were used in both groups. Additionally, the volume and vasopressor/inotropic support were based on dynamic preload parameters in the LiDCO group in the case of circulatory instability and oligouria. Statistical analysis was done using t-tests. Within the first 24 hours postburn, a significantly lower consumption of crystalloids was registered in LiDCO group ($P = .04$). The fluid balance under LiDCO control in combination with hourly diuresis contributed to reducing the cumulative fluid balance approximately by 10% compared with fluid management based on standard monitoring parameters. The amount of applied solutions in the LiDCO group got closer to Brooke formula whereas the urine output was at the same level in both groups (0.8 ml/kg/hr). The new finding in this study is that when a fluid resuscitation is based on the arterial waveform analysis, the initial fluid volume provided was significantly lower than that delivered on the basis of physician-directed fluid resuscitation (by urine output and mean arterial pressure) (Table 2).

▶ The new finding in this study is that when a fluid responsiveness methodology based on the arterial waveform analysis is used in the Fluid Therapy LiDCO Controlled Trial algorithm (Table 2 included in this selection), the crystalloid fluid volume provided was significantly lower than that delivered on the basis of physician-directed fluid. The biggest benefit of the LiDCO technology and the algorithm of volume/inotropic support based on protocolized functional hemodynamic monitoring may be the assessment of volume responsiveness before administration of fluid. This method to assess preload responsiveness, which includes monitoring changes in central venous pressure during spontaneous inspiration, variations in arterial pulse pressure, systolic pressure, and aortic flow variations in response to vena cava collapse during positive pressure ventilation, was combined with hourly urine output in this study. This prospective controlled trial presents a circulation surveillance technique (stroke volume variation, pulse pressure variation, systolic pressure variation) in combination with hourly urine output, which does not, unlike what was previously described in central circulation monitoring techniques, lead to fluid overresuscitation in early resuscitation of significant burns. An implementation of a randomized multicenter study would be appropriate.

D. W. Mozingo, MD

A randomized comparison study of Aquacel Ag and Alginate Silver as skin graft donor site dressings

Ding X, Shi L, Liu C, et al (The Hosp Affiliated to Jiangsu Univ, Zhenjiang, Jiangsu Province, PR China)

Burns 39:1547-1550, 2013

Objective.—This study was conducted to compare pain, healing time, infection rate, and cosmetic outcome between Aquacel Ag (convatec) and Alginate Silver (coloplast) as donor site dressings.

Materials and Methods.—We conducted a prospective randomized controlled trial of donor site dressings, comparing Aquacel Ag with Alginate Silver. Patients were randomly allocated to donor site dressing with one of these materials. Outcome measures included pain scores at rest and during dressing changes, time to re-epithelialization, cosmetic outcome and infection rate. Results were assessed for significance using the independent t-test (non-parametric data) and the chi-square test (parametric data).

Results.—A total of 20 subjects were enrolled in this study. Subjects included in both groups were comparable with no significant differences in demographic data of age, gender, location of burn and type of burns ($P > 0.05$ evaluated by paired t-test) between both groups. The pain scores were found to be higher in Aquacel Ag group than in Alginate Silver group. Time to re-epithelialization was longer in Aquacel Ag group than in Alginate Silver group. There were no significant differences between the two treatment groups with respect to cosmetic outcome and infection rate.

Conclusions.—Based on these results, we find that Alginate Silver is better than Aquacel Ag to cover the skin graft donor site.

► In patients with major body surface burns, the use and reuse of donor sites is important to cover the burn sites quickly and completely. Thus, it is valuable to be able to manage the donor sites so that they can be used again. This prospective, randomized trial compared 2 silver compounds (Aquacel Ag vs Alginate Ag) on donor sites. The Alginate Ag group healed on average 1 day sooner. More importantly, the patients had significantly less pain at the time points measured using the Alginate Ag compound.

It is critically important that studies such as these be conducted in a prospective, randomized fashion. Although only small numbers of patients were included in this study, the 1-day average difference in healing time was statistically (even if not clinically) different. It would be valuable for the authors to continue the study with larger numbers of patients evaluating issues of pain and reuse of donor sites to determine clinically significant outcomes.

J. M. Daly, MD

A comparative study of 1% silver sulphadiazine (Flammazine®) versus an enzyme alginogel (Flaminal®) in the treatment of partial thickness burns

Hoeksema H, Vandekerckhove D, Verbelen J, et al (Ghent Univ Hosp, Belgium)

Burns 39:1234-1241, 2013

Introduction.—In the conservative treatment of burns, rapid wound healing is desirable to obtain good aesthetic and functional results. The aim of this study was to compare the efficacy of 1% Silversulfadiazine (SSD/Flammazine®) and an enzyme alginogel (Flaminal® or Flaminal® Forte) on the healing of superficial and intermediate partial thickness burns.

Methods.—In this retrospective cohort study comparable burn wounds treated with Flaminal® or with 1% SSD were included. Outcome parameters included: length of hospital stay, bacterial burden and time to wound closure. Significance was tested using SPSS package.

Results.—44 wounds in the Flaminal® group, and 39 wounds in the 1% SSD group were included. Wounds treated with Flaminal® showed a significantly higher bacterial load ($p = 0.024$) and contained significantly more bacterial species ($p = 0.010$) but showed a significantly shorter healing time of 17 vs. 24 days ($p < 0.0001$).

Conclusion.—A significantly shorter healing time was demonstrated in partial thickness burn wounds treated with Flaminal® versus 1% SSD, which may lead to a shorter length of hospital stay and better scar quality. The possibility of accurate burn depth assessment and the results in this study corroborate the change in treatment protocol made in the year 2000 when we switched from 1% SSD to Flaminal®.

▶ Prompt healing of burn wounds in patients is critical both for the safety of the patient and the ultimate cosmetic and functional outcomes after burn injury. The authors have presented a retrospective cohort study of patients treated between 1998 and 2003 with either 1% silversulfadiazine (SSD) or alginogel. The authors chose the latter product because it allowed for better determination of the degree of burn injury, was less messy, and might reduce the emergence of bacterial species resistant to silver. They have noted that the alginogel had its primary efficacy via the creation of peroxides and then local oxygen species that were predicted to have better antibacterial effects. All patients treated between the above dates were assessed, but only 60 patients (30 per group) were included, and a total of 83 wounds were treated.

The results of the study suggested that healing time was shorter after treatment with alginogel compared with SSD. However, one must remember that this was a retrospective review with no randomization to therapy. In addition, it is unclear how many patients were actually treated in their burn unit during that time. Finally, there was some disparity between healing time (shorter in the alginogel group), while this group had higher bacterial counts.

The rationale behind using the alginogel is clear, and it may indeed be a better product compared with SSD. Unfortunately, the authors have allowed their practice of burn wound care to continue these last 10 years without a much-needed clinical trial in which they randomly assign patients between the 2 treatments or randomly divide the wounds between the 2 treatments. They decided on a clinical product years ago and have used this cohort study to confirm their bias for burn wound care.

J. M. Daly, MD

Antimicrobial efficacy of a novel silver hydrogel dressing compared to two common silver burn wound dressings: Acticoat™ and PolyMem Silver®

Boonkaew B, Kempf M, Kimble R, et al (The Univ of Queensland, Brisbane, Australia; et al)

Burns 40:89-96, 2014

A novel burn wound hydrogel dressing has been previously developed which is composed of 2-acrylamido-2-methylpropane sulfonic acid sodium salt with silver nanoparticles. This study compared the antimicrobial efficacy of this novel dressing to two commercially available silver dressings; Acticoat™ and PolyMem Silver®. Three different antimicrobial tests were used: disc diffusion, broth culture, and the Live/Dead® Baclight™ bacterial viability assay. Burn wound pathogens (*P. aeruginosa*, MSSA, *A. baumannii* and *C. albicans*) and antibiotic resistant strains (MRSA and VRE) were tested. All three antimicrobial tests indicated that Acticoat™ was the most effective antimicrobial agent, with inhibition zone lengths of 13.9–18.4 mm. It reduced the microbial inocula below the limit of detection (10^2 CFU/ml) and reduced viability by 99% within 4 h. PolyMem Silver® had no zone of inhibition for most tested micro-organisms, and it also showed poor antimicrobial activity in the broth culture and Live/Dead® Baclight™ assays. Alarmingly, it appeared to promote the growth of VRE. The silver hydrogel reduced most of the tested microbial inocula below the detection limit and decreased bacterial viability by 94–99% after 24 h exposure. These results support the possibility of using this novel silver hydrogel as a burn wound dressing in the future.

▶ Both silver nitrate and silver sulfadiazine have been used for many years to reduce the incidence of burn wound infection. They each have clinical toxicities and laboratory adverse side effects but in general have been very effective reducing the mortality of major body surface burns. Newer agents are clearly needed, and the authors have utilized nanotechnology to create a burn wound hydrogel compound with silver nanoparticles. *In vitro* testing found remarkable antimicrobial effectiveness against common burn wound pathogens compared with 2 other commercially available silver dressings.

Clearly, this *in vitro* study is a first step in a long process before this agent is used routinely in vivo in patients. It will have to undergo extensive testing in animal models of burn wound injury and then safety testing in humans if safety and efficacy are shown in the preclinical models. Nevertheless, the use of nanotechnology to create new antimicrobials is an exciting possibility to improve drug effectiveness with potentially fewer associated harmful side effects.

J. M. Daly, MD

Efficacy of debridement and wound cleansing with 2% hydrogen peroxide on graft take in the chronic-colonized burn wounds; a randomized controlled clinical trial

Mohammadi AA, Seyed Jafari SM, Kiasat M, et al (Shiraz Univ of Med Sciences, Iran)

Burns 39:1131-1136, 2013

Background.—Severe burns are associated with dramatic outcomes which are potentially detrimental. Nowadays the standard treatment for deep partial thickness and full-thickness burn is early excision and grafting, which is not always feasible this leads to chronicity and microbial colonization of burn wounds. Interesting properties of hydrogen peroxide 2% soaked gauze convinced us to use it in management of chronic burn wounds.

Methods.—From January 2009 to September 2011, in a prospective clinical trial, 49 patients (98 limbs) with chronic-colonized burn wounds in both limbs were included in this study. Tissue cultures were taken from all the wounds. For the right, after debridement of granulation tissue and washing with hydrogen peroxide 2% soaked gauze for 5 min followed by normal saline irrigation, grafting was done; debridement and skin grafting was performed in the conventional method in left limb wounds. The success rate of graft take was compared between two groups, after 21 days by the surgeon using the formula:

$$\frac{\text{Graft surface area (cm}^2\text{)} \times 100\%}{\text{Total grafted area (cm}^2\text{)}}$$

Results.—The study group was composed of 98 limbs in 49 patients with mean age of 26.44 ± 5.66 and burn in 28.3 ± 7.23% TBSA. The most common causes of the burn wounds chronicity was delayed admission associated with poor compliance. (44.8%) *Staphylococcus* was the most frequent isolate bacterial wounds colonization in our patients. (59.2%) Mean graft take was 82.85% in right limbs, and 65.61% in left limbs; which was significantly different ($P < 0.05$).

Conclusions.—Our study showed that, administration of hydrogen peroxide intraoperatively appears to be safe and significantly increases the mean success rate graft take in chronic-colonized wounds. Therefore, it can be recommended in management of chronic burn wounds management.

▶ This is an excellent study that evaluated the treatment of chronic burn wounds. Generally, patients treated soon after burn injury undergo excision of the burned area with immediate grafting. However, when admission is delayed and the burn wound has become colonized, engraftment does not occur as well. Patients in this study had one leg treated with a 2% hydrogen peroxide solution after debridement of granulation tissue, while the opposite leg received normal saline solution. As expected, *Staphylococcus* was most commonly found after culture. Graft take was significantly better on the legs treated with hydrogen peroxide (83%) compared with saline controls (65%).

This is an important study because the patients acted as their own controls, the methodology required little cost or effort with readily available solutions, and the endpoints measured were relatively clear. The study should be replicated, but if similar findings occur, this method will change the care of chronically burned areas in patients.

J. M. Daly, MD

4 Critical Care

Executive Summary: Developing a New, National Approach to Surveillance for Ventilator-associated Events

Magill SS, Klompas M, Balk R, et al (Ctrs for Disease Control and Prevention, Atlanta, GA; Harvard Med School and Harvard Pilgrim Health Care Inst, Boston, MA; Rush Univ School of Medicine, Chicago, IL; et al)

Ann Am Thorac Soc 10:S220-S223, 2013

In September 2011, the CDC convened a Ventilator-Associated Pneumonia (VAP) Surveillance Definition Working Group to organize a formal process for leaders and experts of key stakeholder organizations to discuss the challenges of VAP surveillance definitions and to propose new approaches to VAP surveillance in adult patients (Table 1). The charges to the Working Group were to:

- Critically review a draft, streamlined VAP surveillance definition developed for use in adult patients;
- Suggest modifications to enhance the reliability and credibility of the surveillance definition within the critical care and infection prevention communities;
- Propose a final adult surveillance definition algorithm, to be implemented in the CDC's National Healthcare Safety Network (NHSN), taking into consideration the potential future use of the definition algorithm in public reporting, interfacility comparisons, and pay-for-reporting and pay-for-performance programs.

▶ The Ventilator-Associated Pneumonia (VAP) Surveillance Definition Working Group's new approach to surveillance in mechanically ventilated adults acknowledges the current limitations in VAP diagnosis and the potential benefit in focusing surveillance on an objective, reliable, but more general measure of significant conditions and complications that occur in patients requiring mechanical ventilation. Ventilator-associated events (VAE) surveillance was implemented by the Centers for Disease Control in January 2013. Although much work remains, this innovative approach to surveillance has significant potential to increase the validity of comparisons among health care facilities and, more importantly, to improve measurement and patient safety in the intensive care unit. An iterative process for refining the definitions must be ensured as experience using the definition algorithm accumulates in coming years. Although there was clearly a need to establish a new surveillance approach, there is also an urgent need to advance the science of surveillance for VAP and other VAE. The VAE surveillance definition algorithm should be studied, validated, and improved in an ongoing manner.

D. W. Mozingo, MD

The impact of intensivists' base specialty of training on care process and outcomes of critically ill trauma patients

Matsushima K, Goldwasser ER, Schaefer EW, et al (Penn State Milton S. Hershey Med Ctr, Hershey, PA)

J Surg Res 184:577-581, 2013

Background.—The care of the critically ill trauma patients is provided by intensivists with various base specialties of training. The purpose of this study was to investigate the impact of intensivists' base specialty of training on the disparity of care process and patient outcome.

Methods.—We performed a retrospective review of an institutional trauma registry at an academic level 1 trauma center. Two intensive care unit teams staffed by either board-certified surgery or anesthesiology intensivists were assigned to manage critically ill trauma patients. Both teams provided care, collaborating with a trauma surgeon in house. We compared patient characteristics, care processes, and outcomes between surgery and anesthesiology groups using Wilcoxon tests or chi-square tests, as appropriate.

Results.—We identified a total of 620 patients. Patient baseline characteristics including age, sex, transfer status, injury type, injury severity score, and Glasgow coma scale were similar between groups. We found no significant difference in care processes and outcomes between groups. In a logistic regression model, intensivists' base specialty of training was not a significant factor for mortality (odds ratio, 1.46; 95% confidence interval; 0.79–2.80; $P = 0.22$) and major complication (odds ratio, 1.11; 95% confidence interval, 0.73–1.67; $P = 0.63$).

Conclusions.—Intensive care unit teams collaborating with trauma surgeons had minimal disparity of care processes and similar patient outcomes regardless of intensivists' base specialty of training.

► In this retrospective study of critically ill trauma patients, the authors found no significant differences in care processes or outcomes between the 2 intensive care unit teams run by either surgery intensivists or anesthesiology intensivists. This is the first study to compare care processes and outcomes by intensivists with different base specialties of training that focused only on trauma patients. The authors demonstrated that the intensivists' base specialty of training, surgery versus anesthesiology, was not a significant factor for disparity of care processes and outcomes of critically ill trauma patients in their intensivist-staffed intensive care unit. The study is limited by being performed in a single institution. The use of common care plans and guidelines, as used at this institution, also serves to reduce variability in care. It may also be difficult to find differences if care of the patients is performed by more than 1 specialist as would be encountered for patients with a longer length of intensive care unit stay. Further investigation in a multicenter prospective study will be needed to verify these results.

D. W. Mozingo, MD

Obesity and overweight as a risk factor for pneumonia in polytrauma patients: A retrospective cohort study

Mica L, Keller C, Vomela J, et al (Univ Hosp of Zürich, Switzerland; Univ Hosp of Cologne, Germany; Univ Hosp of Brno, Czech Republic; et al)

J Trauma Acute Care Surg 75:693-698, 2013

Background.—Obesity is a growing problem in western societies. The aim of this retrospective cohort study was to determine the association between the overweight and obese polytrauma patients and pneumonia after injury.

Methods.—A total of 628 patients with an Injury Severity Score (ISS) of 16 or greater and 16 years or older were included in this retrospective study. The sample was subdivided into three groups as follows: body mass index (BMI) of less than 25 kg/m^2; BMI of 25 kg/m^2 to 30 kg/m^2; and BMI more than 30 kg/m^2. The Murray score was assessed at admission and at its maximum during hospitalization to determine pulmonary problems. Pneumonia was defined as bacteriologically positive sputum with appropriate radiologic and laboratory changes (C-reactive protein and interleukin 6). Data are given as mean ± SEM. One-way analysis of variance and the Kruskal-Wallis test were used for the analyses, and the significance level was set at $p < 0.05$; Bonferroni-Dunn test was performed as post hoc analysis.

Results.—The Abbreviated Injury Scale (AIS) score for the thorax was 3.2 ± 0.1 in the group with a BMI of less than 25 kg/m^2, 3.3 ± 0.1 in the group with a BMI of 25 kg/m^2 to 30 kg/m^2, and 2.8 ± 0.2 in the group with BMI of more than 30 kg/m^2 ($p = 0.044$). The Murray score at admission was elevated with increasing BMI (0.8 ± 0.8 for BMI < 25 kg/m^2, 0.9 ± 0.9 for BMI 25–30 kg/m^2, and 1.0 ± 0.8 for BMI > 30 kg/m^2; $p = 0.137$); the maximum Murray score during hospitalization revealed significant differences (1.2 ± 0.9 for BMI < 25 kg/m^2, 1.6 ± 1.0 for BMI 25–30 kg/m^2, and 1.5 ± 0.9 for BMI > 30 kg/m^2; $p < 0.001$). The incidence of pneumonia also increased with increasing BMI (1.6% for BMI < 25 kg/m^2, 2.0% for BMI 25–30 kg/m^2, and 3.1% for BMI > 30 kg/m^2; $p = 0.044$).

Conclusion.—Obesity leads to an increased incidence of pneumonia in a polytrauma situation.

► This study was designed to evaluate the impact of body mass index (BMI) on the development of pneumonia in patients with polytrauma. Understanding the main source of complications in overweight and obese polytrauma patients may play an important role in their multidisciplinary treatment. Obesity increases comorbidities and posttraumatic complications compared with normal-weight patients. This study shows that increasing BMI is associated with a higher incidence of pneumonia in polytrauma patients. The findings of a higher thorax Injury Severity Score (ISS) and Abbreviated Injury Scale (AIS) score, mainly in the overweight BMI group, may indicate a trauma-based etiology of thoracic problems such as pneumonia. However, the obese group showed a significantly lower thorax ISS and AIS score than did the normal-weight group, suggesting that in this group, not only trauma but also obstructive ventilation caused by obesity may have a role in the etiology of pneumonia. These findings are reflected in the increasing incidence of pneumonia in each group with increasing BMI. Ventilation in the supine-laying obese patient is obstructed by the weight of the abdominal fat and may be a predisposing factor in the development of pneumonia in the obese polytrauma patient.

D. W. Mozingo, MD

Innovations in geriatric trauma and resident research education: bridging the gap

Mangram A (John C. Lincoln North Mountain Hosp, Phoenix, AZ)
Am J Surg 206:834-839, 2013

The recent history of changes in the geriatric population in the US, the unique vulnerability to different mechanisms of trauma and the need for innovative management strategies to address them are discussed using the Geriatric "G-60" service as an illustration. The issue is not whether geriatric trauma "G-60" is coming; G-60 is here. A short detour into my own research experience is presented not as prescription but guidance for the development of futures cadres of surgeons. Resident research is not a luxury but key to transforming knowledge from benchside to bedside and back.

▶ With the increasing numbers of geriatric trauma admissions, the author of this selection noticed an increase of geriatric trauma patients with multiple medical problems and an isolated injury, and no dedicated team was willing to accept responsibility for their care. In many trauma systems, this results in disagreement between the hospitalists, orthopedic surgeons, and trauma surgeons as to who would assume overall care of these patients. In an effort to solve these problems, a geriatric trauma service was organized, led by trauma surgeons, and was designed specifically to expedite the care of geriatric patients through a multidisciplinary approach and to systematically measure the process and patient outcomes. This was named the *G-60 geriatric trauma service*. With G-60, the care of the elderly trauma patients was led by the trauma surgeon and handled through a multidisciplinary approach that included collaboration with other specialist and ancillary services. The goals of the service were (1) 30 minutes from emergency department (ED) presentation to trauma service evaluation, (2) 4 hours from ED presentation to inpatient room, (3) 36 hours from ED presentation to operating room, (4) 5 days from ED to safe and appropriate disposition. All of these goals were met or surpassed within 1 year of creation of the service. Additional reductions in intensive care unit length of stay

(LOS) and overall LOS were also accomplished. As the population of patients older than 60 continues to increase, adoption of this model will become a necessity at trauma centers and acute care surgery programs.

D. W. Mozingo, MD

Characterizing vasopressin and other vasoactive mediators released during resuscitation of trauma patients

Cohn SM, Derosa M, McCarthy J, et al (Univ of Texas Health Science Ctr, San Antonio; et al)

J Trauma Acute Care Surg 75:620-628, 2013

Background.—We sought to perform the first characterization of vasopressin and other vasoactive mediators released during resuscitation of hypotensive trauma patients.

Methods.—This institutional review board-approved study was conducted under waiver of consent. Adults with clinical evidence of acute traumatic injury and systolic blood pressure less than or equal to 90 mm Hg within 1 hour of arrival were evaluated at our Level I trauma center. Two hundred three patients were screened with 50 enrolled from February 2010 to February 2011. Demographic information was also collected. Blood samples were obtained at 0, 30, 60, 90, 120, and 240 minutes after arrival, and assays were performed for vasopressin, angiotensin II, epinephrine, and cortisol. We assessed the significance of variation in these vasoactive mediators with injury and transfusion of more than 600 mL, with adjustment for time using repeated-measures linear models in log units.

Results.—We found that vasopressin ($p = 0.005$) and epinephrine ($p = 0.01$) increased significantly with injury, while angiotensin ($p = 0.60$) and cortisol ($p = 0.46$) did not and that vasopressin ($p < 0.001$) and epinephrine ($p = 0.004$) increased significantly in patients requiring transfusion of more than 600 mL but angiotensin II ($p = 0.11$) and cortisol ($p = 0.90$) did not. Relatively low levels of vasopressin (<30 pg/mL) were observed at least once during the first 2 hours in 88% of trauma patients, and abnormally low epinephrine levels (<100 pg/mL) were observed at least once during the first 2 hours in 18% of trauma patients.

Conclusion.—This is the first clinical trial to serially evaluate vasopressin and other vasoactive mediators following trauma during the resuscitation phase. Vasopressin, in particular, and epinephrine seem to be the key mediators produced in the human response to severe injury. A deficiency of vasopressin may contribute to intractable shock after trauma.

Level of Evidence.—Prognostic/epidemiologic study, level III.

► The strength of this study is that it was prospective in nature. As noted by the authors, the weaknesses are that they were unable to align the times of measurement with the time of the injury, and there was no statistical basis for the sample size. The small population size prevented them from fully characterizing the vasoactive mediator response within subsets of homogeneous patients because the trauma population is quite diverse. They found that blood-level vasopressin and epinephrine increase during resuscitation of trauma patients and are related to the severity of injury. Insufficiency of vasopressin was found during the first 2 hours after admission in those trauma patients with documented hypoperfusion in more than 90% of patients, and epinephrine insufficiency was noted in approximately half of these patients. After severe injury, patients may ultimately be found to benefit from administration of a low dose of vasopressin or epinephrine to avoid the development of refractory shock states. This important finding warrants additional study and the consideration of point-of-care testing for vasopressin and epinephrine.

D. W. Mozingo, MD

Predicting the need for urgent intubation in a surgical/trauma intensive care unit

Politano AD, for the Predictive Monitoring in Patients with Trauma (PreMPT) Group (Univ of Virginia Health System, Charlottesville)
Surgery 154:1110-1116, 2013

Background.—Analysis and modeling of data monitoring vital signs and waveforms in patients in a surgical/trauma intensive care unit (STICU) may allow for early identification and treatment of patients with evolving respiratory failure.

Methods.—Between February 2011 and March 2012, data of vital signs and waveforms for STICU patients were collected. Every-15-minute calculations (n = 172,326) of means and standard deviations of heart rate (HR), respiratory rate (RR), pulse-oxygen saturation (SpO_2), cross-correlation coefficients, and cross-sample entropy for HR-RR, RR-SpO_2, and HR-SpO_2, and cardiorespiratory coupling were calculated. Urgent intubations were recorded. Univariate analyses were performed for the periods <24 and ≥24 hours before intubation. Multivariate predictive models for the risk of unplanned intubation were developed and validated internally by subsequent sample and bootstrapping techniques.

Results.—Fifty unplanned intubations (41 patients) were identified from 798 STICU patients. The optimal multivariate predictive model (HR, RR, and SpO_2 means, and RR-SpO_2 correlation coefficient) had a receiving operating characteristic (ROC) area of 0.770 (95% confidence interval [CI], 0.712–0.841). For this model, relative risks of intubation in the next 24 hours for the lowest and highest quintiles were 0.20 and 2.95, respectively (15-fold increase, baseline risk 1.46%). Adding age and days since previous extubation to this model increased ROC area to 0.865 (95 % CI, 0.821–0.910).

Conclusion.—Among STICU patients, a multivariate model predicted increases in risk of intubation in the following 24 hours based on vital sign data available currently on bedside monitors. Further refinement could allow for earlier detection of respiratory decompensation and

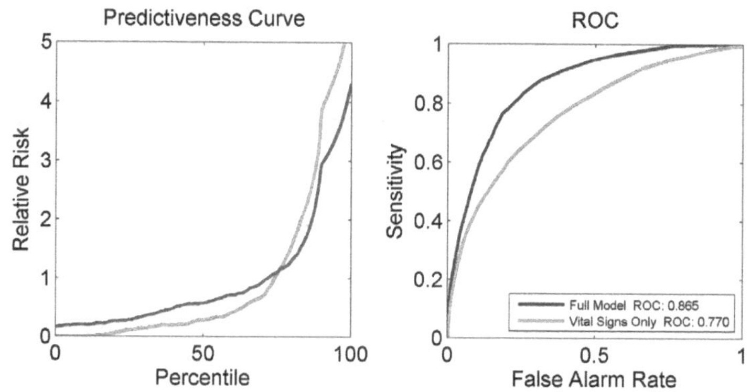

FIGURE 2.—Predictiveness and receiving operating characteristic curves for vital signs only and full model. (Reprinted from Politano AD, for the Predictive Monitoring in Patients with Trauma (PreMPT) Group. Predicting the need for urgent intubation in a surgical/trauma intensive care unit. *Surgery.* 2013;154:1110-1116, Copyright 2013, with permission from Elsevier.)

intervention to decrease preventable morbidity and mortality in surgical/ trauma patients (Fig 2).

▶ The findings in this selection show the feasibility of a developing an internally validated, predictive model from complex vital sign analysis in patients requiring urgent, unplanned intubation in a surgical trauma population. The relatively small number of events in this single-center study may limit the ability to generalize these findings, and the specific vital sign parameters may vary in more diverse patient populations. Also, although this analysis was restricted to a surgical intensive care unit patient population, there was still heterogeneity among patients with regard to their physiologic condition and age. Larger, multicenter studies will be required to validate these findings. The additions of clinical variables improved the performance of the model as defined by the predictiveness curves and receiving operating characteristic area and are included as Fig 2. The clinical importance of the full model, however, should be interpreted cautiously, because the relative contribution of the days since extubation variable to the model potentially overshadows the more clinically relevant vital sign variables.

D. W. Mozingo, MD

Mild Obesity Is Protective After Severe Burn Injury

Jeschke MG, Finnerty CC, Emdad F, et al (Univ of Toronto, Ontario, Canada; Univ of Texas Med Branch, Galveston; et al)
Ann Surg 258:1119-1129, 2013

Objective.—To assess the impact of obesity on morbidity and mortality in severely burned patients.

Background.—Despite the increasing number of people with obesity, little is known about the impact of obesity on postburn outcomes.

Methods.—A total of 405 patients were prospectively enrolled as part of the multicenter trial Inflammation and the Host Response to Injury Glue Grant with the following inclusion criteria: 0 to 89 years of age, admitted within 96 hours after injury, and more than 20% total body surface area burn requiring at least 1 surgical intervention. Body mass index was used in adult patients to stratify according to World Health Organization definitions: less than 18.5 (underweight), 18.5 to 29.9 (normal weight), 30 to 34.9 (obese I), 35 to 39.9 (obese II), and body mass index more than 40 (obese III). Pediatric patients (2 to ≤18 years of age) were stratified by using the Centers for Disease Control and Prevention and World Health Organization body mass index-for-age growth charts to obtain a percentile ranking and then grouped as underweight (<5th percentile), normal weight (5th percentile to <95th percentile), and obese (≥95th percentile). The

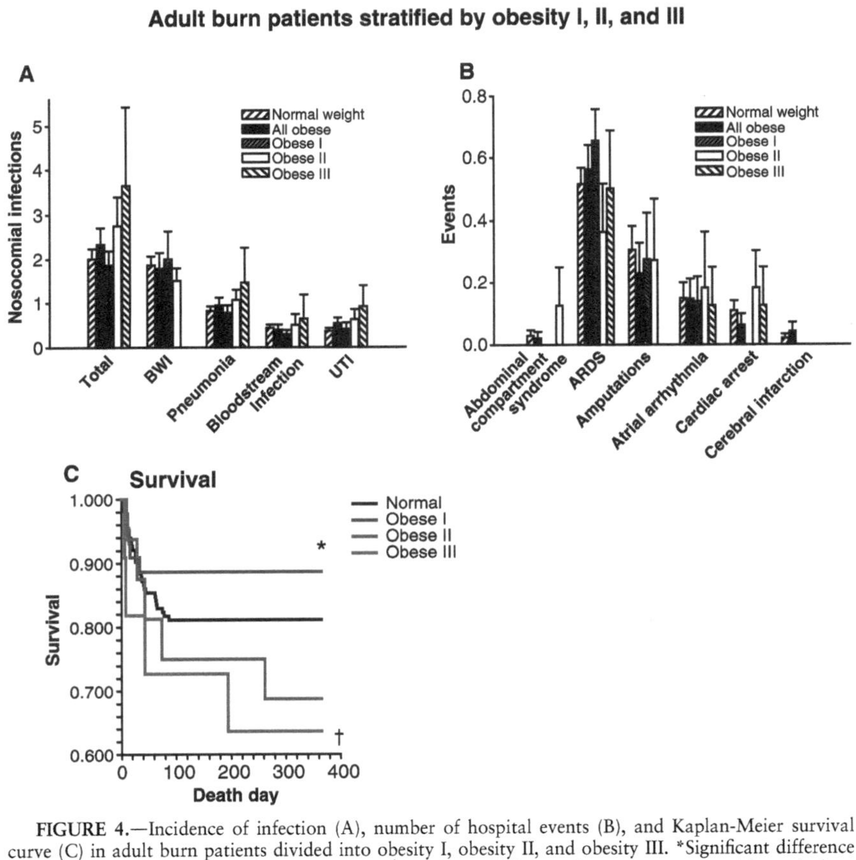

FIGURE 4.—Incidence of infection (A), number of hospital events (B), and Kaplan-Meier survival curve (C) in adult burn patients divided into obesity I, obesity II, and obesity III. *Significant difference between normal weight and obese I, $P < 0.05$. †Significant difference between normal weight and obese II, $P < 0.05$. ARDS indicates acute respiratory distress syndrome; BWI, burn wound infection; UTI, urinary tract infection. (Reprinted from Jeschke MG, Finnerty CC, Emdad F, et al. Mild obesity is protective after severe burn injury. *Ann Surg*. 2013;258:1119-1129, Copyright 2013, with permission from Southeastern Surgical Congress.)

primary outcome was mortality and secondary outcomes were clinical markers of patient recovery, for example, multiorgan function, infections, sepsis, and length of stay.

Results.—A total of 273 patients had normal weight, 116 were obese, and 16 were underweight; underweight patients were excluded from the analyses because of insufficient patient numbers. There were no differences in primary and secondary outcomes when normal weight patients were compared with obese patients. Further stratification in pediatric and adult patients showed similar results. However, when adult patients were stratified in obesity categories, log-rank analysis showed improved survival in the obese I group and higher mortality in the obese III group compared with obese I group ($P < 0.05$).

Conclusions.—Overall, obesity was not associated with increased morbidity and mortality. Subgroup analysis revealed that patients with mild obesity have the best survival, whereas morbidly obese patients have the highest mortality. (NCT00257244) (Fig 4).

▶ In the United States, obesity is the second leading cause of preventable deaths after smoking. Recent increases in adult and childhood obesity have caused health professionals to address this serious public health problem. In general, obesity leads to severe health consequences such as coronary heart disease, osteoarthritis, obstructive sleep apnea, type II diabetes, and others. Given the additional associated morbidities, including insulin resistance, heightened proinflammatory state, increased triglycerides, and high blood pressure, obesity depicts a metabolic syndrome that is associated with chronic inflammation and impaired recovery. In this study, obesity (body mass index [BMI] > 30) was not associated with increased morbidity and mortality after a severe burn injury. Subgroup analysis, depicted in Fig 4, found that mildly obese patients have the best survival rates, whereas morbidly obese patients have the highest postburn mortality. These data indicate that in states of catabolic stress, the existence of energy reserves may in fact confer a survival advantage in patients with BMIs between 30 and 34.9. Confirmatory studies with larger patient numbers need to be conducted to develop better predictors of metabolic risk after severe burn injury. However, this study shows the need for the development of therapeutic strategies for use in morbidly obese patients after a severe burn injury.

D. W. Mozingo, MD

The Frequency and Cost of Treatment Perceived to Be Futile in Critical Care

Huynh TN, Kleerup EC, Wiley JF, et al (Univ of California Los Angeles; et al)
JAMA Intern Med 173:1887-1894, 2013

Importance.—Physicians often perceive as futile intensive care interventions that prolong life without achieving an effect that the patient can appreciate as a benefit. The prevalence and cost of critical care perceived to be futile have not been prospectively quantified.

Objective.—To quantify the prevalence and cost of treatment perceived to be futile in adult critical care.

Design, Setting, and Participants.—To develop a common definition of futile care, we convened a focus group of clinicians who care for critically ill patients. On a daily basis for 3 months, we surveyed critical care specialists in 5 intensive care units (ICUs) at an academic health care system to identify patients whom the physicians believed were receiving futile treatment. Using a multivariate model, we identified patient and clinician characteristics associated with patients perceived to be receiving futile treatment. We estimated the total cost of futile treatment by summing the charges of each day of receiving perceived futile treatment and converting to costs.

Main Outcome and Measure.—Prevalence of patients perceived to be receiving futile treatment.

Results.—During a 3-month period, there were 6916 assessments by 36 critical care specialists of 1136 patients. Of these patients, 904 (80%) were never perceived to be receiving futile treatment, 98 (8.6%) were perceived as receiving probably futile treatment, 123 (11%) were perceived as receiving futile treatment, and 11 (1%) were perceived as receiving futile treatment only on the day they transitioned to palliative care. The patients with futile treatment assessments received 464 days of treatment perceived to be futile in critical care (range, 1-58 days), accounting for 6.7%of all assessed patient days in the 5 ICUs studied. Eighty-four of the 123 patients perceived as receiving futile treatment died before hospital discharge and 20 within 6 months of ICU care (6-month mortality rate of 85%), with survivors remaining in severely compromised health states. The cost of futile treatment in critical care was estimated at $2.6 million.

Conclusions and Relevance.—In 1 health system, treatment in critical care that is perceived to be futile is common and the cost is substantial (Table 3).

▶ The authors of this selection prospectively identified patients perceived as receiving futile treatment in critical care to avoid post hoc bias in labeling patients receiving treatments that were only later judged to be inappropriate.

TABLE 3.—Survival During Hospitalization and up to 6 Months After Intensive Care Unit (ICU) Care

	Death, No. (%) (N = 1136)	
Patient Group	In-Hospital	Within 6 mo of ICU Care
Never received futile treatment (n = 904)	42 (4.6)	66 (7.3)
Received probably futile treatment (n = 98)	23 (23)	33 (34)
Received futile treatment (n = 123)	84 (68)	104 (85)
Futile treatment only on day transitioned to palliative care (n = 11)	9 (82)	11 (100)

In the critical care units that they studied, the authors found that treatment perceived by physicians to be futile is common and that more than 1 in 10 patients received such treatment during their intensive care unit (ICU) stay. The outcomes of this cohort are presented in Table 3. The outcomes of these patients were uniformly poor, with two-thirds dying during the hospitalization and 85% dying within 6 months. The cost of perceived futile treatment, although sizable, accounted for only a small percentage of critical care expenditures at their health system during the study period. Critical care physicians frequently perceive that they are providing futile treatment, and the cost is substantial. Identifying and quantitating ICU treatment that is perceived as futile, as was accomplished in this study, is a first step toward refocusing care on treatments that are more likely to benefit patients.

D. W. Mozingo, MD

Cause and timing of death in massively transfused trauma patients

Cripps MW, Kutcher ME, Daley A, et al (Univ of Texas Southwestern Med Ctr, Dallas; Univ of California, San Francisco)

J Trauma Acute Care Surg 75:S255-S262, 2013

Background.—The purpose of this study was to characterize the cause of death in severely injured trauma patients to define potential responses to resuscitation.

Methods.—Prospective analysis of 190 critically injured patients who underwent massive transfusion protocol (MTP) activation or received massive transfusion (>10 U of packed red blood cells [RBC] per 24 hours). Cause of death was adjudicated into one of four categories as follows: (1) exsanguination, (2) early physiologic collapse, (3) late physiologic collapse, and (4) nonsurvivable injury.

Results.—A total 190 patients underwent massive transfusion or MTP with 76 deaths (40% mortality), of whom 72 deaths were adjudicated to one of four categories: 33.3% died of exsanguination, 16.6% died of early physiologic collapse, 11.1% died of late physiologic collapse, while 38.8% died of nonsurvivable injuries. Patients who died of exsanguination were younger and had the highest RBC/fresh frozen plasma ratio (2.97 [2.24]), although the early physiologic collapse group survived long enough to use the most blood products ($p < 0.001$). The late physiologic collapse group had significantly fewer penetrating injuries, was older, and had significantly more crystalloid use but received a lower RBC/fresh frozen plasma ratio (1.50 [0.42]). Those who were determined to have a nonsurvivable injury had a lower presenting Glasgow Coma Scale (GCS) score, fewer penetrating injuries, and higher initial blood pressure reflecting a preponderance of nonsurvivable traumatic brain injury. The average survival time for patients with potentially survivable injuries was 2.4 hours versus 18.4 hours for nonsurvivable injuries ($p < 0.001$).

Conclusion.—Severely injured patients requiring MTP have a high mortality rate. However, no studies to date have addressed the cause of death

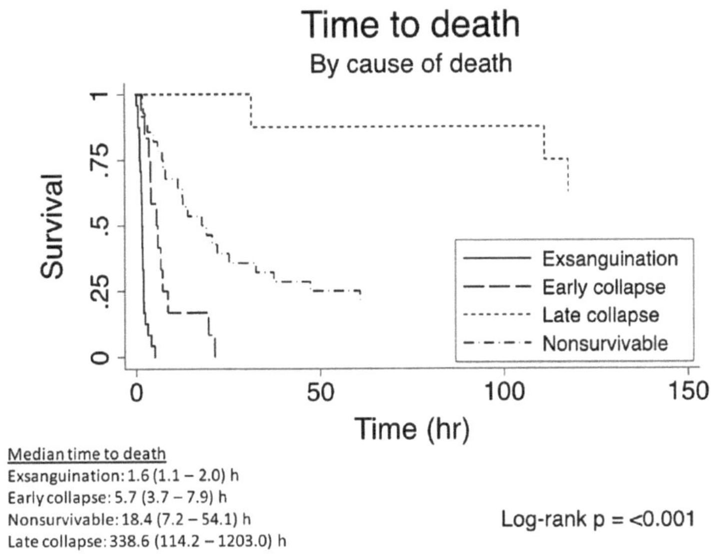

FIGURE 1.—Time-to-death analysis. Those who died of exsanguination died the earliest at a median time of 1.6 hours, while those who died of late physiologic collapse died at a median time of approximately 2 weeks (338.6 hours). (Reprinted from Cripps MW, Kutcher ME, Daley A, et al. Cause and timing of death in massively transfused trauma patients. *J Trauma Acute Care Surg.* 2013;75:S255-S262, with permission from Lippincott Williams & Wilkins.)

after MTP. Characterization of cause of death will allow targeting of surgical and resuscitative conduct to allow extension of the physiologic reserve time, therefore rendering previously nonsurvivable injury potentially survivable (Fig 1).

▶ Much interest exists regarding optimal resuscitation of the severely injured trauma patient. The early use of a balanced resuscitation via a massive transfusion protocol decreases mortality in these patients. Despite data that overwhelmingly support these plasma-based advances in resuscitation, there is considerable disparity in effectiveness from center to center and from study to study. The high mortality rate lends to a large population of potentially preventable deaths, and the lack of data on the cause of early death after injury makes it difficult to determine the true effectiveness of balanced resuscitation protocols on patients with severe survivable injuries. As a result of their analysis, the authors of this selection believe that a staged approach to the goals of resuscitation should be considered in discussions of trauma epidemiology. Patients who die of uncontrolled hemorrhage are ultimately best served by injury prevention efforts and optimization of evacuation to definitive surgical treatment. Those who die of early physiologic collapse require better-targeted resuscitation. Those who die of late physiologic collapse need improvements in critical care. However, the early resuscitation of these patients may also play a critical role in their long-term trajectory. Fig 1 is included depicting the time to death analysis in this cohort. This article supports the need for a multi-institutional study and the start of a national data bank that documents the cause of death in trauma patients to specifically identify risk factors and better-targeted therapy for exsanguination, physiologic collapse, and unsurvivable injuries. The inclusion of these data into quality improvement programs could help identify areas of improvement in trauma resuscitation.

D. W. Mozingo, MD

Improving Mortality Following Emergent Surgery in Older Patients Requires Focus on Complication Rescue

Sheetz KH, Waits SA, Krell RW, et al (Univ of Michigan, Ann Arbor)

Ann Surg 258:614-618, 2013

Objective.—To determine whether a hospital's ability to rescue patients from major complications underlies variation in outcomes for elderly patients undergoing emergent surgery.

Background.—Perioperative mortality rates in elderly patients undergoing emergent general/vascular operations are high and vary widely across Michigan hospitals.

Methods.—We identified 23,224 patients undergoing emergent general/vascular surgical procedures at 41 hospitals within the Michigan Surgical Quality Collaborative between 2006 and 2011. Hospitals were ranked by risk- and reliability-adjusted 30-day mortality rates and grouped into tertiles. We stratified patients by age (<75 and ≥75 years). Risk-adjusted major complication and failure-to-rescue (ie, mortality after major complication) rates were determined for each tertile of hospital mortality.

Results.—Risk-adjusted mortality rates in elderly patients varied 2-fold across all hospitals. Complication rates correlated poorly with mortality. Failure-to-rescue rates, however, were markedly higher in high-mortality hospitals (29% lowest tertile vs 41% highest tertile; $P < 0.01$). When

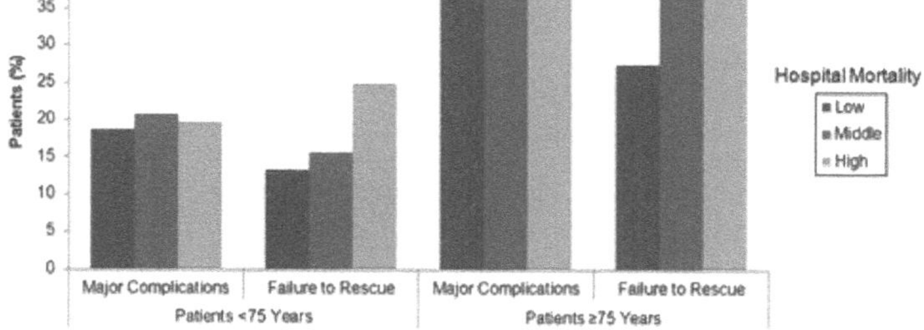

FIGURE 1.—Major complications and failure-to-rescue rates for young (<75 years) and elderly (≥75 years) patients across hospitals ranked by overall mortality. Major complication rates are not significantly different between tertiles of hospital mortality. Failure to rescue correlates with mortality and is significantly higher in elderly patients. (Reprinted from Sheetz KH, Waits SA, Krell RW, et al. Improving mortality following emergent surgery in older patients requires focus on complication rescue. *Ann Surg.* 2013;258:614-618, Copyright 2013, with permission from Southeastern Surgical Congress.)

compared with younger patients, overall failure-to-rescue rates were almost 2-fold greater in the elderly (36.1% ≥75 vs 18.7% <75; $P < 0.01$).

Conclusions.—A hospital's failure to rescue patients from major complications seems to underlie the variation in mortality rates across Michigan hospitals after emergent surgery. Although higher failure-to-rescue rates in the elderly may signify their diminished physiological reserve for surviving critical illness, the wide variation across hospitals also highlights the importance of systems aimed at the early recognition and effective management of major complications in this vulnerable population (Fig 1).

▶ This study adds to the limited body of literature detailing the importance of failure to rescue in evaluating hospital quality for emergency surgery. It further highlights that elderly patients are uniquely vulnerable to poor outcomes after emergency procedures. Mortality rates for these patients are significantly higher and more variable across hospitals than for younger patients, as depicted in Fig 1. This observation is not correlated with morbidity because major complication rates did not differ. Rather, death after major complication, or failure to rescue, is a major driver of mortality differences between hospitals. An age disparity persists; failure-to-rescue rates in elderly patients are significantly higher after emergency surgery than in younger patients. This study elucidates several critical issues regarding surgical care in the elderly. A large proportion of emergency surgery cases are performed in patients older than 75 years, and this is likely to increase as the baby boom generation ages. Implications of this surge must be appreciated by providers at the point of care and by policy makers nationally. First, for surgeons, it is important that care teams establish practice measures specifically for complication rescue. In the elderly, emergency surgical patient, this requires prompt identification of major complications and appropriate management. It is likely that elderly patients possess diminished physiological reserve and are more likely to have poor surgical outcomes.

D. W. Mozingo, MD

Critical Care Medicine in the United States: Addressing the Intensivist Shortage and Image of the Specialty

Halpern NA, Pastores SM, Oropello JM, et al (Memorial Sloan-Kettering Cancer Ctr, NY; Mount Sinai School of Medicine, NY; et al)

Crit Care Med 41:2754-2761, 2013

Intensivists are increasingly needed to care for the critically ill and manage ICUs as ICU beds, utilization, acuity of illness, complexity of care and costs continue to rise. However, there is a nationwide shortage of intensivists that has occurred despite years of well publicized warnings of an impending workforce crisis from specialty societies and the federal government. The magnitude of the intensivist shortfall, however, is difficult to determine because there are many perspectives of optimal ICU administration, patient coverage and intensivist availability and a lack of national data on intensivist practices. Nevertheless, the intensivist shortfall is quite real as evidenced by the alternative solutions that hospitals are deploying to provide care for their critically ill patients. In the midst of these manpower struggles, the critical care environment is dynamically changing and becoming more stressful. Severe hospital bed availability and fiscal constraints are forcing ICUs to alter their approaches to triage, throughput and unit staffing. National and local organizations are mandating that hospitals comply with resource intensive and arguably unproven initiatives to monitor and improve patient safety and quality, and informatics systems. Lastly, there is an ongoing sense of professional dissatisfaction among intensivists and a lack of public awareness that critical care medicine is even a distinct specialty. This article offers proposals to increase the adult intensivist workforce through expansion and enhancements of internal medicine based critical care training programs, incentives for recent graduates to enter the critical care medicine field, suggestions for improvements in the critical care profession and workplace to encourage senior intensivists to remain in the field, proactive marketing of critical care, and expanded engagement by the critical care societies in the challenges facing intensivists (Table 2).

▶ The need for comprehensive and cutting-edge critical care medicine continues to grow in the midst of a nationwide shortage of critical care physicians and ongoing increases in the number of critically ill patients, intensive care unit (ICU) beds, and costs. The intensivist shortage has occurred despite decade-long warnings of a workforce crisis from specialty societies and the federal government. Recommendations drafted to increase the number of intensivists, enhance the critical care medicine field for new physicians and improve its

TABLE 2.—Proposals to Address the Intensivist Shortfall and Image of the CCM Specialty

CCM database
- Create one national CCM fellow database that tracks fellows into the ICU workplace

Expand the pipeline and enhance the training of medical intensivists
- Lift restrictive Accreditation Council on Graduate Medical Education mandates on IM-based CCM programs
- Community hospitals should financially support hospitalists with CCM interests to train in existing CCM programs and assure them intensivist jobs after training
- Publicize the "CCM only" track within Pulmonary/Critical Care programs
- Broaden perioperative critical care training of IM-based CCM fellows
- Create an inpatient-dedicated track in 3-yr IM residency programs with extensive ICU exposure and procedural experiences to prepare these IM trainees for CCM fellowships

Shifting CCM-certified physicians in the ICU
- Government to incentivize recent CCM graduates to work in underserved ICU areas
- Hospitals to incentivize CCM-certified specialists to increase their time in ICU

Enhance the CCM specialty
- Improve professional environment
- Proactively refine and market the CCM-intensivist brand
- Early exposure of medical students to CCM

Better utilization of ICU beds
- Public and physician education on appropriate use of ICU beds, advanced care directives, and shifting goals of care from cure to comfort when further aggressive ICU care is futile

CCM = critical care medicine, IM = internal medicine.

cohesiveness, and engage and educate hospital administrators and the public to the benefits of critical care were not implemented. In this selection, the authors offer proposals (Table 2) to increase the adult intensivist workforce through expansion and enhancements of internal medicine–based critical care training programs; incentives for recent critical care medicine graduates to stay in the ICU; improvements in the critical care medicine profession, workplace, and utilization of ICU beds; proactive marketing of critical care; and enhanced engagement by the critical care medicine organizations in the challenges facing intensivists.

D. W. Mozingo, MD

Effects of Fluid Resuscitation With Colloids vs Crystalloids on Mortality in Critically Ill Patients Presenting With Hypovolemic Shock: The CRISTAL Randomized Trial

Annane D, for the CRISTAL Investigators (Raymond Poincaré Hosp, Garches, France; et al)

JAMA 310:1809-1817, 2013

Importance.—Evidence supporting the choice of intravenous colloid vs crystalloid solutions for management of hypovolemic shock remains unclear.

Objective.—To test whether use of colloids compared with crystalloids for fluid resuscitation alters mortality in patients admitted to the intensive care unit (ICU) with hypovolemic shock.

Design, Setting, and Participants.—A multicenter, randomized clinical trial stratified by case mix (sepsis, trauma, or hypovolemic shock without sepsis or trauma). Therapy in the Colloids Versus Crystalloids for the Resuscitation of the Critically Ill (CRISTAL) trial was open label but outcome assessment was blinded to treatment assignment. Recruitment began in February 2003 and ended in August 2012 of 2857 sequential ICU patients treated at 57 ICUs in France, Belgium, North Africa, and Canada; follow-up ended in November 2012.

Interventions.—Colloids (n = 1414; gelatins, dextrans, hydroxyethyl starches, or 4% or 20% of albumin) or crystalloids (n = 1443; isotonic or hypertonic saline or Ringer lactate solution) for all fluid interventions other than fluid maintenance throughout the ICU stay.

Main Outcomes and Measures.—The primary outcome was death within 28 days. Secondary outcomes included 90-day mortality; and days alive and not receiving renal replacement therapy, mechanical ventilation, or vasopressor therapy.

Results.—Within 28 days, there were 359 deaths (25.4%) in colloids group vs 390 deaths (27.0%) in crystalloids group (relative risk [RR], 0.96 [95% CI, 0.88 to 1.04]; *P* = .26). Within 90 days, there were 434 deaths (30.7%) in colloids group vs 493 deaths (34.2%) in crystalloids group (RR, 0.92 [95% CI, 0.86 to 0.99]; *P* = .03). Renal replacement therapy was used in 156 (11.0%) in colloids group vs 181 (12.5%) in crystalloids group (RR, 0.93 [95% CI, 0.83 to 1.03]; $P = .19$). There were more days alive without mechanical ventilation in the colloids group vs the crystalloids group by 7 days (mean: 2.1 vs 1.8 days, respectively; mean difference, 0.30 [95% CI, 0.09 to 0.48] days; $P = .01$) and by 28 days (mean: 14.6 vs 13.5 days; mean difference, 1.10 [95% CI, 0.14 to 2.06] days; $P = .01$) and alive without vasopressor therapy by 7 days (mean: 5.0 vs 4.7 days; mean difference, 0.30 [95% CI, −0.03 to 0.50] days; $P = .04$) and by 28 days (mean: 16.2 vs 15.2 days; mean difference, 1.04 [95% CI, −0.04 to 2.10] days; $P = .03$).

Conclusions and Relevance.—Among ICU patients with hypovolemia, the use of colloids vs crystalloids did not result in a significant difference in 28-day mortality. Although 90-day mortality was lower among patients receiving colloids, this finding should be considered exploratory and requires further study before reaching conclusions about efficacy.

Trial Registration.—clinicaltrials.gov Identifier: NCT00318942

▶ In recent studies of general intensive care unit patient populations, fluid replacement with 5% albumin or 6% hydroxyethyl starch showed similar effects on mortality compared with isotonic saline. Although there was a suggestion that the subset of patients with severe sepsis might benefit from resuscitation with albumin, the current Surviving Sepsis Campaign guidelines recommended crystalloids as the preferred fluid therapy and against the use of hydroxyethyl starches. The Colloids versus Crystalloids for the Resuscitation of the Critically Ill (CRISTAL) trial was designed to test whether colloids altered mortality compared with crystalloids for fluid resuscitation in critically ill patients. There was no significant difference in mortality rates at 28 days. The authors did report that there were fewer deaths at 90 days among patients treated with colloids than among patients treated with crystalloids. The mortality curves are included as Fig 2 in the original article. Resuscitation with colloids was also associated with more rapid weaning from life-support treatments as shown by significantly more days alive without mechanical ventilation or vasopressor therapy. The authors caution that their findings should be considered exploratory and require further study before reaching conclusions about efficacy.

D. W. Mozingo, MD

5 Wound Healing

Wound Complications in 1145 Consecutive Transumbilical Single-Incision Laparoscopic Procedures

Weiss HG, Brunner W, Biebl MO, et al (Saint John of God Hosp Salzburg, Austria; et al)

Ann Surg 259:89-95, 2014

Objective.—To evaluate the wound complication rate in patients undergoing transumbilical single-incision laparoscopic (SIL) surgery.

Background.—SIL surgery claims to be less invasive than conventional laparoscopy. Small SIL series have raised concerns toward a higher wound complication rate related to the transumbilical incision.

Methods.—In a 44-month period, 1145 consecutive SIL procedures were included. The outcomes were assessed according to the intention-to-treat analysis principle. All procedures were followed for a minimum of 6 months postoperatively, and wound complications were recorded as bleeding, infection (superficial/deep), or hernia. Patients were classified as having a wound complication or not. For all comparisons, significance level was set at $P < 0.05$.

Results.—Pure transumbilical SIL surgery was completed in 92.84%, and additional trocars were used in 7.16%. After a median follow-up of 22.1 (range, 7.67–41.11) months, 29 wound complications (2.53%) had occurred [bleeding 0%/infection 1.05% (superficial 0.9%/deep 0.17%)/early-onset hernia 0.09%/late-onset hernia 1.40%, respectively]. Factors associated with complications were higher patient body mass index (28.16 ± 4.73 vs 26.40 ± 4.68 kg/m^2; $P = 0.029$), longer skin incisions (3.77 ± 1.62 vs 2.96 ± 1.06 cm; $P = 0.012$), and multiport SIL versus single-port SIL (8.47% vs 2.38%; $P = 0.019$) in complicated versus uncomplicated procedures. Furthermore, a learning curve effect was noted after 500 procedures ($P = 0.015$).

Conclusions.—With transumbilical SIL surgery, the incidence of wound complications is acceptable low and is further reduced once the learning curve has been passed.

► As the authors have noted, single-incision laparoscopic (SIL) procedures were devised to minimize scarring using the umbilicus as at the port site. However, the port diameter is larger than that of multiport procedures. The authors performed a single institution review of consecutive patients undergoing SIL to determine wound complications. Of note, 7% of patients had to undergo multiport procedures to accomplish the operation. When specimen retrieval occurred, the combined hernia and wound infection rate was approximately 3%. The hernia/wound infection was slightly more than 2% without specimen retrieval. Follow-up was for a median of 22 months, which is fine to determine the true wound infection rate but still relatively short to determine the long-term wound hernia rate.

The study has many merits in that it was a prospective evaluation of several patients done at a single institution. However, the true test will be its use in a multi-institutional prospective, randomized trial of SIL versus standard multiport laparoscopy.

J. M. Daly, MD

A Prospective Randomized Evaluation of Cyanoacrylate Glue Devices in the Closure of Surgical Wounds

Maloney J, Rogers GS, Kapadia M (Beverly Hosp Oncology Care Ctr, MA; Tufts Univ School of Medicine, Boston, MA)

J Drugs Dermatol 12:810-814, 2013

Background.—The use of medical adhesives for topical wound closure is gaining in popularity over conventional wound closure materials such as sutures and staples. Adhesives provide advantages in both wound closure and patient management with good cosmetic outcome and surgeon and patient satisfaction reported.

Objective.—To compare the use of two currently marketed medical adhesives; LiquiBand® Flow Control and High Viscosity Dermabond™ for the topical closure of surgical incisions.

Methods.—In a prospective blinded manner, subjects were randomly assigned LiquiBand® or Dermabond™ for topical closure of a surgical incision. Variables compared included ease of use, time taken to close wound, subject and surgeon satisfaction with device and wound closure, cosmetic outcome at 90 days, and complication rates.

Results.—Use of both devices resulted in effective wound closure with similar high levels of cosmesis subject and surgeon satisfaction, with only minor complications reported. There was no statistically significant difference between the devices for all the parameters studied, with the exception that the Liquiband device was found to significantly reduce the amount of time required for closure.

Conclusion.—As the two devices appear substantially equivalent in terms of key surgeon and patient variables, product cost should be the primary determinant in selection of the tissue glue device.

▶ The use of adhesives has become much more popular in recent times for closure of skin incisions based on similar cosmetic outcomes and faster closure times compared with suture techniques. The authors should be complimented for the conduct of this randomized, controlled trial comparing 2 different adhesive products. No significant differences were noted in outcomes except for closure time—an average of 54.5 vs 80 seconds, a clinically insignificant difference.

The cosmetic outcomes were similar between groups as judged by a panel of experts.

As the authors noted, in this era, the cost of surgical products is a critical determinant of use, especially when there are no clinical outcome differences. Despite the few patients studied (N = 43), with little difference noted between groups, it is unlikely that larger numbers of patients would have made a difference in the trial. It would be valuable for the authors to perform a comparison of suture or other techniques of closure with either of these adhesives.

J. M. Daly, MD

Impact of Preoperative Local Water-Filtered Infrared A Irradiation on Postoperative Wound Healing: A Randomized Patient-and Observer-Blinded Controlled Clinical Trial

Künzli BM, Liebl F, Nuhn P, et al (Universität München, Germany)

Ann Surg 258:887-894, 2013

Objective.—In addition to a preoperative antibiotic single-shot prophylaxis, we tested the impact of a one-time preoperative water-filtered infrared A irradiation (wIRA) on postoperative wound healing of patients.

Background.—wIRA improves wound healing in postoperative settings.

Methods.—A total of 400 consecutive patients undergoing gastrointestinal surgery were randomly assigned to the treatment group (A) or placebo group (B). We applied wIRA for 20 minutes while patients were prepared for surgery. Patients and observer were blinded to group assignment. Primary endpoints were surgical site infections (SSIs), wound healing, and rate and level of pain within 30 days after surgery. Primary efficacy analysis was carried out on the basis of an intention-to-treat (ITT) population and a full-analysis set (FAS). Missing values of primary outcome variables were considered as SSIs and maximum pain levels in the ITT analysis, respectively.

Results.—FAS: The incidence of SSI was 9 of 178 patients (5.1%) within group A compared with 22 of 182 (12.1%) within group B [$P = 0.018$; relative risk (RR) = 0.42; 95% CI: 0.18–0.93]. ITT: 32 of 200 (16%) SSIs occurred within group A and 39 of 200 (20%) within group B ($P = 0.248$) with an RR of 0.74 (95% CI: 0.43–1.28). The wIRA group showed lower postoperative pain at both the ITT ($P = 0.092$) and the FAS analysis ($P = 0.045$).

Conclusions.—This trial indicates a clinically relevant benefit of one-time application of preoperative wIRA as a supportive addition to prophylactic antibiotics. wIRA contributes to both reduced SSI rates and postoperative pain but also effectively decreases morbidity and related expenses in the health care system.

► The ability to decrease surgical site infections (SSIs) is critical to the care of surgical patients. Currently, preoperative administration of intravenous antibiotics within 30 minutes of the incision start, warming of the patient, control of blood glucose levels, administration of supplemental oxygen in the immediate perioperative period, and other means are used to decrease infectious complications. As pointed out by the authors, warming of the postoperative hernia repair site for 2 hours can substantially decrease wound infection rates. They noted that administration of water-filtered infrared A irradiation (wIRA) would penetrate 2 to 3 cm into the subcutaneous tissues and increase vasculation and oxygen distribution to the tissues. Their randomized, controlled study enrolled 400 patients, and their intent-to-treat analysis was done properly showing a significant benefit (reducing SSIs) using wIRA (5.1%) compared with controls (12.1%). All patients received preoperative antibiotics. In addition, postoperative pain was reduced in the treated group.

Importantly, the cost to treat each patient was estimated to be 60 cents. This report is important in that there was greater than 50% reduction in SSIs, which normally would translate to decreased hospital costs and length of stay.

The study should be replicated using other types of patients with different diagnoses and wounds. If these results are repeated, it would be a major breakthrough in the care of surgical patients.

J. M. Daly, MD

Systemic Review and Meta-analysis of Randomized Clinical Trials Comparing Primary vs Delayed Primary Skin Closure in Contaminated and Dirty Abdominal Incisions

Bhangu A, Singh P, Lundy J, et al (Royal Centre for Defence Medicine, Birmingham, England; San Antonio Military Med Ctr, Fort Sam Houston, TX)
JAMA Surg 148:779-786, 2013

Importance.—Surgical site infection remains a major challenge in surgery. Delayed primary closure of dirty wounds is widely practiced in war surgery; we present ameta-analysis of evidence to help guide application of the technique in wider context.

Objective.—To determine using meta-analysis whether delayed primary skin closure (DPC) of contaminated and dirty abdominal incisions reduces the rate of surgical site infection (SSI) compared with primary skin closure (PC).

Data Sources.—A systematic review of the literature published after 1990 was conducted of the Medline, PubMed, Current Controlled Trials, and Cochrane databases. The last search was performed on October 6, 2012. No language restrictions were applied.

Study Selection.—Randomized clinical trials comparing PC vs DPC were included.

Data Extraction and Synthesis.—Two of us independently selected studies based on quality assessment using the Cochrane Collaboration tool for assessing risk of bias in randomized trials. Data were pooled using fixed- and random-effects models.

Main Outcome and Measure.—Rate of SSI, as defined by the individual study.

Results.—The final analysis included 8 studies randomizing 623 patients with contaminated or dirty abdominal wounds to either DPC or PC. The most common diagnosis was appendicitis (77.4%), followed by perforated abdominal viscus (11.5%), ileostomy closure (6.5%), trauma (2.7%), and intra-abdominal abscess/other peritonitis (1.9%). The time to first review for DPC was provided at between 2 and 5 days postoperatively. All studies were found to be at high risk of bias, with marked deficiencies in study design and outcome assessment. When SSI was assessed across all studies using a fixed-effect model, DPC significantly reduced the chance of SSI (odds ratio, 0.65; 95% CI, 0.40-0.93; $P = .02$). However, heterogeneity was high (72%), and using a random-effects model, the effect was no longer significant (odds ratio, 0.65; 95% CI, 0.25-1.64; $P = .36$).

Conclusions and Relevance.—Delayed primary skin closure may reduce the rate of SSI, but current trials fail to provide definitive evidence because of poor design.Well-designed, large-numbered randomized clinical trials are warranted.

▶ As the authors note, delayed primary closure of contaminated wounds became a fundamental tenet of wartime injuries. These wounds, often caused by high-velocity weapons, led to tissue necrosis, which was not determined at initial inspection. In the elective surgical setting, too often primary closure of contaminated wounds is performed, sometimes with drains or wicks between loosely placed sutures. Although the surgeon often thinks of "getting away" with it in most cases, serious infections in some often overwhelm any positive results.

This meta-analysis points out several issues. First, the authors were appropriately critical of the quality of the previous randomized, controlled clinical trials comparing primary closure with delayed primary closure. Second, the appropriate time for delayed closure is between 2 and 5 days after the initial operation. Third, the statistical methodology led to the conclusion that delayed closure was better than primary closure, but the heterogeneity of the studies obviated that conclusion. Once again, we as surgeons can be criticized for the poor quality of the clinical trials we perform.

J. M. Daly, MD

Preoperative Smoking Status and Postoperative Complications: A Systematic Review and Meta-analysis

Grønkjær M, Eliasen M, Skov-Ettrup LS, et al (Univ of Southern Denmark, Copenhagen, Denmark)

Ann Surg 259:52-71, 2014

Objective.—To systematically review and summarize the evidence of an association between preoperative smoking status and postoperative complications elaborated on complication type.

Background.—The conclusions of studies examining the association between preoperative smoking and postoperative complications are inconsistent, thus there is a need for a review and meta-analysis to summarize the existing evidence.

Methods.—A systematic review and meta-analysis based on a search in MEDLINE, EMBASE, CINAHL, and PsycINFO. Included were original studies of the association between smoking status and postoperative complications occurring within 30 days of operation. In total, 9354 studies were identified and reviewed for eligibility and data were extracted. Forest plots and summarized relative risks (RR) including 95% confidence intervals (CIs) were estimated for various complication types.

Results.—Of the 9354 identified studies, 107 studies were included in the meta-analyses and based on these, 157 data sets were extracted. Preoperative smoking was associated with an increased risk of various postoperative complications including general morbidity (RR = 1.52, 95% CI: 1.33–1.74), wound complications (RR = 2.15, 95% CI: 1.87–2.49), general infections (RR = 1.54, 95% CI: 1.32–1.79), pulmonary complications (RR = 1.73, 95% CI: 1.35–2.23), neurological complications (RR = 1.38, 95% CI: 1.01–1.88), and admission to intensive care unit (RR = 1.60, 95% CI: 1.14–2.25). Preoperative smoking status was not observed to be associated with postoperative mortality, cardiovascular complications, bleedings, anastomotic leakage, or allograft rejection.

Conclusions.—Preoperative smoking was found to be associated with an increased risk of the following postoperative complications: general morbidity, wound complications, general infections, pulmonary complications, neurological complications, and admission to the intensive care unit.

▶ It has generally been assumed that preoperative smoking history is associated with postoperative complications usually caused by other comorbidities such as chronic obstructive pulmonary disease and cardiovascular problems. The authors identified more than 9000 studies of smoking and perioperative morbidity but only selected 107 studies for inclusion (approximately, 0.1%). As noted, general morbidity, wound, pulmonary, and neurologic complications were more common in smokers than nonsmokers.

This year marks 50 years since the Surgeon General's report identifying smoking as a major cause of morbidity and early mortality in the United States. As surgeons, we have a major obligation to counsel our patients against smoking. It has been found that counseling by the surgeon has a major positive effect on patients stopping smoking (10%–15%) compared with very few that stop on their own. In addition, there is clear evidence that the adverse effects of smoking (primarily due to nicotine on wounds, immune function, lung function, vascular supply) can be reversed after as little as 6 to 8 weeks of abstinence from smoking.

Thus, it is incumbent upon us as surgeons to spend time with our patients to encourage them strongly to quit smoking before their operation.

J. M. Daly, MD

Negative pressure wound therapy in infants and children: a single-institution experience

Rentea RM, Somers KK, Cassidy L, et al (Med College of Wisconsin, Milwaukee)

J Surg Res 184:658-664, 2013

Background.—Information regarding the use of negative pressure wound therapy (NPWT) in the pediatric population is limited. Because of adverse outcomes in adult patients, the Food and Drug Administration issued a warning in 2011 about the use of NPWT in infants and children.

Methods.—We performed an institutional review board–approved, single-institution, retrospective review of pediatric patients who had undergone NPWT from 2007–2011. We collected the types of wounds for which NPWT was initiated, the NPWT outcomes, and the complications encountered.

Results.—The data from 290 consecutive patients were reviewed. Their average age was 9.3 y (range 12 d to 18 y), and their average weight was 46.5 kg (range 1.1–177). Of the wounds, 66% were classified as acute, 10% as chronic, and 24% as traumatic. The two most common indications were surgical wound dehiscence ($n = 47$) and skin grafting ($n = 41$). NPWT was used in 15 wounds containing surgical hardware, with 2 devices requiring eventual removal. NPWT was used for a median of 9 d per patient (two dressing changes). Complications occurred in 5 patients (1.7%). Documentation problems were noted in 44 patients. After NPWT, about one-third of the patients ($n = 95$ patients) were able to undergo delayed primary closure.

Conclusions.—NPWT is an effective adjunct in wound healing and closure in the pediatric population, with no mortality ascribed to NPWT. Also, the complication rates were low.

► Negative pressure wound therapy (NPWT) is such a simple concept, one can wonder why it took so long for us to figure it out. Randomized trials in adults have clearly found benefit in faster, more complete healing of difficult soft tissue and abdominal wounds. It is a therapy that can be used both in the hospital and at home with quieter, more portable devices coming on the market to improve patient satisfaction. Great care must be taken, however, in the exact dressing of the wound and protection of underlying intestine in the case of open abdominal wounds.

This retrospective review of NPWT in pediatric patients found very few complications (1.7%), which is encouraging. The treatment was used a median of 9 days. It is unclear what happened to the patients that were unable to undergo delayed primary closure (two-thirds of patients). Presumably they had closure of their wounds spontaneously.

Although it may be difficult to draw too many conclusions from this retrospective review, it is clear that the pediatric population, like the adult, benefits from NPWT when it is necessary.

J. M. Daly, MD

A pilot trial using topical regular crystalline insulin vs. aqueous zinc solution for uncomplicated cutaneous wound healing: Impact on quality of life

Attia EAS, Belal DMI, El Samahy MH, et al (Ain Shams Univ, Cairo, Egypt)

Wound Repair Regen 22:52-57, 2014

When wounds are treated with regular insulin, they are also being treated with zinc; used in the formula to crystallize insulin molecules. It is not clear if regular insulin-accelerated wound healing is due to insulin, the zinc it contains, or both. Thus, we aimed to compare topical regular crystalline insulin (containing zinc) vs. aqueous zinc chloride solution to controls, on healing of open uncomplicated cutaneous wounds. In this randomized controlled pilot study, 90 nondiabetic patients were randomly assigned to one of three groups depending on the twice daily applications received; group I: regular insulin; group II: aqueous zinc chloride solution, and group III: 0.9% saline (control). A questionnaire was used to determine the effect of wounds on the quality of life. Both topical regular crystalline insulin (containing zinc) and aqueous zinc chloride solution enhanced healing of uncomplicated cutaneous wounds of nondiabetic patients, than control ($p < 0.001$), and hence improved patients' quality of life. However, regular insulin showed better results than aqueous zinc solution ($p = 0.015$), probably due to synergistic effect between insulin and zinc of its formulation. Healing rate was significantly higher in acute than chronic wounds ($p < 0.001$), in those ≤ 40 years than those >40 ($p = 0.004$), and in upper body wounds than lower body ($p = 0.015$).

► It is well known that there are many growth factors, nutrients, and other substances that may enhance the healing rate of wounds. Among these is insulin. It has been questioned as to whether the potential improvement in healing is caused by the insulin itself or by the zinc present in the solution. This nicely presented study randomly assigned 90 nondiabetic patients to receive a topical insulin solution, a topical zinc solution, or saline as a control solution. The rate of healing and patient satisfaction was best with the insulin solution and second with the zinc solution. Both the rate of healing and patient satisfaction were better after the treatment of acute wounds compared with those more chronic in nature.

Clearly, this study needs to be replicated with a larger patient population because it has major overtones in our care of the surgical patient.

J. M. Daly, MD

Frequency of Debridements and Time to Heal: A Retrospective Cohort Study of 312 744 Wounds

Wilcox JR, Carter MJ, Covington S (Healogics, Jacksonville, FL; Strategic Solutions Inc, Cody, WY)

JAMA Dermatol 149:1050-1058, 2013

Importance.—Chronic wounds usually get trapped in the inflammatory stage of wound healing; however, aggressive debridement transforms chronic wounds to acute wounds and therefore complete healing.

Objective.—To investigate healing outcomes and debridement frequency in a large wound data set.

Design.—Retrospective cohort study.

Setting.—Data collected from 525 wound care centers from June 1, 2008, through June 31, 2012, using a web-based clinical management system.

Patients.—Referred sample of 154 644 patients with 312 744 wounds of all causes (of an initial data set of 364 534 wounds) participated. A total of 47.1%were male. Median age was 69 years (age range, 19-112 years), with 59.2%having one wound. Eligibility criteria included age older than 18 years, receiving at least 1 debridement, and having been discharged from the system. Advanced therapeutic treatment was ineligible. Because of incomplete, questionable, or ineligible data, 57 190 wounds were not included. Most wounds were diabetic foot ulcers (19.0%), venous leg ulcers (26.1%), and pressure ulcers (16.2%).

Intervention.—Debridement (removal of necrotic tissue and foreign bodies from the wound) at different frequencies.

Main Outcome and Measure.—Wound healing (completely epithelialized with dimensions at 0 × 0 × 0 cm).

Results.—A total of 70.8% of wounds healed. The median number of debridements was 2 (range, 1-138). Frequent debridement healed more wounds in a shorter time ($P < .001$). In regression analysis, significant variables included male sex, physician category, wound type, increased patient age, and increased wound age, area, and depth. The odds ratio varied considerably for each variable.

Conclusions and Relevance.—The more frequent the debridements, the better the healing outcome. Although limited by retrospective data, this study's strength was the analysis of the largest wound data set to date.

▶ Wilcox et al used data from a web-based clinical data management system to evaluate factors that might be associated with improved healing of chronic wounds. Their initial data set for this retrospective study was more than 150 000 patients from 525 wound centers. Importantly, most wounds healed (70%), and there were associations including patient gender, wound type, and patient age. In their analysis, frequency of debridements led to faster healing.

This is an interesting concept in that the treating health care professional wants to remove necrotic tissue with each debridement but does not want to remove viable healing tissue. Although this is a very large series, often data sets are incomplete. For example, nearly 20% of cases were not included in the analyses. Thus, these are associations and not definitive conclusions, which could only be reached by a randomized, controlled, prospective trial.

J. M. Daly, MD

Laparoscopic component separation reduces postoperative wound complications but does not alter recurrence rates in complex hernia repairs

Fox M, Cannon RM, Egger M, et al (Univ of Louisville, KY)

Am J Surg 206:869-875, 2013

Background.—The purpose of this study was to evaluate and compare the incidence of wound complications after laparoscopic component separation (LCS) vs open component separation (OCS) in patients with complex abdominal wall hernias.

Methods.—A retrospective review was performed of all patients who underwent LCS or OCS for repair of a complex abdominal wall hernia at a single institution between 2009 and 2011. Charts were reviewed to identify postoperative wound complications. A computed tomographic scan or physical examination was used for the determination of hernia recurrence. Categoric variables were compared using the Fisher exact test. Univariate and multivariate analyses were performed using linear and Cox regression. Recurrence rates were compared using log-rank tests (Kaplan-Meier method).

Results.—A total of 44 patients underwent LCS (n = 18) or OCS (n = 26). There was no statistically significant difference between categoric variables. Multivariate analysis using wound complications as the dependent variable showed a statistically significantly lower rate of wound complications in the LCS group.

Conclusions.—LCS is associated with a lower rate of wound complications when compared with OCS but yields comparable recurrence rates.

▶ This retrospective review of a small number of patients (N = 44) compared laparoscopic abdominal wall component separation with that of open abdominal wall component separation. They noted fewer wound infections in the laparoscopic group compared with the open group. The study suffers from the small number of patients included and its retrospective nature. However, the results are similar to those of other prospective trials that compared open vs laparoscopic ventral hernia repair with or without component separation. Its results are also similar to those of studies in obese patients undergoing bariatric surgery showing reduced postoperative wound complications using the laparoscopic approach vs the open procedures. Taken together, laparoscopic methods should be used in these patients whenever possible.

J. M. Daly, MD

Human Acellular Dermis Seeded with Autologous Fibroblasts Enhances Bronchial Anastomotic Healing in an Irradiated Rodent Sleeve Resection Model

Roessner E, Vitacolonna M, Schulmeister A, et al (Univ Med Centre Mannheim, Germany; et al)

Ann Surg Oncol 20:S709-S715, 2013

Background.—The combination of neoadjuvant radiochemotherapy and parenchyma-preserving sleeve resection for lung cancer remains controversial because of potentially increased rate of anastomotic breakdown. We analyzed the effects of applying a decellularized human dermis transplant seeded with autologous fibroblasts in a rodent sleeve resection model with neoadjuvant radiotherapy.

Materials and Methods.—A total of 64 male Fisher rats underwent a transsection and surgical anastomosis of the left main bronchus and were randomized to receive plus/minus radiation treatment and plus/minus augmentation of the anastomosis with a fibroblast-seeded dermis transplant (2 × 2 factorial design). A μCT scan was performed at postoperative days 7 and 14, and the animals were sacrificed on day 14. Anastomotic bursting pressure and hydroxyproline concentration were measured.

Results.—In the irradiated groups, the anastomotic bursting pressure was significantly higher in the augmented group at day 7 (100.9 ± 18.3 vs 141.3 ± 18.0 kPa, $p = 0.0005$) but not at day 14. Hydroxyproline levels showed a similar pattern in the irradiated group with significant differences at day 7 (7 days postoperative 158 ± 11.6 vs 198.2 ± 10.9 nmol/mg, $p < 0.0001$) but not at day 14 postoperatively.

Conclusions.—Augmentation of a bronchial anastomosis by a dermal matrix, seeded with autologous, viable fibroblasts improves early wound breaking strength. Fibroblast-enhanced dermal matrices provide a new and easily usable tool to prevent early anastomotic leakage after neoadjuvant chemoradiation in locally advanced lung cancer.

▶ Bronchial disruption after major pulmonary surgery subsequent to radiochemotherapy is a major complication that can occur too often. The ability to bolster the anastomosis either internally or externally can be very beneficial. Some have used pleura or other viable tissue not as a sealant but a means to provide fibroblasts and other cells to the area to stimulate local wound healing. In this animal study, the authors used a fibroblast-seeded dermis transplant to augment the bronchial anastomosis. They found that the augmented anastomosis showed better early healing compared with the controls.

Many studies of wound healing using impaired healing animal models (eg, diabetes, radiation therapy, chemotherapy) are used to control for the healing process across groups and to allow for precise physiologic (bursting and breaking strengths) and biochemical (hydroxyproline) measurements to reflect collagen deposition. Often, these studies show improvement in early healing while later healing is similar to that of controls. It is as though the host eventually "gets it right," although it is a slower process. The average time for an intestinal anastomosis to develop leakage is 7 days. Thus, improvement in early healing is a significant benefit.

This material should undergo further testing to potentially allow it to be used within investigational trials in humans.

J. M. Daly, MD

Development of a wound healing index for patients with chronic wounds

Horn SD, Fife CE, Smout RJ, et al (Inst for Clinical Outcomes Res, Salt Lake City, UT; Intellicure Inc, Woodlands, TX)

Wound Repair Regen 21:823-832, 2013

Randomized controlled trials in wound care generalize poorly because they exclude patients with significant comorbid conditions. Research using real-world wound care patients is hindered by lack of validated methods to stratify patients according to severity of underlying illnesses. We developed a comprehensive stratification system for patients with wounds that predicts healing likelihood. Complete medical record data on 50,967 wounds from the United States Wound Registry were assigned a clear outcome (healed, amputated, etc.). Factors known to be associated with healing were evaluated using logistic regression models. Significant variables ($p < 0.05$) were determined and subsequently tested on a holdout sample of data. A different model predicted healing for each wound type. Some variables predicted significantly in nearly all models: wound size, wound age, number of wounds, evidence of bioburden, tissue type exposed (Wagner grade or stage), being nonambulatory, and requiring hospitalization during the course of care. Variables significant in some models included renal failure, renal transplant, malnutrition, autoimmune disease, and cardiovascular disease. All models validated well when applied to the holdout sample. The "Wound Healing Index" can validly predict likelihood of wound healing among real-world patients and can facilitate comparative effectiveness research to identify patients needing advanced therapeutics.

▶ The ability to more precisely predict the healing of wounds has been sought by many. This study used the United States Wound Registry, including a database of more than 50 000 wounds. Like most registries, it included several patient and wound characteristics that could be measured soon after wounding and as the wound healed. Using logistic regression methodologies, the authors sought to develop formulas to predict the healing time of these wounds. They compared their predictive models with a "holdout sample of wounds" and found good correlation. However, it will be incumbent for these authors to use another large prospective, perhaps multi-institutional, sample of wounded patients to determine if their predictive models truly work outside of the registry, which will help create the formulas for prediction of healing.

J. M. Daly, MD

6 Transplantation

The Impact of Meeting Donor Management Goals on the Development of Delayed Graft Function in Kidney Transplant Recipients

Malinoski DJ, on behalf of the United Network for Organ Sharing (UNOS) Region 5 Donor Management Goals (DMG) Workgroup (Portland Veterans Affairs Med Ctr, OR; et al)

Am J Transplant 13:933-1000, 2013

Many organ procurement organizations (OPOs) utilize preset critical care endpoints as donor management goals (DMGs) in order to standardize care and improve outcomes. The objective of this study was to determine the impact of meeting DMGs on delayed graft function (DGF) in renal transplant recipients. All eight OPOs of the United Network for Organ Sharing Region 5 prospectively implemented nine DMGs in every donor after neurologic determination of death (DNDD). "DMGs met" was defined a priori as achieving any seven of the nine DMGs and this was recorded at the time of consent for donation to reflect donor hospital ICU management, 12–18 h later, and prior to organ recovery. Multivariable analyses were performed to identify independent predictors of DGF (dialysis in the first week after transplantation) with a $p < 0.05$. A total of 722 transplanted kidneys from 492 DNDDs were included. A total of 28% developed DGF. DMGs were met at consent in 14%, 12–18 h in 32% and prior to recovery in 38%. DGF was less common when DMGs were met at consent (17% vs. 30%, $p = 0.007$). Independent predictors of DGF were age, Cr and cold ischemia time, while meeting DMGs at consent was significantly protective. The management of potential organ donors prior to consent affects outcomes and should remain a priority in the intensive care unit.

► The gap between organ availability and demand continues to grow. Despite the excessive need, the numbers of organs discarded for quality remains high. The Department of Health and Human Services (DHHS) has proposed donor management goals as an effort to improve the transplant organ function and subsequent utilization. The impact of achieving these donor management goals was assessed across multiple organ procurement organizations. Interestingly, no single management goal was associated with improved graft function; rather, how quickly the goals were reached stipulated the outcome (prevention of delayed graft function). Although intuition would have ultimate achievement of basic donor management goals resulting in improved organ function, the critical variable was whether there were management goals that needed correction at the time of consent. Perhaps there are different elements that determine outcomes.

T. Pruett, MD

Comparing Molecular Assessment of Implantation Biopsies With Histologic and Demographic Risk Assessment

Kreepala C, Famulski KS, Chang J, et al (Alberta Transplant Applied Genomic Centre, Edmonton, Canada)

Am J Transplant 13:415-426, 2013

We hypothesized that measurement of previously defined acute kidney injury-induced transcripts at the time of implantation would add a new dimension to existing methods based on donor factors, histology and recipient factors. We analyzed microarray results from implantation biopsies taken after reperfusion from 70 kidneys from 53 deceased donors. We used two definitions of early dysfunction: serum creatinine > 265 umol/L at day 7 posttransplant; and dialysis in the first week. The strongest correlate with early dysfunction was the mean expression of 30 injury transcripts. Older donor and recipient age were associated with early dysfunction, but histologic lesions were not. Prediction was best when the injury transcript expression was combined with donor or recipient age, particularly in standard criteria donors. In contrast, although extended criteria donor kidneys had a high risk of early dysfunction, no variables tested, including injury transcripts, predicted risk significantly, probably because these kidneys were allocated preferentially to old, high risk recipients. The injury transcripts did not predict late function, which was mainly associated with donor age. Thus, measurement of injury-induced transcripts at the time of implantation improves the prediction of early kidney dysfunction, but risk prediction may fail when old kidneys are transplanted into old recipients.

▶ This article demonstrated that meeting donor management goals after gaining consent did not improve subsequent kidney transplant early function. Although somewhat counterintuitive, taken in context with this gene array analysis of kidneys immediately after reimplantation, it makes some sense. In this study from Edmonton, an expression of acute kidney injury gene patterns within the kidney immediately after reperfusion was the best predictor of immediate graft function. Although the precise time course is not articulated, some intriguing issues are raised by the findings. Can the injury response be altered after it is initiated? Assuming that a graded response is possible, is the time course the same for all varieties? Clinical experience dictates a heterogeneous response and one that will require understanding of the biological repair mechanisms. In the meantime, this sort of understanding gives new impetus to use organs that may possess sufficient capacity for recovery so that potential recipients can benefit from transplantation.

T. Pruett, MD

Renal Transplantation After *Ex Vivo* Normothermic Perfusion: The First Clinical Study

Nicholson ML, Hosgood SA (Univ of Leicester, UK)

Am J Transplant 13:1246-1252, 2013

Ex vivo normothermic perfusion (EVNP) is a novel method of preservation that restores circulation and allows an organ to regain function prior to transplantation. The aim of this study was to assess the effects of EVNP in kidneys from marginal donors. Eighteen kidneys from extended criteria donors (ECD) underwent a period of EVNP immediately before transplantation. Kidneys were perfused with a plasma free red-cell based solution at a mean temperature of 34.6°C. The outcome of these kidneys was compared to a control group of 47 ECD kidneys that underwent static cold storage (CS). The mean donor age was 61 ± 1 years in the EVNP and 62 ± 6 years in the CS group ($p = 0.520$). EVNP kidneys were perfused for an average of 63 ± 16 min and all were transplanted successfully. The delayed graft function rate (DGF), defined as the requirement for dialysis within the first 7 days was 1/18 patients (5.6%) in the EVNP group versus 17/47 (36.2%) in the CS group ($p = 0.014$). There was no difference in graft or patient survival at 12 months ($p = 0.510$, 1.000). This first series of EVNP in renal transplantation demonstrates that this technique is both feasible and safe. Our preliminary data suggests that EVNP offers promise as a new technique of kidney preservation.

▶ The hallmark of organ preservation has be hypothermia to decrease cell metabolism during the hypoxic/anoxic state after removal from the body. The notion of normothermic preservation with oxygen delivery has recently been found to be feasible. A clinical study of marginal, extended criteria donor kidney using normothermic perfusion is reported in this report. It is noteworthy that the average length of cold ischemia was around 11 hours, and the duration of normothermic perfusion occurred for only 60 minutes. However, of the 18 kidneys treated with ex vivo normothermic preservation, only one experienced delayed graft function, significantly less than would have been expected. Additionally, intrarenal resistance was fairly consistent with what would be expected with hypothermic machine perfusion. Although the logistics of this sort of preservation would not be cost efficient for many kidneys, the possibility of recovering kidneys for the purpose of transplantation is attractive. This would especially be so if one could correlate change in protein expression/oxygen utilization/gene array with duration of recovery and time on pump. The data would have been much more convincing had the authors compared outcomes of one kidney placed on *ex vivo* normothermic perfusion and the other kidney kept in static, cold traditional storage.

T. Pruett, MD

Strategies for Successful Left-Lobe Living Donor Liver Transplantation in 250 Consecutive Adult Cases in a Single Center

Ikegami T, Shirabe K, Soejima Y, et al (Kyushu Univ, Fukuoka, Japan)

J Am Coll Surg 216:353-362, 2013

Background.—Living donor liver transplantation (LDLT) using left-lobe grafts was not generally recognized as feasible due to the problem of graft size.

Study Design.—We retrospectively evaluated strategies for successful left-lobe LDLT in 250 consecutive cases stratified into 2 eras: Era 1 (n = 121), in which surgical procedures were continually refined, and Era 2 (n = 129), in which established procedures were used.

Results.—Graft volume (GV) did not affect the incidence of graft function or survival. Era 2 patients had decreased portal vein (PV) pressure at closure (16.0 ± 3.5 mm Hg vs 19.1 ± 4.6 mm Hg, $p < 0.01$), increased PV flow/GV (301 ± 125 mL/min/100g vs 391 ± 142 mL/min/100 g, $p < 0.01$), and improved graft survival rate (1-year: 90.6% vs 81.8%. $p < 0.01$) despite the smaller GV/standard volume (SLV) ratio (36.2% ± 5.2% vs 41.2% ± 8.8%, $p < 0.01$) compared with Era 1. Patients in Era 2 had lower PV pressure and greater PV flow (y = 598-5.7x, $p = 0.02$) at any GV/SLV compared with cases in Era 1 (y = 480-4.3x, $p < 0.01$), representing greater graft compliance. Univariate analysis for graft survival showed that Era 1, Model for End-Stage Liver Disease (MELD) score ≥20, inpatient status, closing portal venous pressure ≥20 mm Hg, no splenectomy, and operative blood loss ≥10 L were the risk factors for graft loss, and multivariate analysis showed that Era 1 was the only significant factor ($p < 0.01$). During Era 2, development of primary graft dysfunction was associated with inpatient recipient status ($p = 0.02$) and donor age ≥45 years ($p < 0.01$).

Conclusions.—The outcomes of left-lobe LDLT were improved by accumulated experience and technical developments.

▶ A shortage of deceased organ donors limits the ability to care for those with chronic kidney and liver failure. However, the tradition of using organs from living donors should be able to fill the shortfall if disincentives and risks could be minimized. Adult liver recipients have traditionally been thought to require a significant liver mass, and therefore, the full right lobe has been the predominant graft taken from the living donor. The right hepatectomy is associated with greater morbidity for the donor, prompting the community to expand into a less "risky" procedure to obtain a graft for a recipient. The left lobe has been attempted over the years, with less than optimal results. However, recent donor events have led many to reinvigorate its use. This report from Japan explains many of the technical modifications that have resulted in significant improvements in transplant outcomes from left lobe grafts. Much knowledge has been gained by understanding the relationship between blood flow to the liver and outcomes. Small grafts that are exposed to high blood volumes and pressures do not do well. Using pressure and flow as well as liberal techniques to diminish portal flow (absent portosystemic shunt) and maximize hepatic outflow, the authors demonstrate a current 5-year survival in excess of 90%. Many steps need to be taken to perform procedures with an acceptable morbidity for the donor, yet still provide sufficient benefit to the recipient to justify any procedure.

T. Pruett, MD

Demographic, Metabolic, and Blood Pressure Characteristics of Living Kidney Donors Spanning Five Decades

Taler SJ, for the RELIVE Study Group (Mayo Clinic, Rochester, MN; et al)
Am J Transplant 13:390-398, 2013

While cautious criteria for selection of living kidney donors are credited for favorable outcomes, recent practice changes may include acceptance of less than ideal donors. To characterize trends in donor acceptance, the Renal and Lung Living Donors Evaluation (RELIVE) Study evaluated 8,951 kidney donors who donated between 1963 and 2007 at three major U.S. transplant centers. Over the study interval, there was an increase in the percentage of donors >40 years old from 38% to 51%; donors >60 years varied between 1% and 4%. The proportion of donors with obesity increased from 8% to 26% and with glucose intolerance from 9% to 25%. The percentage of hypertensive donors was consistent (5–8%). Accepted donors ≥60 years old were more likely to have obesity, glucose intolerance, and/or hypertension compared to younger donors ($p < 0.0001$). Our results demonstrate important trends in acceptance of older and more obese donors. The fraction of older donors accepted with glucose intolerance or hypertension remains small and for the majority includes mild elevations in glucose or blood pressure that were previously classified as within normal limits.

▶ The greatest population of live organ donors has been for the purpose of kidney transplantation. The RELIVE study has provided significant insights into the behavior and outcomes of kidney donors from 3 large kidney centers. The cumulative experience from the last 5 decades of live kidney donation was evaluated. They showed that over the years, the donors have gotten older and, had a higher body mass index and a higher incidence of a few acceptable comorbidities. It was also found that non–biologic-related donors increased in frequency, a trend that will certainly continue with the expansion of paired kidney exchanges. A registry, such as RELIVE, will prove very useful in identifying patterns of donor acceptance and outcomes that will be necessary to aid in the decision-making process associated with caring for those with end-stage renal disease.

T. Pruett, MD

Preventive Intervention for Living Donor Psychosocial Outcomes: Feasibility and Efficacy in a Randomized Controlled Trial

Dew MA, DiMartini AF, DeVito Dabbs AJ, et al (Univ of Pittsburgh, PA; Univ of Pittsburgh School of Nursing, PA; et al)

Am J Transplant 13:2672-2684, 2013

There are no evidence-based interventions to prevent adverse psychosocial consequences after living donation. We conducted a single-site randomized controlled trial to examine the postdonation impact of a preventive intervention utilizing motivational interviewing (MI) to target a major risk factor for poor psychosocial outcomes, residual ambivalence (i.e. lingering hesitation and uncertainty) about donating. Of 184 prospective kidney or liver donors, 131 screened positive for ambivalence; 113 were randomized to (a) the MI intervention, (b) an active comparison condition (health education) or (c) standard care only before donation. Ambivalence was reassessed postintervention (before donation). Primary trial outcomes—psychosocial variables in somatic, psychological and family interpersonal relationship domains—were assessed at 6 weeks and 3 months postdonation. MI subjects showed the greatest decline in ambivalence ($p = 0.050$). On somatic outcomes, by 3 months postdonation MI subjects reported fewer physical symptoms ($p = 0.038$), lower rates of fatigue ($p = 0.021$) and pain ($p = 0.016$), shorter recovery times ($p = 0.041$) and fewer unexpected medical problems ($p = 0.023$). Among psychological and interpersonal outcomes, they had a lower rate of anxiety symptoms ($p = 0.046$) and fewer unexpected family-related problems ($p = 0.045$). They did not differ on depression, feelings about donation or family relationship quality. The findings suggest that the intervention merits testing in a larger, multisite trial.

▶ There are many impediments to living donation. Although the medical community focuses on medical morbidities and outcomes, many other barriers persist. The study design in this report is intriguing in that a very low threshold for donor ambivalence was set. More than 60% of potential donors we identified as being ambivalent toward donation. Even with this very low threshold, psychosocial interventions resulted in significant improvements in somatic return. Interestingly, the incidence of depression was unaffected by the psychosocial intervention.

It is pivotal that donation teams treat donors' issues in totality and not restrict interests to somatic issues. This study suggests an interrelated connection between physical recovery and psychosocial factors. Although hardly a startling conclusion, the study was performed in a prospective and randomized fashion showing the strength of the relationship.

T. Pruett, MD

Rate of Renal Graft Function Decline After One Year Is a Strong Predictor of All-Cause Mortality

Moranne O, Maillard N, Fafin C, et al (Hôpital Pasteur et Larchet, France; Université Jean MONNET, France)

Am J Transplant 13:695-706, 2013

The slope of GFR associates with an increased risk for death in patients with native CKD but whether a similar association exists in kidney transplantation is not known. We studied an inception cohort of 488 kidney transplant recipients (mean follow-up of 12 ± 4 years) for whom GFR was longitudinally measured by inulin clearance (mGFR) at 1 year and then every 5 years. Association of mGFR at 1 year posttransplant and GFR slope after the first year with all-cause mortality was studied with a Cox regression model and a Fine and Gray competing risk model. While in Crude analysis, the mGFR value at 1 year posttransplant and the rate of mGFR decline were both associated with a higher risk of all-cause mortality, only the slope of mGFR remained a significant and strong predictor of death in multivariate analysis. Factors independently associated with a more rapid mGFR decline were feminine gender, higher HLA mismatch, retransplantation, longer duration of transplantation, CMV infection during the first year and higher rate of proteinuria. Our data suggest that the rate of renal graft function decline after 1 year is a strong predictor of all-cause mortality in kidney transplantation.

► A clear problem with chronic kidney failure is the increased mortality associated with the progressively failing kidney. It is not clear what will be the impact of a failing kidney transplant because recipients will have survived the initial decline in kidney function—the transplant population may represent a biased population. This single-center study assessed the rate of decline of glomerular filtration rate (GFR) after kidney transplantation and correlated it with all-cause mortality. It was shown in this study that the risk of death is higher with a failing transplanted kidney, compared with individuals with more stable function. Although the greatest single cause of death associated with rapidly declining renal function was cardiovascular, infection and neoplasia were significant etiologies of death before the resumption of dialysis. Whether this is the consequence of causality or association is unclear (those with infections or malignancy had immunosuppression, lost renal function, and succumbed from a combination of causes). There are some significant deficits in both data collection and conclusions; however, this study reports the importance of maintaining adequate GFR to promote quantity of life.

T. Pruett, MD

Kidney Transplants With Progressing Chronic Diseases Express High Levels of Acute Kidney Injury Transcripts

Famulski KS, Reeve J, de Freitas DG, et al (Dept of Laboratory Medicine and Pathology, Manchester, UK; Alberta Transplant Applied Genomic Centre, Manchester, UK)

Am J Transplant 13:634-644, 2013

We previously reported that kidney transplants with early acute injury express transcripts indicating injury repair—the acute kidney injury signal. This study investigated the significance of this signal in transplants with other conditions, including rejection and recurrent disease. The injury signal was elevated in biopsies in many different conditions, including T cell-mediated rejection and potentially progressive diseases such as antibody-mediated rejection and glomerulonephritis. A high injury signal correlated with poor function and with inflammation in areas of fibrosis, but not with fibrosis without inflammation. In multivariate survival analysis, the injury signal in late kidney transplant biopsies strongly predicted future graft loss, similar to a published molecular risk score derived in late kidneys. Indeed, the injury signal shared many individual transcripts with the risk score, e.g. ITGB6, VCAN, NNMT. The injury signal was a better predictor of future graft loss than fibrosis, inflammation or expression of collagen genes. Thus the acute injury signal, first defined in early reversible injury, is present in many diseases as a reflection of parenchymal distress, where its significance is dictated by the inducing insult, i.e. treatable/self-limited versus untreatable and sustained. Progression in troubled transplants is primarily a function of ongoing parenchymal injury by disease, not fibrogenesis.

▶ Long-term organ function is a central goal for organ transplantation. However, there are many recognized events that alter the ability of the transplanted organ to function. Building off previous work that the authors did with acute kidney injury and prediction of early function, they extended their interests to acute rejection, recurrent disease, antibody-mediated graft damage, and ability to project graft loss. Not surprisingly, the finding of ongoing acute injury pattern gene response is associated with a shortened graft loss. The prospect of following a gene pattern to discern efficacy of therapy would be beneficial. This study promises newer sophistication in the assessment of therapeutics efficacy.

T. Pruett, MD

Five-Year Outcomes in Living Donor Kidney Transplants With a Positive Crossmatch

Bentall A, Cornell LD, Gloor JM, et al (Mayo Clinic, Rochester, MN)

Am J Transplant 13:76-85, 2013

Renal transplant candidates with high levels of donor-specific anti-HLA antibodies have low transplantation rates and high mortality rates on dialysis. Using desensitization protocols, good short-term outcomes are possible in "positive crossmatch kidney transplants (+XMKTx)", but long-term outcome data are lacking. The aim of the current study was to determine *actual* 5-year graft outcomes of +XMKTx. We compared graft survival and the functional and histologic status of 102 +XMKTx to 204 −XMKTx matched for age and sex. Actual 5-year death-censored graft survival was lower in the +XMKTx group (70.7% vs. 88.0%, $p < 0.01$) and chronic injury (glomerulopathy) was present in 54.5% of surviving grafts. Graft survival was higher in recipients with antibody against donor class I only compared with antibody against class II (either alone or in combination with class I) (85.3% vs. 62.6%, $p = 0.05$) and was similar to −XMKTx (85.3 vs. 88.0%, $p = 0.64$). Renal function and proteinuria ranged across a wide spectrum in all groups reflecting the different histological findings at 5 years. We conclude that when compared to −XMKTx, +XMKTx have inferior outcomes at 5 years, however, almost half of the surviving grafts do not have glomerulopathy and avoiding antibodies against donor class II may improve outcomes.

▶ Antibodies that are directed against the human leukocyte antigens (HLAs) that reside on other peoples' cells have long been known to negatively impact kidney transplant outcomes. Detection of these alloantibodies was the foundation of the screening cross match that would inform the providers of the risk for hyperacute rejection of the graft. As time and numbers of people with alloantibodies have increased, attempts to get around humoral immunity have evolved. There are several confounders, such as increasing capacity to determine the presence of alloantibody (either against donor cells or single antigen beads). Additionally, a plethora of techniques involving plasmapheresis to reduce antibody levels, intravenous immunoglobulin infusion with or without agents to inhibit B or plasma cell function. It is clear that people can gain benefit from kidneys that would have been thought untransplantable in the past for immunologic reasons. This review further refines the Mayo experience with positive cross match live kidney transplants stratified by how the antibody was detected and by whether the recipient had antibody to HLA class 1, 2, or both. The results are not surprising in that cytotoxic antibodies confer worse outcomes than fluorescent detectable antibodies, and antibodies against the type of HLA antigen confer differential outcomes. It behooves the transplant community to address the manner in which one reacts to these preexisting barriers to repeat transplantation, as the numbers of people reentering the national waitlist is continuing to rise.

T. Pruett, MD

Complement-Binding Anti-HLA Antibodies and Kidney-Allograft Survival

Loupy A, Lefaucheur C, Vernerey D, et al (Université Paris Descartes, France; et al)

N Engl J Med 369:1215-1226, 2013

Background.—Anti-HLA antibodies hamper successful transplantation, and activation of the complement cascade is involved in antibody-mediated rejection. We investigated whether the complement-binding capacity of anti-HLA antibodies plays a role in kidney-allograft failure.

Methods.—We enrolled patients who received kidney allografts at two transplantation centers in Paris between January 1, 2005, and January 1, 2011, in a population-based study. Patients were screened for the presence of circulating donor-specific anti-HLA antibodies and their complement-binding capacity. Graft injury phenotype and the time to kidney-allograft loss were assessed.

Results.—The primary analysis included 1016 patients. Patients with complement-binding donor-specific anti-HLA antibodies after transplantation had the lowest 5-year rate of graft survival (54%), as compared with patients with non—complement-binding donor-specific anti-HLA antibodies (93%) and patients without donor-specific anti-HLA antibodies (94%) ($P < 0.001$ for both comparisons). The presence of complement-binding donor-specific anti-HLA antibodies after transplantation was associated with a risk of graft loss that was more than quadrupled (hazard ratio, 4.78; 95% confidence interval [CI], 2.69 to 8.49) when adjusted for clinical, functional, histologic, and immunologic factors. These antibodies were also associated with an increased rate of antibody-mediated rejection, a more severe graft injury phenotype with more extensive microvascular inflammation, and increased deposition of complement fraction C4d within graft capillaries. Adding complement-binding donor-specific anti-HLA antibodies to a traditional risk model improved the stratification of patients at risk for graft failure (continuous net reclassification improvement, 0.75; 95% CI, 0.54 to 0.97).

Conclusions.—Assessment of the complement-binding capacity of donor-specific anti-HLA antibodies appears to be useful in identifying patients at high risk for kidney-allograft loss.

▶ Alloantibody by itself does necessarily portend a poor outcome for the kidney recipient. This article goes past the detection of donor-specific alloantibody and ties outcome to the capacity of the antibody to bind complement. Over a significant observation period, those recipients that developed complement-binding alloantibody had the worst long-term graft survival, whereas outcomes were similar between groups with no donor antibody and those that developed non—complement-binding antibody. The complexity of the immune response to the transplanted organ suggests that the fluidity and durability of the immune response has a significant impact on outcomes.

T. Pruett, MD

Higher Risk of Kidney Graft Failure in the Presence of Anti-Angiotensin II Type-1 Receptor Antibodies

Taniguchi M, Rebellato LM, Cai J, et al (Terasaki Foundation Laboratory, Los Angeles, CA; East Carolina Univ (ECU), Greenville, NC; et al)
Am J Transplant 13:2577-2589, 2013

Reports have associated non-HLA antibodies, specifically those against angiotensin II type-1 receptor (AT1R), with antibody-mediated kidney graft rejection. However, association of anti-AT1R with graft failure had not been demonstrated. We tested anti-AT1R and donor-specific HLA antibodies (DSA) in pre- and posttransplant sera from 351 consecutive kidney recipients: 134 with biopsy-proven rejection and/or lesions (abnormal biopsy group [ABG]) and 217 control group (CG) patients. The ABG's rate of anti-AT1R was significantly higher than the CG's (18%vs. 6%, $p < 0.001$). Moreover, 79% of ABG patients with anti-AT1R lost their grafts (vs. 0%, CG), anti-AT1R levels in 58% of those failed grafts increasing posttransplant. With anti-AT1R detectable before DSA, time to graft failure was 31 months—but 63 months with DSA detectable before anti-AT1R. Patients with both anti-AT1R *and* DSA had lower graft survival than those with DSA alone (log-rank $p = 0.007$). Multivariate analysis showed that *de novo* anti-AT1R was an independent predictor of graft failure in the ABG, alone (HR: 6.6), and in the entire population (HR: 5.4). In conclusion, this study found significant association of anti-AT1R with graft failure. Further study is needed to establish causality between anti-AT1R and graft failure and, thus, the importance of routine anti-AT1R monitoring and therapeutic targeting.

▶ Immunologic damage to the transplanted organ is predominantly thought to be the consequence of self/nonself immune responses. However, immunologic responses against other cell proteins have been long known in autoimmunity. Antiendothelial antibodies are recognized to be associated with kidney dysfunction, and this report suggests that the presence of antibodies to angiotensin II type-1 receptors is associated with accelerated graft loss. A disproportionate percentage of these recipients were retransplants, suggesting that exposure to prior human antigens may be an impetus to generate immunity against those antigens. The world of autoimmunity should serve as a guide to the transplant community to seek out some of these mechanisms for the purpose of discovery of pathways for graft injury. It is not clear that autoimmune responses require a significantly different therapeutic pathway from controlling alloimmunity, but the possibility exists.

T. Pruett, MD

Urinary-Cell mRNA Profile and Acute Cellular Rejection in Kidney Allografts

Suthanthiran M, for the Clinical Trials in Organ Transplantation 04 (CTOT-04) Study Investigators (Weill Cornell Med College, NY; et al)
N Engl J Med 369:20-31, 2013

Background.—The standard test for the diagnosis of acute rejection in kidney transplants is the renal biopsy. Noninvasive tests would be preferable.

Methods.—We prospectively collected 4300 urine specimens from 485 kidney-graft recipients from day 3 through month 12 after transplantation. Messenger RNA (mRNA) levels were measured in urinary cells and correlated with allograft-rejection status with the use of logistic regression.

Results.—A three-gene signature of 18S ribosomal (rRNA)—normalized measures of CD3ϵ mRNA and interferon-inducible protein 10 (IP-10) mRNA, and 18S rRNA discriminated between biopsy specimens showing acute cellular rejection and those not showing rejection (area under the curve [AUC], 0.85; 95% confidence interval [CI], 0.78 to 0.91; $P < 0.001$ by receiver-operating-characteristic curve analysis). The cross-validation estimate of the AUC was 0.83 by bootstrap resampling, and the Hosmer—Lemeshow test indicated good fit ($P = 0.77$). In an external-validation data set, the AUC was 0.74 (95% CI, 0.61 to 0.86; $P < 0.001$) and did not differ significantly from the AUC in our primary data set ($P = 0.13$). The signature distinguished acute cellular rejection from acute antibody-mediated rejection and borderline rejection (AUC, 0.78; 95% CI, 0.68 to 0.89; $P < 0.001$). It also distinguished patients who received anti—interleukin-2 receptor antibodies from those who received T-cell—depleting antibodies ($P < 0.001$) and was diagnostic of acute cellular rejection in both groups. Urinary tract infection did not affect the signature ($P = 0.69$). The average trajectory of the signature in repeated urine samples remained below the diagnostic threshold for acute cellular rejection in the group of patients with no rejection, but in the group with rejection, there was a sharp rise during the weeks before the biopsy showing rejection ($P < 0.001$).

Conclusions.—A molecular signature of CD3ϵ mRNA, IP-10 mRNA, and 18S rRNA levels in urinary cells appears to be diagnostic and prognostic of acute cellular rejection in kidney allografts. (Funded by the National Institutes of Health and others.)

► Diagnosing the etiology of kidney dysfunction has always been a challenge for the transplant physician. The gold standard for the allograft dysfunction diagnosis has been the kidney biopsy (including routine histology but also immunohistochemistry and often electron microscopy). With the growing spectrum of gene amplification techniques, the prospect that one may use these for diagnostic assessments has grown. This report addresses the use of mRNA within the urine to discern processes within the kidney. Using a handful of amplified genes, the authors found that they were able to detect rejection episodes within the kidney with a reasonable degree of accuracy. The limitations of this technology will be (1) reliable RNA within the sample (almost 20% of samples were inadequate for analysis) and (2) discriminating the gene profile from nonalloimmune inflammatory processes within the kidney. Remembering the conclusions found in report 7,[1] the kidney injury pattern seems to be fairly limited. Are the genes found in the urine donor or recipient in origin? Although most gene targets appear to be from recipient immune responses, the specificity and differentiation of alloimmune versus other inflammatory responses is certainly a major issue that must be clarified.

T. Pruett, MD

Reference

1. Famulski K, Reeve J, de Freitas D, Kreepala C, Chang J, Halloran P. Kidney Transplants With Progressing Chronic Diseases Express High Levels of Acute Kidney Injury Transcripts. *Am J Transplant.* 2013;13:634-644.

Predicting End-Stage Renal Disease After Liver Transplant

Israni AK, Xiong H, Liu J, et al (Univ of Minnesota, Minneapolis; Minneapolis Med Res Foundation, MN; et al)
Am J Transplant 13:1782-1792, 2013

Few equations have been developed to predict end-stage renal disease (ESRD) after deceased donor liver transplant. This retrospective observational cohort study analyzed all adult deceased donor liver transplant recipients in the Scientific Registry of Transplant Recipients (SRTR) database, 1995–2010. The prediction equation for ESRD was developed using candidate predictor variables available in SRTR after implementation of the allocation policy based on the model for end-stage liver disease. ESRD was defined as initiation of maintenance dialysis therapy, kidney transplant or registration on the kidney transplant waiting list. We used Cox proportional hazard models to develop separate equations for assessing risk of ESRD by 6 months posttransplant and between 6 months and 5 years posttransplant. Variables in the 6-month equation included recipient age, history of diabetes, history of dialysis before liver transplant, history of malignancy, body mass index, serum creatinine and liver donor risk index. Variables in the 6-month to 5-year equation included recipient race, history of diabetes, hepatitis C status, serum albumin, serum bilirubin and serum creatinine. The prediction equations have good calibration and discrimination (C statistics 0.74–0.78). We have produced risk prediction equations that can be used to aid in understanding the risk of ESRD after liver transplant.

▶ End-stage renal disease (ESRD) is a consistent morbidity after extrarenal organ transplant. Liver transplantation has presented a particular wrinkle in that kidney dysfunction is a major contributor to the Model for End-Stage Liver Disease

(MELD) score and hence allocation. Additionally, the observation that survival after liver transplantation is lower in individuals staying on dialysis after transplantation has resulted in a focus on a patient's persistent need for renal replacement therapy and the use of combination liver-kidney transplantation. This review of the US national experience sought to derive short- and long-term predictors of renal replacement therapies after liver transplantation. It was disturbing that the studies did not define what was being assessed. Were the authors looking only at recipients who required dialysis indefinitely after transplantation or at those who "only" required support at the time of discharge? Some liver recipients are on dialysis at the time of transplantation as described in the equation for the 6-month need. The variables associated with early ESRD and development of a requirement for permanent renal replacement therapies include pretransplant dialysis and an elevated serum creatinine. Variables associated with a later risk for ESRD development are those that are used to measure chronic disease, residual renal function, nutrition, ongoing inflammation, diabetes, age, and body mass index. However, the real value is discerning those variables that would reliably predict renal recovery (at least temporarily). Due to the shortage of kidneys that are available for kidney alone recipients, there is grave concern regarding which patients should or should not receive a combined liver-kidney transplant. What is not clear from this analysis is whether the authors could identify indices that will predictably discern at the time a liver offer was made, whether renal function will recover, or whether the recipient would optimally be treated with a combined liver-kidney transplant.

T. Pruett, MD

Class II Alloantibody and Mortality in Simultaneous Liver–Kidney Transplantation

O'Leary JG, Gebel HM, Ruiz R, et al (Baylor Univ Med Ctr, Dallas, TX; Emory Univ, Atlanta, GA)

Am J Transplant 13:954-960, 2013

Hyperacute kidney rejection is unusual in crossmatch positive recipients of simultaneous liver–kidney transplants (SLKT). However, recent data suggest that these patients remain at risk for antibody-mediated kidney rejection. To further investigate the risk associated with donor-specific alloantibodies (DSA) in SLKT, we studied 86 consecutive SLKT patients with an available pre-SLKT serum sample. Serum samples were analyzed in a blinded fashion for HLA DSA using single antigen beads (median florescence intensity ≥ 2,000 = positive). Post-SLKT samples were analyzed when available (76%). Thirty patients had preformed DSA, and nine developed *de novo* DSA. Preformed class I DSA did not change the risk of rejection, patient or allograft survival. In contrast, preformed class II DSA was associated with a markedly increased risk of renal antibody mediated rejection (AMR) ($p = 0.006$), liver allograft rejection ($p = 0.002$), patient death ($p = 0.02$), liver allograft loss ($p = 0.02$) and renal allograft loss ($p = 0.045$). Multivariable modeling showed class II

DSA (preformed or *de novo*) to be an independent predictor of patient death (HR = 2.2; p = 0.043) and liver allograft loss (HR = 2.2; p = 0.044). These data warrant reconsideration of the approach to DSA in SLKT.

▶ Alloantibodies against donor antigens are a significant barrier to early and long-term renal function. Their role in liver transplantation has been of such little impact that most liver programs do not run crossmatches before transplantation. However, the culture clash has routinely occurred in those instances in which the kidney and liver are transplanted simultaneously. The Baylor group has been archiving serum on liver transplant patients for years and had a ready group of patients. In a retrospective analysis, they demonstrated that donor-specific alloantibody by itself was not an outcome predictor. However, the presence of class II antibody against donor major histocompatibility complex affected kidney and liver survival and was associated with more rejection irrespective of whether the antibody was detected before or after the transplants. Unfortunately, the authors did not describe in the 8 patients who developed de novo antibodies the time after procedure, patient noncompliance with immunosuppressive regimens, or whether rejections occurred before or after antibody detection. Because therapies for alloantibody are substantial in effort and cost, it is necessary that some of these issues are resolved before embracing the specific relevance of class II antibodies in liver-kidney transplantation.

T. Pruett, MD

Monocytic Myeloid-Derived Suppressor Cells Accumulate in Renal Transplant Patients and Mediate CD4⁺ Foxp3⁺ Treg Expansion

Luan Y, Mosheir E, Menon MC, et al (Ichan School of Medicine at Mount Sinai, NY)

Am J Transplant 13:3123-3131, 2013

Myeloid-derived suppressor cells (MDSC) are negative regulators of the immune response and are in part responsible for the inhibition of the T cell–mediated immune responses. While MDSC have been demonstrated to participate in the induction of prolonged allograft survival in animal models of transplantation, little is known about their immune regulatory function in human transplant recipients. Here, we report that two subsets of human MDSC expressing $CD11b^+$, $CD33^+$ and HLA-DR^- develop in renal patients posttransplantation. We found that $CD14^+$ expressing monocytic MDSC isolated from transplant recipients were highly efficient in suppressing the proliferation of $CD4^+$ T cells in mixed leukocyte reactions. In addition, we observed that $CD11b^+$ $CD33^+$ HLA-DR^- MDSC are capable of expanding Treg *in vitro*, and their accumulation overtime after transplantation linearly correlated with an increase in Treg *in vivo*. This is the first study to link the presence of MDSC with the emergence of Treg *in vivo* in transplant recipients, and to define the subpopulation of MDSC derived from transplant recipients responsible for generation of

Treg. Further studies are necessary to determine the alloimmune regulatory function of MDSC in human transplant recipients.

▶ An increasing field of transplant interest resides with understanding the regulatory elements of the immune response to antigens. Although attention has been paid to T regulator cells (Tregs), this report describes the role of another population of regulatory cells, the myeloid-derived suppressor cells. Their role in attenuating $CD4^+$ T cells and potential association with expanded Tregs is notable. Although not definitive, this study shows that attenuation of the human immune response is multipronged. The finding that $CD14^+$ cells were a key indicator of these cells makes one query whether the innate and protein/allospecific distinctions of immune responses may be a bit artificial. This study was done on a small number of patients and is worthy of repeat validation in other centers.

T. Pruett, MD

MicroRNA Signature at the Time of Clinical HCV Recurrence Associates With Aggressive Fibrosis Progression Post-Liver Transplantation

Gehrau RC, Mas VR, Villamil FG, et al (Univ of Virginia, Charlottesville; British Hosp, Buenos Aires, Argentina; et al)
Am J Transplant 13:729-737, 2013

Diagnosis and prediction of the severity of hepatitis C virus recurrence (HCV*rec*) after liver transplantation (LT) remain a challenge. MicroRNAs have been recently recognized as potential disease biomarkers. Archival liver biopsy samples from 43 HCV+ LT recipients were collected at clinical HCV*rec* time and at 3 years post-LT. Patients were classified as progressors (P = F0/F1) or nonprogressors (NP = F3/F4) according to the severity of fibrosis on the 3-year biopsy. Training (n = 27) and validation (n = 16) sets were defined. RNA was isolated from all biopsies at clinical HCV*rec* time, labeled and hybridized to miRNA-arrays. Progressors versus nonprogressors were compared using the two-sample *t*-test. A p-value ≤ 0.01 was considered significant. The ingenuity pathway analysis tool was used for microRNA and miRNA:mRNA ontology data integration. Nine microRNAs were differentially expressed between groups. A supervised cluster analysis separated samples in two well-defined groups (progressors vs. nonprogressors). Pathway analysis associated those microRNAs with hepatitis, steatosis, fibrosis, cirrhosis and T cell-related immune response. Data integration identified 17 genes from a previous genomic study as 9-microRNAs signature targets. Seven microRNAs were successfully validated in the validation set using QPCR. We have identified a 9-microRNA signature able to identify early post-LT patients at high risk of severe HCV*rec* during long-term follow-up.

▶ The use of gene arrays of transplanted organs can and will be confounded by alloimmunity, ischemia reperfusion, and other variables. The impact of the "other" variables is represented in this article in which liver recipients' liver gene arrays were assessed when the clinical activity of hepatitis C virus was recognized after transplantation. Not surprisingly, the gene arrays found in the liver were different in those livers that progressed toward fibrosis, compared with those that were less damaged by the virus/immune response.

This article highlights some of the difficulties associated with the clinical use of gene arrays. It is incontrovertible that the gene array within the transplanted organ is malleable, but the predictability of the response to injury or other stimuli remains ill defined. One of the significant limitations of gene technology resides in incomplete information about the normal spectrum of gene transformation in normal states and with (significant) stress. Until we have such information, much gene data will continue to be difficult to decipher.

T. Pruett, MD

Subclinical Epstein–Barr Virus Viremia Among Adult Renal Transplant Recipients: Incidence and Consequences

Bamoulid J, Courivaud C, Coaquette A, et al (INSERM, Besançon, France; CHU Besançon, France)

Am J Transplant 13:656-662, 2013

The natural history and clinical significance of posttransplant Epstein-Barr virus (EBV) infection remain largely unknown. The aims of this study are to describe the incidence, risk factors and consequences of EBV infection after kidney transplantation. A total of 383 consecutive patients having received a kidney transplant between January 2002 and December 2010 were included. EBV polymerase chain reaction (PCR) was performed every 2 weeks for 3 months, and every 4 weeks for the next 9 months. A total of 155 of the 383 patients (40%) had at least one positive viremia during the first year posttransplant. The median time to viremia was day 31 posttransplant (14–329). A total of 73 (47%) had EBV viremia > 10^3 log and 23 (15%) had positive viremia for more than 6 months. EBV D+/R− patients (12/18 (67%) versus 143/365 (39%), $p = 0.02$) and those having received antithymocyte globulins (ATG) (54% vs. 35%; $p < 0.001$) were more likely to develop EBV infection. EBV infection (hazard ratio [HR], 3.03; 95% confidence interval [CI], 1.72–8.29; $p = 0.01$) was associated with the occurrence of opportunistic infections. A positive EBV PCR during the first 6 months posttransplant was associated with graft loss (HR, 3.04; 95% CI, 1.36–6.79; $p = 0.014$). EBV reactivation is frequent after transplantation and reflects overimmunosuppression. Prospective studies should examine the association between EBV and graft loss.

► Humans are exposed to many organisms and viruses, some of which can reactivate with immunosuppression or be transmitted through organ transplantation. Epstein-Barr virus (EBV) is a common DNA virus associated with posttransplant lymphoproliferative disease. However, serial surveillance of kidney recipients from France revealed that 40% of recipients developed subclinical viremia. It was not demonstrated how much of this was reactivation of virus from the recipient or what was a donor strain/superinfection. However, in the seronegative recipients receiving a seropositive graft, there was a 67% incidence of viremia despite prophylactic therapy. All recipients received antivirals, and none developed posttransplant lymphoma or clinical EBV disease. Death-censored graft loss was higher in patients with viremia, although the authors did not delineate the reasons. Opportunistic infections were also more frequent in viremic recipients. This article demonstrates that subclinical events are common in transplant recipients and that some may affect recipient morbidity and graft function. The need to stratify recipient risk proves to be more difficult as more is learned about clinical and subclinical events.

T. Pruett, MD

Raccoon Rabies Virus Variant Transmission Through Solid Organ Transplantation

Vora NM, the Transplant-Associated Rabies Virus Transmission Investigation Team (Cts for Disease Control and Prevention, Atlanta, GA; et al)
JAMA 310:398-407, 2013

Importance.—The rabies virus causes a fatal encephalitis and can be transmitted through tissue or organ transplantation. In February 2013, a kidney recipient with no reported exposures to potentially rabid animals died from rabies 18 months after transplantation.

Objectives.—To investigate whether organ transplantation was the source of rabies virus exposure in the kidney recipient, and to evaluate for and prevent rabies in other transplant recipients from the same donor.

Design.—Organ donor and all transplant recipient medical records were reviewed. Laboratory tests to detect rabies virus–specific binding antibodies, rabies virus neutralizing antibodies, and rabies virus antigens were conducted on available specimens, including serum, cerebrospinal fluid, and tissues from the donor and the recipients. Viral ribonucleic acid was extracted from tissues and amplified for nucleoprotein gene sequencing for phylogenetic comparisons.

Main Outcomes and Measures.—Determination of whether the donor died from undiagnosed rabies and whether other organ recipients developed rabies.

Results.—In retrospect, the donor's clinical presentation (which began with vomiting and upper extremity paresthesias and progressed to fever, seizures, dysphagia, autonomic dysfunction, and brain death) was consistent with rabies. Rabies virus antigen was detected in archived autopsy brain tissue collected from the donor. The rabies viruses infecting the donor and the deceased kidney recipient were consistent with the raccoon rabies virus variant and were more than 99.9% identical across the entire *N* gene (1349/1350 nucleotides), thus confirming organ transplantation as the route of transmission. The 3 other organ recipients remained asymptomatic, with rabies virus neutralizing antibodies detected in their serum after completion of postexposure prophylaxis (range, 0.3-40.8 IU/mL).

Conclusions and Relevance.—Unlike the 2 previous clusters of rabies virus transmission through solid organ transplantation, there was a long incubation period in the recipient who developed rabies, and survival of 3 other recipients without pretransplant rabies vaccination. Rabies should be considered in patients with acute progressive encephalitis of unexplained etiology, especially for potential organ donors. A standard evaluation of potential donors who meet screening criteria for infectious encephalitis should be considered, and risks and benefits for recipients of organs from these donors should be evaluated.

▶ Contrary to the prior report, uncommon disease transmission events can be devastating. The report of raccoon rabies transmission is important for several reasons. Correct attribution of death in organ donors can be difficult. Even after pathologic examination of the brain, donor rabies was undiagnosed until after the recipient succumbed to rabies. The time to disease recognition in the recipient was extraordinarily long—almost a year. This implies that the transplant clinician should recognize that donor disease transmission can become clinically relevant long after the usual first few months.

Disease penetration did not occur in all recipients. Three other recipients of organs from this donor did get rabies, although they were vaccinated a year after their transplants and generated antirabies antibodies. Disease transmission through organ transplantation is a recognized risk, requiring systems approaches for techniques of risk assessment and communications to individuals at risk.

T. Pruett, MD

Islet Survival and Function Following Intramuscular Autotransplantation in the Minipig

Sterkers A, Hubert T, Gmyr V, et al (INSERM, Lille, France; et al)

Am J Transplant 13:891-898, 2013

The liver may not be an optimal site for islet transplantation due to obstacles by an instant blood-mediated inflammatory response (IBMIR), and low revascularization of transplanted islets. Therefore, intramuscular islet transplantation (IMIT) offers an attractive alternative, based on its simplicity, enabling easier access for noninvasive graft imaging and cell explantation. In this study, we explored the outcome of autologous IMIT in the minipig (n = 30). Using the intramuscular injection technique, we demonstrated by direct histological evidence the rapid revascularization of islets autotransplanted into the gracilius muscle. Islet survival assessment was performed using immunohistochemistry staining for insulin and glucagon up to a period of 6 months. Furthermore, we showed the crucial role of minimizing mechanical trauma to the myofibers and limiting exocrine contamination. Intramuscular islet graft function after transplantation was confirmed by documenting the acute insulin response to intravenous glucose in 5/11 pancreatectomized animals. Graft function after IMIT remained however significantly lower than the function measured in 12 out of 18 minipigs who received a similar islet volume in the liver through intraportal infusion. Collectively, these results demonstrated in a clinically relevant preclinical model, suggest IMIT as a promising alternative to intraportal infusion for the transplantation of β cells in certain medical situations.

▶ Cell transplantation is a less-morbid therapy than organ transplantation, especially as it relates to glycemic control. A significant issue for islet transplantation has been purity of cells, ability to engraft, placement of islets, and durability of subsequent function. Intraportal injection has been the preferred site for clinical islet transplantation but has some theoretical and practical limitations. The use of an intramuscular injection site proved to be a useful and successful, clinically and in an experimental model. However, the interplay between isolation technique, cell recovery, and implantation site is not as simple as this report suggests. However, as time progresses, the multiple variables will become understood, and cell-based therapies (differentiated and undifferentiated cells) will become increasingly useful.

T. Pruett, MD

Cyclosporine A Drives a Th17- and Th2-Mediated Posttransplant Obliterative Airway Disease

Lemaître PH, Vokaer B, Charbonnier L-M, et al (Université Libre de Bruxelles, Gosselies, Belgium; et al)

Am J Transplant 13:611-620, 2013

Calcineurin-inhibitor refractory bronchiolitis obliterans (BO) represents the leading cause of late graft failure after lung transplantation. T helper (Th)2 and Th17 lymphocytes have been associated with BO development. Taking advantage of a fully allogeneic trachea transplantation model in mice, we addressed the pathogenicity of Th cells in obliterative airway disease (OAD) occurring in cyclosporine A (CsA)-treated recipients. We found that CsA prevented $CD8^+$ T cell infiltration into the graft and downregulated the Th1 response but affected neither Th2 nor Th17 responses *in vivo*. In secondary mixed lymphocyte cultures, CsA dramatically decreased donor-specific IFN-γ production, enhanced IL-17 production and did not affect IL-13. As $CD4^+$ depletion efficiently prevented OAD in CsA-treated recipients, we further explored the role of Th2 and Th17 immunity *in vivo*. Although IL-4 and IL-17 deficient untreated mice developed an OAD comparable to wild-type recipients, a single cytokine deficiency afforded significant protection in CsA-treated recipients. In conclusion, CsA treatment unbalances T helper alloreactivity and favors Th2 and Th17 as coexisting pathways mediating chronic rejection of heterotopic tracheal allografts.

▶ Animal models have been used to discern pathologic mechanisms of many diseases. This article purports to describe cellular immunologic mechanisms of the very real problem of post–lung transplantation bronchiolitis obliterans.

The authors utilized a free tracheal graft placed within a subcutaneous pocket and drew extrapolations from observations around histologic and cellular assessment of free tracheal placement. It was concluded that cyclosporine A attenuated early rejection but did little to modify collagen deposition long term (28 days). It was observed that syngeneic tracheas did not elicit a Th2 or IL-17 response, whereas allotransplanted tracheas elicited significant Th2 and IL-17 lymphocytic response that was not suppressed by cyclosporine A administration. Although these findings are intriguing and may be important in the understanding of an extraordinarily important clinical entity, it is very unclear whether the model is in any fashion reflective of clinical chronic airway disease seen after lung transplantation. What is the role of hypoxia, lack of vascularization, and injury recovery after placement of the trachea in the pouch? Is 28 days appropriate? Conclusions should be drawn after some semblance of verification that pathologic mechanisms are similar to those seen clinically.

T. Pruett, MD

7 Surgical Infections

Introduction

Surgical site infection (SSI) will occur at some frequency after surgical procedures. There are many factors that can increase the risk and some that have been shown to diminish the risk of these unwanted events. Now that SSI is part of "quality" metrics for payment, the scrutiny of the community is on processes that can impact the occurrence of SSI. However, the real issue is that SSI is an unintended outcome that affects a person. Paper 1 describes the straight financial cost to an institution of SSI. Resource consumption is dramatically increased by the occurrence of the infection and institutional financial margins are decreased, but the real financial cost for the system is in the loss of capacity due to people occupying beds that could otherwise be used to generate new dollars. Assuming that a hospital is in a high-demand environment, SSI is a significant cause of inefficiency and revenue loss. Understanding the relevant variables that predispose an individual to SSI is central to appropriate risk adjustment that is pivotal in understanding deviations from baseline. The risk for SSI is not the same for all individuals. In paper 2, the "homogeneous" population of colon resection surgery was assessed for differences and variables that were associated with the incidence of SSI. This was accomplished by analyzing the NSQIP database of over 27 000 colon resections for deep and superficial SSI. What became apparent was that, despite the common procedure of "colon resection," SSI outcomes were different. Resection for benign lesions had a lesser incidence than those for malignant lesions and inflammatory bowel disease. Procedures that could be performed laprascopically had a lower incidence of SSI than those done open. Increasing BMI was associated with increasing incidence of SSI, mostly the superficial variant. Disseminated cancer and irradiation increased the risk of deep infections, but not superficial. This is a very insightful analysis when generating expected outcomes after performance of a "homogenous" procedure. Unfortunately, normalizing the data for outcomes turns out to involve a large number of variables. The complexity mandates that disease-specific analyses be performed, and the authors suggest that quality metrics not be overly simplified to meet reductionist administrative needs.

Antibiotic prophylaxis was recognized as an effective tool to decrease SSI after colon surgery in the 1940s, and solid microbiology was applied to the process in the 1970s, so why is this still an issue in 2013? Paper 3 assessed the impact of oral antibiotics upon hospital resources. It was found that, compared to no bowel preparation or mechanical bowel prep, the oral antibiotic bowel preparation reduced length of stay, readmission and overall cost, predominantly through decreasing the SSI rate. It is remarkable that this study was even performed, as the surgical literature is so painfully replete with studies demonstrating the efficacy of microbe reduction in the risk for SSI. They reported that, without oral antibiotics, the rate of SSI was more than doubled. What the authors didn't describe was the use of parenteral antibiotics when oral agents were or were not given. There are ample reports of the efficacy of parenteral agents reducing the risk of SSI. It seems that many lessons of the past need to be relearned today. In 1961, Burke published that antibiotics needed to be administered within a given time window if there was to be effectiveness in reducing skin infections induced by inoculation of bacteria. This and other clinical data has led to the Surgical Care Improvement Project (SCIP) recommendations that prophylactic antibiotics should be administered within an hour of a surgical incision. This recommendation has taken on a life of its own and is now widely measured as a quality parameter by CMS. Virtually all hospitals expend considerable time and effort to comply with this quality metric. Sadly, compliance with this metric was not associated with a reduction in SSI in paper 4. It was reaffirmed that the antibiotics had to be active against bacteria that contaminate a wound to effectively reduce the incidence of SSI. The use of the quality metric of time of antibiotic administration relative to incision is misplaced energy. If one focuses very hard on this single variable, it is possible to show that timing of antibiotic administration is associated with a reduction in infection rate. Paper 5 did an analysis that calculated that an 11.3% reduction in the risk of SSI if antibiotics were administered within 4 minutes before incision vs an hour before. Assuming a clean case infection rate of 1.7%, the SSI rate could be reduced to 1.52%, having to have appropriate confidence limits. Other clinical variables can and do overwhelm this effect. There is a need to find the most significant variable(s) rather than the one most easily measured for the establishment of quality metrics.

The above studies are all predicated upon analyses of large databases (NSQIP and VA system). Paper 6 looks at how database entries of a well-established process, wound classification (clean, clean/contaminated, contaminated and dirty) as the basis of SSI risk stratification are influenced by who generates the data. Surgeons, OR nurses, and NSQIP data extractors disagreed on wound classification in 48% of cases performed in a single hospital. Such a high frequency of discrepancy must make one question the confidence that can be placed in interinstitutional comparisons and expected outcomes, where the variables used are much less understood. Finally, the Surgical Infection Prevention project was started in 2002 and efforts have been made with the purpose of improved compliance with antibiotic prophylaxis to reduce SSI and promote "evidence-based" policy and procedure. Paper 7 reviewed 46 papers published since the SIP project started and were evaluated by the modified criteria for evaluating quality improvement studies (Standards for Quality Improvement

Reporting Excellence). This review focused upon the consistency of methodology, intrinsic bias, randomization or blinding of groups, sample size calculation, factors affecting generalization, assessment of SSI, and implementation barriers. It was found that deficits in methodology and design precluded application of the findings of the papers to specific, individual practices. In other words, evidence-based practice for one of the most common adverse events was not feasible. While evidence-based, quality-driven performance is an excellent goal, these papers describe many of the limitations of the existing literature and our failure to embrace the process.

"Best" treatment for specific diseases has also been generated from large databases and will likely be used in hospitals in order to generate policy. Paper 8 proposes to tailor surgical therapy for appendicitis based on the NSQIP database. The outcomes from over 61 000 NSQIP appendectomy records were reviewed. In uncomplicated appendectomy, the laprascopic approach was associated with lower risk for superficial SSI, while the open approach was less likely to result in organ space infection (deep SSI). The intriguing part about this type of report is all the things that were not included within the analysis: surgical difficulty with mobilization of the appendix, spillage of enteric contents, damage to mesentery, and blood left in the wound that could become infected. Also not reported in this analysis but in the database was the type of antibiotic given (adequacy) and the timeliness of administration. There are large numbers of variables associated with adverse clinical outcomes, and capturing them in a relevant clinical database is pivotal to appropriate analysis. The difficulty in making evidence-based decisions was addressed by the Canadian Association of General Surgeons and the ACS, where they perform a joint Evidence-based Review in Surgery. Paper 9 is an analysis of literature about therapy for acute appendicitis. Unlike analysis of NSQIP data, this review addressed antibiotics vs surgical removal of the appendix when there is a clinical diagnosis of appendicitis. The discussion is excellent regarding the limitations and application of Standards for Quality Improvement Reporting Excellence to the existing literature. The conclusion that sufficient ambiguity exists to warrant a randomized double-blind study is an indictment of the process after years of data collection.

There were a number of the "lesser" issues that were addressed in the 2013 literature. Paper 10 reports a double-blind randomized trial on the duration of antibiotics after thoracic surgery. Many surgeons articulate the need for continuation of antibiotics as therapy and not prophylaxis after a surgical procedure, especially thoracic surgery where chest tubes are required. The randomized, blinded study had patients receive either preoperative antibiotics only or continued perioperative agents for 48 hours or until the chest tubes were removed, whichever was shorter. Findings demonstrated no benefit for protracted administration. While the study did not achieve the required numbers of the power analysis, the authors discussed the limitations reasonably. However, whether the evidence was sufficient to change practice could not be made due to underpowering. Paper 11 addresses the univariate aspect of SSI and number of blood transfusions in peripheral vascular reconstruction. The authors rightly state in the conclusion that the population that requires blood is not really the same as the one that can undergo revascularization without blood and that blood usage as a single measure is probably not sufficient. While there may be surgeon-specific blood requirements, the patient populations are not the same. Yes, SSI is higher in those people requiring >3 u PRBC, but the complexity of the procedure and patients may be more relevant than the single element of blood transfusion. Skin antisepsis has been a foundational piece of surgery for over a century.

Reduction of skin flora in hospitalized patients may diminish the incidence of nosocomial infections. Paper 12 reports the effect of chlorhexidine bathing upon such hospital-acquired infections. It was associated with a diminution of blood stream infections in medical, but not surgical ICUs. Acquisition of VRE and MRSA was diminished during the use of the swabs. The study did not assess the efficacy of the bathing in reducing skin flora at the site, of application, did not state effect upon skin around intravenous catheter sites, nor address issue of SSI in surgical ICUs. Antiseptic skin bathing is a simple process that may be beneficial. However, the necessary supporting data, power calculations, discussion of inclusion and exclusion of data, potential bias, and general applicability were not provided. Management of the contaminated wound continues to be controversial. Primary closure vs delayed primary closure was the topic of paper 13. This meta-analysis was performed on papers published since 1990. This review was written under the auspices of the military, one of the major proponents of the use of DPC. As with the other meta-analyses of common problems, the literature suggests that there is benefit, but the literature is not written in such a fashion that it can be reliably applied to specific clinical indications. Management of ventral or incisional hernias involves complex decision making.

Paper 14 is a manifestation of many of our clinical biases, with the purpose of demonstrating that repair of the contaminated hernia can be done with synthetic mesh (contrasted to the need for biologic material). What is not discussed within the manuscript is patient management strategies other than surgical technique and management of surgical sequelae. Were antibiotics used and for how long? Was additional imaging and subsequent drainage done? All of these may (or not) be important management strategies that become necessary to achieve good patient outcomes. The cost analysis at the end of the discussion is an eye opener.

Takedown of an enteric stoma is another common procedure with a significant risk for SSI. A report from the VA (paper 15) noted the associated SSI rate of 36%. As stoma reversal is a totally elective procedure, there seems to be much room for improvement. Associated variables with SSI were consistent with surgical principles, but the question remains whether any intervention would have diminished the likelihood of SSI. If seroma was associated with SSI, would a drain have reduced the occurrence and did these occur more frequently in the obese patients? Would different antibiotic selection and duration have modified the clinical occurrence of SSI? Was bowel preparation (with or without oral antibiotics) used in the case of colostomy takedown? There are certainly many relevant clinical elements that would have helped discern risk for SSI development. Management of trauma victims is a surgical responsibility, and the consequence of intra-abdominal infection/abscess or enteric fistula is an unwanted SSI that should be avoided. Paper 16 draws from the American Association of Surgery for Trauma (AAST) database to discern the variables associated with surgical site infectious consequences after damage control laparotomy. The variables associated with these complications were again common sense: colon resection, need for multiple laparotomies, and large volume resuscitation (severe injury). What was not discussed was what could have been done to lessen the risk. Were infections associated with staple breakdown, missed injuries, or infected hematomas? Our literature (and databases) needs to reflect not only "problems" but also complete variables associated with the generation. The failure of databases is not that the people who established them didn't know; rather, there is limited ability to collect and enter data. Cost and lack of reliability escalate with more and more elements that are essential to quality metrics.

Necrotizing soft tissue infections also fall within the surgeon's domain, and stratifying outcome likelihood is an important exercise. Using the NSQIP data, a calculator was generated for likelihood of mortality after necrotizing soft tissue infection (paper 17). While useful, again information about important clinical variables is not included in the analysis (time from symptoms to debridement, adequacy of debridement, use/not of hyperbaric oxygen, appropriateness of antimicrobial spectrum). The current emphasis upon clinical outcomes analysis is severely limited by therapeutic data that is not analyzed. Finally, a paper is included to represent the impact of FDA standards on clinical trials to license indications for antibiotic usage. Paper 18 reports the results of the ESTABLISH-1 trial to obtain approval for a new antibiotic with the indication for soft tissue infections, where it failed to achieve the non-inferiority status. This failure is an extraordinarily expensive proposition, one that the makers of these agents want to avoid. The discussion describes how study design and accountability drive the evolution of new therapies.

The final three papers address new biologic issues/therapies that may/not be applied to surgical patients. While experimental models of sepsis have shown utility for anti-LPS products, their utility in clinical infections has not been borne out. The most recent iteration is reported in paper 19. In a randomized fashion, patients were randomized to either LPS antagonist or placebo. About 50% of the patients were lung infections, about a quarter abdominal and another fifth urinary. With this patient mix, there was no associated benefit. About 40% had measurable endotoxin, of a subset where the assay was performed. The quest for anti-toxin therapy may well be over, now that there have been repeated studies that have failed to achieve efficacy. Paper 20 is another disappointing study where the use of an anti-*Staphylococcus* vaccine failed to provide protection against deep SSI and mediastinitis after cardiac surgery. In fact, there was an associated increased risk of death associated with *Staphylococcus* infection in those people who had received the vaccine. The final manuscript assesses the impact of telomere chromosomal length on propensity to develop infection. While the report is very controlled and about acquisition of viral infections, the observation that telomere length can change with season and age suggests that there may be more biologic phenomena in surgical healing and infection than we surmised.

It would be great if biologics could be introduced into clinical practice that would modify the course of clinical infections. The changing regulatory standards and cost of doing clinical studies may make newer therapies cost prohibitive. The overall theme of this year's surgical articles stresses the limitations of large databases and the regulatory impact upon surgical practice.

Timothy L. Pruett, MD

Financial Impact of Surgical Site Infections on Hospitals: The Hospital Management Perspective

Shepard J, Ward W, Milstone A, et al (The Johns Hopkins Health System, Baltimore, MD; Johns Hopkins Univ, Baltimore, MD; The Johns Hopkins Hosp, Baltimore, MD; et al)

JAMA Surg 148:907-914, 2013

Importance.—Surgical site infections (SSIs) may increase health care costs, but few studies have conducted an analysis from the perspective of hospital administrators.

Objective.—To determine the change in hospital profit due to SSIs.

Design.—Retrospective study of data from January 1, 2007, to December 31, 2010.

Setting.—The study was performed at 4 of The Johns Hopkins Health System acute care hospitals in Maryland: Johns Hopkins Bayview (560 beds); Howard County General Hospital (238 beds); The Johns Hopkins Hospital (946 beds); and Suburban Hospital (229 beds).

Participants.—Eligible patients for the study included those patients admitted to the 4 hospitals between January 1, 2007, and December 31, 2010, with complete data and the correct *International Classification of Diseases, Ninth Revision* code, as determined by the infection preventionist. Infection preventionists performed complete medical record review using National Healthcare Safety Network definitions to identify SSIs. Patients were stratified using the All Patient Refined Diagnosis Related Groups to estimate the change in hospital profit due to SSIs.

Exposure.—Surgical site infections.

Main Outcomes and Measures.—The outcomes of the study were the difference in daily total charges, length of stay (LOS), 30-day readmission rate, and profit for patients with an SSI when compared with patients without an SSI. The hypothesis, formulated prior to data collection, that patients with an SSI have higher daily total costs, a longer LOS, and higher 30-day readmission rates than patients without an SSI, was tested using a nonpaired

Mann-Whitney *U* test, an analysis of covariance, and a Pearson χ^2 test. Hospital charges were used as a proxy for hospital cost.

Results.—The daily total charges, mean LOS, and 30-day readmission rate for patients with an SSI compared with patients without an SSI were \$7493 vs \$7924 ($P = .99$); 10.56 days vs 5.64 days ($P < .001$); and 51.94 vs 8.19 readmissions per 100 procedures ($P < .001$). The change in profit due SSIs was \$2 268 589.

Conclusions and Relevance.—The data suggest that hospitals have a financial incentive to reduce SSIs, but hospitals should expect to see an increase in both cost and revenue when SSIs are reduced.

► Surgical site infections (SSIs) are undesired outcomes after the performance of a surgical procedure. To the surgeon and patient, it may prove to be on the continuum from an inconvenience to a life-threatening event. However, to the payment and health care delivery system, SSI proves to be an expensive proposition. The impact was discussed regarding the impact on the Johns' Hopkins delivery system. SSIs added cost to the system at the same time as impairing efficiency. The added costs of SSI per occurrence were an increased length of stay (up almost 90% over control) and total charges (almost 64% increase). Efforts to control SSI have, therefore, moved to the fore in systems to control quality and care delivery. Surgeons are caught in the middle of compliance and economic forces. The importance of understanding the elements essential for positive effect is central to developing appropriate metrics.

T. Pruett, MD

Risk Factors for Superficial vs Deep/Organ-Space Surgical Site Infections: Implications for Quality Improvement Initiatives

Lawson EH, Hall BL, Ko CY (Univ of California, Los Angeles; Washington Univ School of Medicine, St Louis, MO)

JAMA Surg 148:1-10, 2013

Importance.—Surgical site infections (SSIs) are the focus of numerous quality improvement initiatives because they are a common and costly cause of potentially preventable patient morbidity. Superficial and deep/organ-space SSIs differ in terms of anatomical location and clinical severity.

Objective.—To identify risk factors that are uniquely predictive of superficial vs deep/organ-space SSIs occurring after colectomy procedures.

Design.—Retrospective cohort study.

Setting.—American College of Surgeons National Surgical Quality Improvement Program.

Participants.—Patients undergoing colectomy procedures in 2011 were identified by *Current Procedural Terminology* codes.

Intervention.—Colectomy procedures.

Main Outcomes and Measures.—We compared rates of superficial SSI and deep/organ-space SSI associated with perioperative variables of interest: demographics; preoperative clinical severity, risk factors, and comorbidities and variables related to the hospitalization or procedure. Hierarchical multivariable logistic regression models were developed to identify risk-adjusted predictors of each SSI type.

Results.—Among 27 011 patients identified from 305 hospitals, 6.2% developed a superficial SSI and 4.7% developed a deep/organ-space SSI. Risk factors common to the occurrence of both SSI types were identified: open surgery (vs laparoscopic) and current smoker. Risk factors with differential effects on each SSI type included specific postoperative diagnoses, disseminated cancer, and irradiation therapy, which were all associated with increased odds of deep/organ-space SSI only. The graded relationship between increasing body mass index and SSI occurrence appeared to be stronger for superficial SSI.

Conclusions and Relevance.—Risk factors for superficial SSI and deep/organ-space SSI vary in terms of magnitude and significance, suggesting that these SSI types are somewhat different disease processes. Groups interested in preventing SSIs might improve success by considering these SSI types independently for root-cause analyses and development of best practices and interventions.

▶ Identifying the variables associated with development of surgical site infection (SSI) after a procedure sounds simple and has been the focus of years of clinical and basic research. However, generating systems approaches to prevention of SSI may vary according to the individual patient. An examination of the National Surgical Quality Improvement Program (NSQIP) assessed SSIs after colon surgery and divided results into superficial and deep infections. In this comprehensive database, the development of SSI was not uniform across all types of colon surgery. Many disease-specific, comorbidity, and behavioral findings were found to be associated with increased likelihood of perioperative SSI. To the end that risk adjustment is required to assess measures associated with reduced risk (laparoscopic vs open) or more interesting time of procedure (shorter times associated with less infection), the question is begged whether these measures are real or an epiphenomenon that simpler cases are less likely to have problems. That which must be done open or takes a bit longer may just be more diseased and require special attention. All of these measures attempt to find a surrogate for good surgical judgment, an entity that has been notoriously difficult to measure.

T. Pruett, MD

Oral Antibiotic Bowel Preparation Reduces Length of Stay and Readmissions after Colorectal Surgery

Toneva GD, Deierhoi RJ, Morris M, et al (Birmingham Veterans Affairs Hosp, AL; et al)

J Am Coll Surg 216:756-763, 2013

Background.—Oral antibiotic bowel preparation (OABP) before colorectal resection has been shown to reduce surgical site infections. We examined whether OABP decreases length of stay (LOS) and readmissions for colorectal surgery.

Study Design.—This retrospective study used national Veterans Affairs Surgical Quality Improvement Program preoperative risk and outcomes data linked to Veterans Affairs Administrative and Pharmacy Benefits Management data on patients undergoing elective colorectal resections from 2005 to 2009. Exclusion criteria were preoperative LOS >2 days, American Society of Anesthesiologists class 5, or death before discharge. Patient and surgery characteristics, bowel preparation use, presence of an ostomy, indication for surgery, and indication for readmission using ICD-9 codes were determined. Negative binomial regression was used to model LOS. Logistic regression analyses modeled 30-day readmission.

Results.—Of the 8,180 patients, 1,161 (14.2%) were readmitted within 30 days. Length of stay and readmissions varied significantly by bowel preparation, procedure, presence of an ostomy, and American Society of Anesthesiologists class. Oral antibiotic bowel preparation was associated with a below-median postoperative LOS (negative binomial regression estimate = −0.1159; $p < 0.0001$) and fewer 30-day readmissions (adjusted odds ratio = 0.81; 95% CI, 0.68–0.97). Overall, 4.9% were readmitted for infections (ICD-9 codes) and this varied by bowel preparation (no preparation 6.1%, mechanical 5.4%, OABP 3.9%; $p = 0.001$). The readmission rate for noninfectious reasons was 9.3% and did not differ significantly by bowel preparation (no preparation 9.9%, mechanical 9.6%, OABP 8.8%; $p = 0.38$).

Conclusions.—Oral antibiotic bowel preparation before elective colorectal surgery is associated with shorter postoperative LOS and lower 30-day readmission rates, primarily due to fewer readmissions for infections. Prospective studies are needed to verify these results.

▶ The Veterans Affairs system has been touted as an exemplar of data repository and evidence-based improvement system. This review of a large series of colon resections is important for what it doesn't report. The conclusion was that antibiotic bowel preparation results in fewer infectious complications than either mechanical preparation or no bowel preparation. The missing elements were information as to the effectiveness of prophylactic antimicrobial agents for the enteric flora. An abundance of information has shown that optimization of infection risk reduction is only accomplished by administration of agents with empiric activity against aerobic gram-negative bacteria and anaerobic organisms. The review did not comment on timely administration of other antimicrobial agents in any of the groups. Abundant inconclusive reports state equal efficacy of intravenous antimicrobials and oral/topical bowel decontamination. The putative length of stay and readmission benefit of the oral regimen is almost certainly the consequence of the reduction in SSI, although the key variable of efficiency of antimicrobial prophylaxis was left decidedly vague. Although the authors conclude that a randomized trial should be performed to confirm their conclusion of retrospective information, they neglected to include data within their own data repository, which would have to be included in a prospective study.

T. Pruett, MD

Timing of Surgical Antibiotic Prophylaxis and the Risk of Surgical Site Infection

Hawn MT, Richman JS, Vick CC, et al (Birmingham Veterans Administration Hosp, AL; et al)

JAMA Surg 148:649-657, 2013

Importance.—Timing of prophylactic antibiotic administration for surgical procedures is a nationally mandated and publicly reported quality metric sponsored by the Centers for Medicare and Medicaid Services Surgical Care Improvement Project. Numerous studies have failed to demonstrate that adherence to the Surgical Care Improvement Project prophylactic antibiotic timely administration measure is associated with decreased surgical site infection (SSI).

Objective.—To determine whether prophylactic antibiotic timing is associated with SSI occurrence.

Design.—Retrospective cohort study using national Veterans Affairs patient-level data on prophylactic antibiotic timing for orthopedic, colorectal, vascular, and gynecologic procedures from 2005 through 2009.

Setting.—National Veterans Affairs Surgical Care Improvement Project data from 112 Veterans Affairs hospitals and matched Veterans Affairs Surgical Quality Improvement Program data.

Patients.—Patients undergoing hip or knee arthroplasty, colorectal surgical procedures, arterial vascular surgical procedures, and hysterectomy.

Intervention.—Timing of prophylactic antibiotic administration with respect to surgical incision time.

Main Outcomes and Measures.—Data for prophylactic antibiotic agent, prophylactic antibiotic timing with respect to surgical incision, and patient and procedure risk variables were assessed for their relationship with the occurrence of a composite superficial or deep incisional SSI within 30 days after the procedure. Nonlinear generalized additive models were used to examine the association between antibiotic timing and SSI.

Results.—Of the 32 459 operations, prophylactic antibiotics were administered at a median of 28 minutes (interquartile range, 17-39 minutes) prior to surgical incision, and 1497 cases (4.6%) developed an SSI. Compared with procedures with antibiotic administration within 60 minutes prior to incision, higher SSI rates were observed for timing more than 60 minutes prior to incision (unadjusted odds ratio [OR] = 1.34; 95% CI, 1.08-1.66) but not after incision (unadjusted OR = 1.26; 95% CI, 0.92-1.72). In unadjusted generalized additive models, we observed a significant nonlinear relationship between prophylactic antibiotic timing and SSI when considering timing as a continuous variable (P =.01). In generalized additive models adjusted for patient, procedure, and antibiotic variables, no significant association between prophylactic antibiotic timing and SSI was observed. Vancomycin hydrochloride was associated with higher SSI occurrence for orthopedic procedures (adjusted OR = 1.75; 95% CI, 1.16-2.65). Cefazolin sodium and quinolone in combination with an anaerobic agent were associated with fewer SSI events (cefazolin: adjusted OR = 0.49; 95% CI, 0.34-0.71; quinolone: adjusted OR = 0.55; 95% CI, 0.35-0.87) for colorectal procedures.

Conclusions and Relevance.—The SSI risk varies by patient and procedure factors as well as antibiotic properties but is not significantly associated with prophylactic antibiotic timing. While adherence to the timely prophylactic antibiotic measure is not bad care, there is little evidence to suggest that it is better care.

▶ Antibiotics must be in contact with bacteria to prevent replication that can reach a critical number resulting in clinical infection/surgical site infection (SSI). This simple concept is the justification for the time boundary within the Surgical Care Improvement Project (SCIP) parameters. The results of a retrospective study bring the timeliness factor into question as contrasted with the efficacy of the specific agents delivered against pathogenic bacteria that contaminate the surgical wound. The recommendations were initially made based on pharmacokinetics and blood elimination, but the clinical effect of administration of prophylactic antibiotics will be dependent on tissue concentrations that will reduce bacterial proliferation. A problem associated with retrospective data, such as Veterans Affairs information systems used in this report, is the effect of known performance metrics on the recording of data.

To the end that providers are held accountable for timely administration, there will be a tendency to enter data within the known performance time, irrespective of whether the agents were actually given during that proscribed interval. This study reinforces the premise that antimicrobials that can effectively prevent bacterial replication will reduce the incidence of SSI. Common sense states that there must be enough tissue antimicrobial activity to inhibit bacterial proliferation, but the prescription that they must administer within a specific time interval is not supported by this data analysis. In review of this database, appropriateness of antimicrobial agent trumps timing of administration.

T. Pruett, MD

Is It Time to Refine? An Exploration and Simulation of Optimal Antibiotic Timing in General Surgery

Koch CG, Li L, Hixson E, et al (Cleveland Clinic, OH)

J Am Coll Surg 217:628-635, 2013

Background.—Postoperative infections increase morbidity, resource use, and costs. Our objective was to examine whether within guideline recommendations an optimal time exists for an initial dose of antibiotic to reduce postoperative infections in general surgery, and to simulate the magnitude of a reduction in infections should an optimal time be implemented.

Study Design.—The population consisted of 6,731 patients who underwent 7,095 general surgery procedures between January 5, 2006 and June 25, 2012. Patients with pre-existing infections, such as pneumonia and sepsis, and patients with no recorded use of antibiotics were excluded, as were patients on vancomycin and surgical procedures longer than 4 hours in duration. The final analysis dataset included 4,453 patients. The National Surgical Quality Improvement Program was used for perioperative variables and outcomes. The end point was a composite of wound disruption; superficial, deep, organ space, surgical site infections; and sepsis. Semiparametric logistic regression was used to study the association between antibiotic timing and infection.

Results.—There were 444 (10%) patients with a primary end point of infectious complication. A nonlinear "bowl-shaped" relationship between duration of interval from antibiotic administration and surgical incision and infection was observed; lowest risk corresponding to administration time close to incision was 4 minutes before incision (95% one-sided CI, 0–18 minutes). The model suggested optimal timing would result in an 11.3% reduction in the primary infection end point.

Conclusions.—Risk of infectious complications decreased as antibiotic administration moved closer to incision time. These data suggest an opportunity to reduce infections by 11.3% by targeting initial antibiotic administration closer to incision.

▶ Consistent with the premise that antimicrobials must contact bacteria to be effective, this review of the National Surgical Quality Improvement Program database purports that the optimal time of antibiotic administration is 4 minutes before incision. Is that when the infusion starts or ends? How rapidly was it administered? What are the confidence limits around the recording of the data? The conclusion seems logical, but how reliable are the data for such a granular conclusion? Voluntary databases, in which data are entered voluntarily and without safeguards of strict accuracy, have limits to data accuracy. Just as significant digits apply to the measured sciences, these types of reports need explanation regarding the reliability of the data points that are used to generate conclusions. As noted in the prior report, timing may be a less important variable when the agent used has lesser activity against the bacteria in the wound. Although the concept is certainly sound, the data supporting the conclusion are less convincing.

T. Pruett, MD

Wound Classification in Pediatric General Surgery: Significant Variation Exists among Providers

Snyder RA, Johnson L, Tice J, et al (Vanderbilt Univ School of Medicine, Nashville, TN)

J Am Coll Surg 217:819-826, 2013

Background.—Risk-adjusted rates of surgical site infections (SSI) are used as a quality metric to facilitate improvement within a hospital system and allow comparison across institutions. The NSQIP-Pediatric, among others, uses surgical wound classification as a variable in models designed to predict risk-adjusted postoperative morbidity, including SSI rates. The purpose of this study was to measure the level of agreement in wound classification assignment among 3 providers: surgeons, operating room (OR) nurses, and NSQIP surgical clinical reviewers (SCR).

Study Design.—An analysis was performed of pediatric general surgery operations from 2010 to 2011. Wound classification was assigned at the time of operation by the OR nurse and surgeon, and by the NSQIP SCR postoperatively, according to NSQIP methodology. Disagreement was defined as any discrepancy in classification among the 3 providers, and the level of agreement was determined using the kappa statistic.

Results.—For the 374 procedures reviewed, there was an overall disagreement of 48% among all providers, kappa 0.48 (95% CI 0.43 to 0.53). When comparing wound classification by surgeon and NSQIP SCR, 23% of cases were in disagreement, kappa 0.74 (95% CI 0.68 to 0.78). Disagreement between OR nurse and either surgeon or NSQIP SCR was higher: 38%, kappa 0.45 (95% CI 0.38 to 0.53) and 40%, kappa 0.44 (95% CI 0.37 to 0.51). Fundoplication, appendectomy, and cholecystectomy demonstrated the highest overall disagreement (73%, 71%, and 60%, respectively).

Conclusions.—There is significant variation in assigning surgical wound classification among health care providers. For future SSI comparative analyses, it will be critical to improve uniformity and understanding of wound class assignment among providers and institutions.

▶ The likelihood of developing a surgical site infection (SSI) is influenced by the degree of bacterial contamination during the procedure. To appropriately understand the frequency of SSI within a hospital system, it is necessary to appropriately define and then record the wound classification. Reliability of the information with a database is essential for appropriate stratification of operative procedures. This report compares the classification of the same procedure by surgeon or operative nurse of the clinical abstractor for entry into the National Surgical Quality Improvement Program database. Overall, the discordance between the 3 observers was 48%. This introduces a significant element of uncertainty when attempting to predict significance of observed versus expected SSI. The report stresses the vagaries by which data are collected, interpreted, and recorded. As long as a single system collects observations in a consistent fashion, trending is possible. However, institutional comparisons and national oversight become far less certain without attention to methodologic detail.

T. Pruett, MD

What Is the Quality of Reporting of Studies of Interventions to Increase Compliance with Antibiotic Prophylaxis?

Levy SM, Phatak UR, Tsao K, et al (Univ of Texas Med School at Houston)

J Am Coll Surg 217:770-779, 2013

Background.—Despite studies reporting successful interventions to increase antibiotic prophylaxis compliance, surgical site infections remain a significant problem. The reasons for this lack of improvement are unknown. This review evaluates the internal and external validity of quality improvement studies of interventions to increase surgical antibiotic prophylaxis compliance.

Study Design.—Three investigators independently performed systematic literature searches and selected eligible studies that evaluated interventions to improve perioperative antibiotic prophylaxis timing, type, and/or discontinuation. Studies published before the Surgical Infection Prevention project inception in 2002 were excluded. Each study was assessed based on modified criteria for evaluating quality improvement studies (Standards for Quality Improvement Reporting Excellence) and for facilitating implementation of evidence into practice (Reach-Efficacy-Adoption-Implementation-Maintenance).

Results.—Forty-six articles met inclusion criteria; 93% reported improvement in antibiotic prophylaxis compliance. Surgical site infections were evaluated in 50% of studies and 65% reported an improvement. Less than 5% of studies used randomization, allocation concealment, or blinding. Nine percent of studies described efforts to minimize bias in the design results and analysis and 13% described a sample size calculation. Approximately one-third of studies described participant adoption of the intervention (26%), factors affecting generalizability (33%), or implementation barriers (37%). Most studies (80%) used multiple interventions; no single intervention was associated with change in compliance. Studies with the lowest baseline compliance showed the greatest improvement, regardless of the intervention(s).

Conclusions.—The methodology and reporting of quality improvement studies on perioperative antibiotic prophylaxis is suboptimal, and factors that would improve generalizability of successful intervention implementation are infrequently reported. Clinicians should use caution in applying the results of these studies to their general practice.

▶ Evidence-based medicine is the current trend in health care. Improvements in appropriate antibiotic delivery to the surgical patient are a desired end. In an analysis of methodologies reported within the surgical literature, the authors found that significant weakness exists in much of the current literature. This limitation makes application of the recommendations generating from the reported studies very suspect. The authors make the point that studies designed to address better adherence to goals of prophylactic antimicrobials in surgical procedures should adhere to quality improvement principles, such as acknowledgment of methodologic limitations, bias potential in the study design, randomization or blinded studies to diminish likelihood of system adoption of unhelpful or potentially harmful procedures, and finally, specific local issues that had to be addressed to gain (or prevent) effective implementation of the process. This common sense review of the surgical literature puts many issues into process perspective.

T. Pruett, MD

Tailoring the Operative Approach for Appendicitis to the Patient: A Prediction Model from National Surgical Quality Improvement Program Data

Senekjian L, Nirula R (Univ of Utah School of Medicine, Salt Lake City)
J Am Coll Surg 216:34-40, 2013

Background.—Laparoscopic appendectomy (LA) is increasingly being performed in the United States, despite controversy about differences in infectious complication rates compared with open appendectomy (OA). Subpopulations exist in which infectious complication rates, both surgical site and organ space, differ with respect to LA compared with OA.

Study Design.—All appendectomies in the National Surgical Quality Improvement Program database were analyzed with respect to surgical site infection (SSI) and organ space infection (OSI). Multivariate logistic regression analysis identified independent predictors of SSI or OSI. Probabilities of SSI or OSI were determined for subpopulations to identify when LA was superior to OA.

Results.—From 2005 to 2009, there were 61,830 appendectomies performed (77.5% LA), of which 9,998 (16.2%) were complicated (58.7% LA). The risk of SSI was considerably lower for LA in both noncomplicated and complicated appendicitis. Across all ages, body mass index, renal function, and WBCs, LA was associated with a lower probability of SSI. The risk of OSI was considerably greater for LA in both noncomplicated and complicated appendicitis. In complicated appendicitis, OA was associated with a lower probability of OSI in patients with WBC >12 cells × $10^3/\mu L$. In noncomplicated appendicitis, OA was associated with a lower probability of OSI in patients with a body mass index <37.5 when compared with LA.

Conclusions.—Subpopulations exist in which OA is superior to LA in terms of OSI, however, SSI is consistently lower in LA patients.

► Minimally invasive (laparoscopic) surgery is the preferred approach to most simple procedures. However, even simple procedures can become complex so that a modification of approach is warranted. This is the realization of the old axiom "just because you can do it, doesn't mean that you should." The authors took a simple procedure, appendectomy, and attempted to discern (retrospectively) patient characteristics where open appendectomy was associated with fewer complications than laparoscopic appendectomy. On the whole, laparoscopic procedures had fewer wound infections and complications. However, a subset of patients was identified who had an open appendectomy performed, and these individuals had fewer operative site infections than similar people that had a laparoscopic procedure. Using a retrospective, experiential database (National Surgical Quality Improvement Program) does not allow for reasoning that led a surgeon to choose correctly or incorrectly an open procedure. The conclusion must be that some conditions carry higher risk for morbidities than others, and therapeutic approaches may need to vary as conditions necessitate.

T. Pruett, MD

Antibiotics vs Appendectomy for Uncomplicated Acute Appendicitis

Kao LS, for Members of the Evidence-Based Reviews in Surgery Group
J Am Coll Surg 216:501-505, 2013

Background.—Only recently have alternatives to appendectomy been suggested for acute appendicitis because of traditional concerns about progression to perforation and its complications. Advances in diagnostic ability, antibiotic therapies, and surgical techniques have led to laparoscopic appendectomy becoming a safe and viable choice for uncomplicated acute appendicitis. Antibiotic therapy has now been offered as another alternative based on multiple cases series from remote or resource-poor areas. A review of current studies was undertaken to compare the effectiveness and safety of antibiotics with those of appendectomy for the treatment of uncomplicated acute appendicitis.

Methods.—The studies were identified in a search of Medline, Cochrane Controlled Trials Register, Cochrane Library, and Embase. Two articles were selected, with one offering both retrospective and prospective nonrandomized and randomized studies and the other including only randomized controlled trials that were subjected to meta-analysis. Outcome measures were antibiotic failure and recurrent appendicitis. Antibiotic efficacy was defined as a definitive improvement without needing surgical intervention a median of 1 year after the incident. Surgical efficacy was defined as confirmation of acute appendicitis or other appropriate indication for surgery at the time of appendectomy.

Results.—The reported mean antibiotic failure rate was 6.9%, and the mean recurrent appendicitis rate was 14.2%, with a mean of 7.3% of patients having a normal appendix at appendectomy. Treatment efficacy of surgery rather than antibiotic treatment had an odds ratio of 6.01; the odds ratio for complications was 1.92. One study found that antibiotic treatment may fail and recurrence risk is present, but surgically treated patients faced the risks of operative morbidity and mortality. The other study found that a nonsurgical antibiotic approach reduces complications but its lower efficacy prevents it from being a viable alternative to surgery.

Conclusion.—The available evidence does not support changing from a surgical to an antibiotic approach for the treatment of uncomplicated acute appendicitis. Clinicians should consider the evidence in support of antibiotic treatment when deciding the best course for individual patients, along with factors such as surgical risk, compliance with medical therapy, and importance to the patient of returning to work, suffering pain, and experiencing anxiety about the risk of recurrence, as well as other specific preferences. Which patients are most likely to benefit from antibiotic therapy alone has not yet been determined by high-quality randomized clinical trials, nor have clinically relevant, patient-centered guidelines been developed.

▶ Evidence-based therapy is important to delivery of good care. Something as simple as treatment of acute appendicitis is one such subject that is amenable to comparative studies. The Canadian Association of General Surgeons and the American College of Surgeons produced a critical analysis of the evidence-based reviews within the literature. They address how the studies used for the meta-analysis were chosen (bias), endpoint definitions, and how heterogeneity between studies was assessed and stratified. The process is important, as it delineates essential elements of generating meaningful information from disparate reporting. Evidence-based medicine is a wonderful catch phrase; however, despite the plethora of data and clinical investigations on the treatment of acute appendicitis, there is insufficient evidence to make a definitive recommendation on how to treat one of the most common entities in surgery. The conclusion of the discussion is that there are sufficient data to warrant a well-controlled randomized, controlled trial. If after many years and multiple studies to discern the best therapy for acute, uncomplicated appendicitis there is no consistent evidence for a simple disease, how will evidence-based decisions in the more complex entities be made? Perhaps the community has set a standard that is unobtainable.

T. Pruett, MD

Postoperative Antibacterial Prophylaxis for the Prevention of Infectious Complications Associated With Tube Thoracostomy in Patients Undergoing Elective General Thoracic Surgery: A Double-blind, Placebo-Controlled, Randomized Trial

Oxman DA, Issa NC, Marty FM, et al (Brigham and Women's Hosp, Boston, MA)

JAMA Surg 148:440-446, 2013

Objective.—To determine whether extended postoperative antibacterial prophylaxis for patients undergoing elective thoracic surgery with tube thoracostomy reduces the risk of infectious complications compared with preoperative prophylaxis only.

Design.—Prospective, randomized, double-blind, placebo-controlled trial.

Setting.—Brigham and Women's Hospital, an 800-bed tertiary care teaching hospital in Boston, Massachusetts.

Participants.—A total of 251 adult patients undergoing elective thoracic surgery requiring tube thoracostomy between April 2008 and April 2011.

Interventions.—Patients received preoperative antibacterial prophylaxis with cefazolin sodium (or other drug if the patient was allergic to cefazolin). Postoperatively, patients were randomly assigned (at a 1:1 ratio) using a computer-generated randomization sequence to receive extended antibacterial prophylaxis (n = 125) or placebo (n = 126) for 48 hours or until all thoracostomy tubes were removed, whichever came first.

Main Outcome Measures.—The combined occurrence of surgical site infection, empyema, pneumonia, and *Clostridium difficile* colitis by postoperative day 28.

Results.—A total of 245 patients were included in the modified intention-to-treat analysis (121 in the intervention group and 124 in the placebo group). Thirteen patients (10.7%) in the intervention group and 8 patients (6.5%) in the placebo group had a primary end point (risk difference, −4.3% [95% CI, −11.3% to 2.7%]; $P = .26$). Six patients (5.0%) in the intervention group and 5 patients (4.0%) in the placebo group developed surgical site infections (risk difference, −0.93% [95% CI, −6.1% to 4.3%]; $P = .77$). Seven patients (5.8%) in the intervention group and 3 patients (2.4%) in the placebo group developed pneumonia (risk difference, −3.4% [95% CI, −8.3% to 1.6%]; $P = .21$). One patient in the intervention group developed empyema. No patients experienced *C difficile* colitis.

Conclusions.—Extended postoperative antibacterial prophylaxis for patients undergoing elective thoracic surgery requiring tube thoracostomy did not reduce the number of infectious complications compared with preoperative prophylaxis only.

Trial Registration.—clinicaltrials.gov Identifier: NCT00818766.

▶ Duration of antimicrobial prophylaxis is an important topic and one that elicits many reasons and justifications for "exceptions." The boundary between prophylaxis and therapy often becomes blurred in the mind of the practitioner. This is often used as a justification for extended antibiotic use in thoracic surgery procedures that require chest tubes. In an attempt to answer the question of whether preoperative prophylaxis only or the use of extended antimicrobials to either 48 hours or until chest tubes were removed (whichever was shorter) provided better prevention of infectious complications, a randomized, double-blind, controlled study was performed. Although the enrollment goals were not achieved, the authors addressed this limitation with the rationale that it was unlikely the outcomes would have changed even with full enrollment. Other limitations and bias within the study were also addressed. The authors' conclusion that extended use of antibiotics did not afford any infectious prevention benefit should be taken seriously (within the context of the limitations of the study design).

T. Pruett, MD

Blood Transfusion for Lower Extremity Bypass Is Associated with Increased Wound Infection and Graft Thrombosis

Tan TW, Vascular Study Group of New England (Louisiana State Univ Health Sciences Ctr, Shreveport; et al)

J Am Coll Surg 216:1005-1014, 2013

Background.—Packed RBC transfusion has been postulated to increase morbidity and mortality after cardiac/general surgical operations, but its effects after lower extremity bypass (LEB) have not been studied extensively.

Study Design.—Using the Vascular Study Group of New England's database (2003–2010), we examined 1,880 consecutive infrainguinal LEB performed for critical limb ischemia. Perioperative transfusion was categorized as 0 U, 1 to 2 U, and ≥3 U. Cohort frequency group matching was used to compare groups of patients receiving 1 to 2 U and 0 U with patients receiving ≥3 U using age, coronary artery disease, diabetes, urgency, and indication of revascularization. Primary end points were perioperative mortality, wound infection, and loss of primary graft patency at discharge, as well as 1-year mortality and loss of primary graft patency.

Results.—In the study cohort, 1,532 LEBs (81.5%) received 0 U, 248 LEBs (13.2%) received 1 to 2 U, and 100 LEBs (5.3%) received ≥3 U transfusion. In the study cohort and group frequency matched cohort, transfusion was associated with significantly higher perioperative wound infection (0 U:4.8% vs 1 to 2 U: 6.5% vs ≥3 U: 14.0%; $p = 0.0004$) and graft thrombosis at discharge (4.5% vs 7.7% vs 15.3%; $p < 0.0001$). At 1 year, there were no differences in infection or graft patency. In multivariate analysis, transfusion was independently associated with increased perioperative wound infection in the study cohort and group frequency matched cohort (1 to 2 U vs 0 U: adjusted odds ratio [OR] = 1.4; 95% CI, 0.8–2.5; p = 0.263; ≥3 U vs 0 U: OR = 3.5; 95% CI, 1.8–6.7; p = 0.0002; overall p = 0.002) and increased graft thrombosis at discharge (1 to 2 U vs 0 U: OR = 2.1; 95% CI, 1.2–3.6; p = 0.01; ≥3 U vs 0 U: OR = 4.8; 95% CI, 2.5–9.2; p < 0.0001, overall p < 0.0001).

Conclusions.—Perioperative transfusion in patients undergoing LEB is associated with increased perioperative wound infection and graft thrombosis. From this observational study, it appears transfusion does not have major consequences during mid-term follow-up, but the presumed benefits of blood replacement should be weighed carefully because of the increased risk of perioperative complications with transfusion.

► Within the surgical doctrine, the need for blood transfusions has been shown to increase the risk of infections. This is yet another study demonstrating an increased risk, this time in lower-extremity revascularization. The study used a large database to analyze the outcomes after revascularization stratified by amounts of blood transfused. Compared with those people receiving no blood, a significant incidence of infection was found in those patients receiving more than 3 units of blood with the procedure. This study demonstrated that the people requiring blood were different from those who did not. Not surprisingly, more complex patients using more antiplatelet agents may require more dissection with an increased blood use to find an acceptable location for revascularization. What was not reported was the duration of surgery, whether antibiotics were redosed, whether the incisions had to be extended, and other procedures associated with a wound at risk. This article demonstrates many of the complexities surrounding risk stratification. There is likely a surgical site infection rate that one cannot get below. Unfortunately, it is not clear what that is.

T. Pruett, MD

Effect of Daily Chlorhexidine Bathing on Hospital-Acquired Infection

Climo MW, Yokoe DS, Warren DK, et al (Hunter Holmes McGuire Veterans Affairs Med Ctr, Richmond; Brigham and Women's Hosp and Harvard Med School, Boston, MA; Washington Univ School of Medicine, St Louis, MO; et al)

N Engl J Med 368:533-542, 2013

Background.—Results of previous single-center, observational studies suggest that daily bathing of patients with chlorhexidine may prevent hospital-acquired bloodstream infections and the acquisition of multidrug-resistant organisms (MDROs).

Methods.—We conducted a multicenter, cluster-randomized, nonblinded crossover trial to evaluate the effect of daily bathing with chlorhexidine-impregnated washcloths on the acquisition of MDROs and the incidence of hospital-acquired bloodstream infections. Nine intensive care and bone marrow transplantation units in six hospitals were randomly assigned to bathe patients either with no-rinse 2% chlorhexidine–impregnated washcloths or with nonantimicrobial washcloths for a 6-month period, exchanged for the alternate product during the subsequent 6 months. The incidence rates of acquisition of MDROs and the rates of hospital-acquired bloodstream infections were compared between the two periods by means of Poisson regression analysis.

Results.—A total of 7727 patients were enrolled during the study. The overall rate of MDRO acquisition was 5.10 cases per 1000 patient-days with chlorhexidine bathing versus 6.60 cases per 1000 patient-days with nonantimicrobial washcloths ($P = 0.03$), the equivalent of a 23% lower rate with chlorhexidine bathing. The overall rate of hospital- acquired bloodstream infections was 4.78 cases per 1000 patient-days with chlorhexidine bathing versus 6.60 cases per 1000 patient-days with nonantimicrobial washcloths ($P = 0.007$), a 28% lower rate with chlorhexidine-impregnated washcloths. No serious skin reactions were noted during either study period.

Conclusions.—Daily bathing with chlorhexidine-impregnated washcloths significantly reduced the risks of acquisition of MDROs and development of hospital-acquired bloodstream infections. (Funded by the Centers for Disease Control and Prevention and Sage Products; ClinicalTrials.gov number, NCT00502476.)

▶ A significant element associated with reduction of surgical site infection (SSI) has been preoperative use of antiseptic skin preparation. The expansion of the application to intensive care unit patients resulted in fewer blood stream infections. Interestingly, the frequency of colonization of multidrug-resistant organisms was not affected by chlorhexidine daily wash. Although reduction in density of organisms on the skin (not demonstrated in this study) may diminish the overall risk of blood stream infections, it may not significantly modify the type of organisms that contaminate the subsequent surgical wound. Many techniques are now used by hospital infection control that may (or not) alter the frequency and type of organisms that contaminate the surgical wound and result in SSI.

T. Pruett, MD

Systemic Review and Meta-analysis of Randomized Clinical Trials Comparing Primary vs Delayed Primary Skin Closure in Contaminated and Dirty Abdominal Incisions

Bhangu A, Singh P, Lundy J, et al (Royal Centre for Defence Medicine, Birmingham, England; San Antonio Military Med Ctr, Fort Sam Houston, TX)
JAMA Surg 148:779-786, 2013

Importance.—Surgical site infection remains a major challenge in surgery. Delayed primary closure of dirty wounds is widely practiced in war surgery; we present a meta-analysis of evidence to help guide application of the technique in wider context.

Objective.—To determine using meta-analysis whether delayed primary skin closure (DPC) of contaminated and dirty abdominal incisions reduces the rate of surgical site infection (SSI) compared with primary skin closure (PC).

Data Sources.—A systematic review of the literature published after 1990 was conducted of the Medline, PubMed, Current Controlled Trials, and Cochrane databases. The last search was performed on October 6, 2012. No language restrictions were applied.

Study Selection.—Randomized clinical trials comparing PC vs DPC were included.

Data Extraction and Synthesis.—Two of us independently selected studies based on quality assessment using the Cochrane Collaboration tool for assessing risk of bias in randomized trials. Data were pooled using fixed- and random-effects models.

Main Outcome and Measure.—Rate of SSI, as defined by the individual study.

Results.—The final analysis included 8 studies randomizing 623 patients with contaminated or dirty abdominal wounds to either DPC or PC. The most common diagnosis was appendicitis (77.4%), followed by perforated abdominal viscus (11.5%), ileostomy closure (6.5%), trauma (2.7%), and intra-abdominal abscess/other peritonitis (1.9%). The time to first review for DPC was provided at between 2 and 5 days postoperatively. All studies were found to be at high risk of bias, with marked deficiencies in study design and outcome assessment. When SSI was assessed across all studies using a fixed-effect model, DPC significantly reduced the chance of SSI (odds ratio, 0.65; 95% CI, 0.40-0.93; $P = .02$). However, heterogeneity was high (72%), and using a random-effects model, the effect was no longer significant (odds ratio, 0.65; 95% CI, 0.25-1.64; $P = .36$).

Conclusions and Relevance.—Delayed primary skin closure may reduce the rate of SSI, but current trials fail to provide definitive evidence because of poor design. Well-designed, large-numbered randomized clinical trials are warranted.

► Management of a heavily contaminated surgical wound remains a source of disagreement. Although a wound VAC is often used, it is resource-intensive and not feasible in many parts of the world. The 3 "low-tech" options include primary closure, delayed primary closure, and healing by secondary intention. Although the last of these poses almost no risk of surgical site infection (SSI), it is prolonged and often results in a large scar. Therefore, the efficient goal would be to diminish the SSI risk with primary closure. A meta-analysis of existing literature supports delayed primary closure as the most efficient process. It was necessary to review 337 abstracts to find 38 articles for full review before identifying the 8 articles suitable for the meta-analysis. However, controls, bias, and description were not sufficient within the articles to recommend DPC conclusively. The incidence of SSI can be influenced by surgical technique.

T. Pruett, MD

Outcomes of Synthetic Mesh in Contaminated Ventral Hernia Repairs

Carbonell AM, Criss CN, Cobb WS, et al (Greenville Hosp System Univ Med Ctr, SC; Univ Hosps Case Med Ctr, Cleveland, OH)

J Am Coll Surg 217:991-998, 2013

Background.—Given the questionable long-term durability of biologic meshes, additional prosthetic options for ventral hernia repairs (VHR) in contaminated fields are necessary. Recent evidence suggests improved bacterial resistance of reduced-weight, large-pore synthetics, giving a potential mesh alternative for repair of contaminated hernias. We aimed to evaluate the clinical outcomes of 2 institutions' experience implanting lightweight polypropylene synthetic mesh in clean-contaminated and contaminated fields.

Study Design.—Open VHRs performed with polypropylene mesh in the retro-rectus position in cleancontaminated and contaminated fields were evaluated. Primary outcomes parameters included surgical site infection, surgical site occurrence, mesh removal, and hernia recurrence.

Results.—One hundred patients (50 male, 50 female) with a mean age of 60 ± 13 years and a mean body mass index (calculated as kg/m^2) of 32 ± 9.3 met inclusion criteria. There were 42 clean-contaminated and 58 contaminated cases. The incidence of surgical site occurrence was 26.2% in clean-contaminated cases and 34% in contaminated cases. The 30-day surgical site infection rate was 7.1% for clean-contaminated cases and 19.0% for contaminated cases. There were a total of 7 recurrences with a mean follow-up of 10.8 ± 9.9 months (range 1 to 63 months). Mesh removal was required in 4 patients: 2 due to early anastomotic leaks,

1 due to stomal disruption and retraction in a morbidly obese patient, and 1 from a long-term enterocutaneous fistula.

Conclusions.—Although perhaps not yet considered standard of care in the United States, we have demonstrated favorable infection, recurrence, and mesh removal rates associated with the use of synthetic mesh in contaminated VHR.

▶ Repair of a ventral hernia in the face of bacterial contamination is somewhat controversial. Although many consider biologic mesh the optimal material, the authors reviewed their experience with placement of synthetic mesh in 100 ventral hernia repairs with contaminated wounds. No use of synthetic mesh was reported in dirty wounds. There were no controls with biologic mesh usage, but in a comparison of a separate series with biologic mesh, the wound infection rate was lower with the synthetic mesh. Management of the contaminated hernia is complex, and use of materials to repair the abdomen is heavily influenced by surgeon bias.

T. Pruett, MD

Outcomes and Predictors of Incisional Surgical Site Infection in Stoma Reversal

Liang MK, Li LT, Avellaneda A, et al (Michael E. DeBakey Veterans Affairs Med Ctr, Houston, TX; et al)

JAMA Surg 148:183-189, 2013

Importance.—Surgical site infection following stoma reversal (SR) poses a substantial burden to the patient and health care system. Its overall incidence is likely underreported and poorly characterized. Improving our understanding of surgical site infection following stoma reversal may help us identify methods to decrease this complication.

Objective.—To evaluate the incidence of surgical site infection (SSI) and identify predictors of SSI following SR.

Design.—A review of computerized hospital records on SR performed from January 1, 2005, until February 27, 2011.

Setting.—An integrated medical system at the Michael E. DeBakey Veterans Affairs Medical Center.

Participants and Intervention.—All adults undergoing SR during the study period.

Main Outcome Measures.—Rates of SSI and characteristics of patients with and without SSI were compared. A logistic regression model was developed to identify predictors of SSI.

Results.—One hundred twenty-eight patients underwent SR; 46 patients (36.0%) had an SSI. In comparison with no SSI, the infection was associated with seromas (17.4% vs 2.4%, $P = .004$), fascial dehiscence (15.2% vs 2.4%, $P = .01$), intensive care unit admission (34.8% vs 17.1%, $P = .03$), increased hospital length of stay (20 vs 9 days, $P = .02$), readmission (32.6% vs 13.4%, $P = .01$), delayed wound healing (91 vs 66 days,

P =.02), and reoperation (32.6% vs 13.4%, P =.01). On multivariate analysis, history of fascial dehiscence (odds ratio, 16.9; 95% CI, 1.94-387), colostomy (5.07; 2.12-13.0), thicker subcutaneous fat (2.02; 1.33-3.21), and black race (0.35; 0.13-0.86) were associated with incisional SSI. There was no significant difference in patient satisfaction or functional status in late follow-up (1-73 months).

Conclusions and Relevance.—Surgical site infection is common following SR and is associated with significant morbidity. Four factors are strongly associated with increased risk of SSI in SR: history of fascial dehiscence, thicker subcutaneous fat, colostomy, and white race. Patients with none of these risk factors had a 0% SSI risk; patients with all 4 risk factors had a 100% risk of SSI.

▶ Of 128 patients undergoing stoma reversal, there were 46 (36%) surgical site infections (SSIs) in this single-center study. This rate should be able to provide insight into risks and efficacy of interventions to ameliorate this high rate. Unfortunately, the report continued to address those factors associated with SSI development and not compare like groups to discern important variables that alter risk for SSI. The latter is in a large degree due to the plethora of variables that need control. An interesting reporting twist is that despite this type of surgery resulting in at best a clean versus contaminated wound, the documentation that appropriate antibiotics were administered in a timely fashion was not one of the variables assessed. Antibiotics were certainly administered as organisms retrieved from SSI wounds demonstrated antibiotic pressure; *Enterococcus* sp, methicillin-resistant *Staphylococcus aureus*, and *Pseudomonas* sp. In the patient demographics of the 38 hernia repairs, 25 used mesh and 13 did not. SSIs developed in more than half with mesh (16 of 25), but there was no mention of whether biologic or synthetic mesh was used. SSI in repairs without mesh was significantly less (5 of 13), but there was no mention of the extent of additional tissue dissection to mobilize the posterior abdominal wall. This type of article demonstrates many of the shortcomings of database analyses; the context of the clinical event by necessity is overwhelmed by the amount of data points within a broad charge capture electronic medical record. The ability to extract data relevant to the clinical condition is problematic.

T. Pruett, MD

Independent Predictors of Enteric Fistula and Abdominal Sepsis After Damage Control Laparotomy: Results From the Prospective AAST Open Abdomen Registry

Bradley MJ, for the AAST Open Abdomen Study Group (Univ of Maryland Med System, Baltimore; et al)

JAMA Surg 148:947-954, 2013

Importance.—Enterocutaneous fistula (ECF), enteroatmospheric fistula (EAF), and intra-abdominal sepsis/abscess (IAS) are major challenges for surgeons caring for patients undergoing damage control laparotomy after trauma.

Objective.—To determine independent predictors of ECF, EAF, or IAS in patients undergoing damage control laparotomy after trauma, using the AAST Open Abdomen Registry.

Design.—The AAST Open Abdomen registry of patients with an open abdomen following damage control laparotomy was used to identify patients who developed ECF, EAF, or IAS and to compare these patients with those without these complications. Univariate analyses were performed to compare these groups of patients. Variables from univariate analyses differing at $P < .20$ were entered into a stepwise logistic regression model to identify independent risk factors for ECF, EAF, or IAS.

Setting.—Fourteen level I trauma centers.

Participants.—A total of 517 patients with an open abdomen following damage control laparotomy.

Main Outcomes and Measures.—Complication of ECF, EAF, or IAS.

Results.—More patients in the ECF/EAF/IAS group than in the group without these complications underwent bowel resection (63 of 111 patients [57%] vs 133 of 406 patients [33%]; $P < .001$). Within the first 48 hours after surgery, the ECF/EAF/IAS group received more colloids ($P < .03$) and total fluids ($P < .03$) than did the group without these complications. The ECF/EAF/IAS group underwent almost twice as many abdominal reexplorations as did the group without these complications (mean [SD] number, 4.1 [4.1] vs 2.2 [3.4]; $P < .001$). After multivariate analysis, the independent predictors of ECF/EAF/IAS were a large bowel resection (adjusted odds ratio [AOR], 3.56 [95% CI, 1.88-6.76]; $P < .001$), a total fluid intake at 48 hours of between 5 and 10 L (AOR, 2.11 [95% CI, 1.15-3.88]; $P = .02$) or more than 10 L (AOR, 1.93 [95% CI, 1.04-3.57]; $P = .04$), and an increasing number of reexplorations (AOR, 1.14 [95% CI, 1.06-1.21]; $P < .001$).

Conclusions and Relevance.—Large bowel resection, large-volume fluid resuscitation, and an increasing number of abdominal reexplorations were statistically significant predictors of ECF, EAF, or IAS in patients with an open abdomen after damage control laparotomy.

▶ One hundred eleven of 517 laparotomies for traumatic damage control developed abdominal visceral complications leading to either abscess or fistula. The associated variables identified were colon resection, bowel left in discontinuity, and large-volume fluid resuscitation. Although these are not unexpected, the variables associated with prevention of the intraabdominal infectious complications would have been helpful. How many fistulas arose from missed injuries, how many resulted from leaks at resection lines, how many arose from surgical injuries such as packs/repeat laparotomy injury, or how many arose from anastomoses with or without a proximal diverting ostomy? Surgical techniques may not always prevent complications, but experience is a great teacher for what not to do.

T. Pruett, MD

Development and Validation of a Necrotizing Soft-Tissue Infection Mortality Risk Calculator Using NSQIP

Faraklas I, Stoddard GJ, Neumayer LA, et al (Univ of Utah, Salt Lake City)
J Am Coll Surg 217:153-161, 2013

Background.—Necrotizing soft-tissue infections (NSTI) are a group of uncommon, rapidly progressive infections requiring prompt surgical debridement and systemic support. A previous attempt to define risk factors for mortality from NSTI had multiple limitations. The objective of this study was to develop and validate a 30-day postoperative mortality risk calculator for patients with NSTI using NSQIP.

Study Design.—The NSQIP Participant Use Files (2005–2010) were used as the primary data source. Patients diagnosed with NSTI were identified by ICD-9 codes. Multiple logistic regression analysis identified key preoperative variables predicting mortality. Bootstrap analysis was used to validate the model.

Results.—In 1,392 identified NSTI cases, demographics were as follows: 42% were female, median age was 55 years (interquartile range 46 to 63 years), and median body mass index was 32 kg/m^2 (interquartile range 26 to 40 kg/m^2). Thirty-day mortality was 13%. Seven independent variables were identified that correlated with mortality: age older than 60 years (odds ratio [OR] = 2.5; 95% CI 1.7–3.6), functional status (partially dependent: OR = 1.6; 95% CI 1.0–2.7; totally dependent: OR = 2.3; 95% CI 1.4–3.8), requiring dialysis (OR = 1.9; 95% CI 1.2–3.1), American Society of Anesthesiologists class 4 or higher (OR = 3.6; 95% CI 2.3–5.6), emergent surgery (OR = 1.6; 95% CI 1.0–2.3), septic shock (OR = 2.4; 95%CI 1.6–3.6), and lowplatelet count (<50K/μL: OR = 3.5; 95% CI 1.6–7.4; <150K/μL but >50K/μL: OR = 1.9; 95% CI 1.2–2.9). The receiver operating characteristic area was 0.85 (95% CI 0.82–0.87), which indicated a strong predictive model. Using bootstrap validation, the optimism-corrected receiver operating characteristic area was 0.83 (95% CI 0.81–0.86), which represents the model performance in future patients. The model was used to develop an interactive risk calculator.

Conclusions.—This risk calculator has excellent predictive ability for mortality in patients with NSTI. This simple interactive tool can aid physicians and patients in the decision-making process.

▶ Surgical therapy remains the mainstay of therapy of necrotizing soft tissue infection. This review uses the National Surgical Quality Improvement Program (NSQIP) database to generate a score used to predict mortality from necrotizing soft tissue infection. Seven elements were identified within the reported elements with hazard ratios applied, and a calculator generates the risk of death. However, what was not included within the NSQIP was the time from symptom onset to operative debridement and the adequacy of the operative approach. Operative intervention for necrotizing infections must be timely and effective. Significant delays allow for infection expansion, and inadequate debridement or procedures that do not remove necrotic tissue will allow continued infection progression. Surely these are variables that should influence outcomes. The fact that the surgical variables were not included within the data set does mean that they shouldn't be recognized as major contributors to successful interventions. Other variables thought to be important, but not mentioned as important variables, include antibiotic effectiveness against pathogens retrieved from necrotic tissue and application of hyperbaric oxygen. The calculator may give a prediction, but the variables that might alter that outcome may not have been provided.

T. Pruett, MD

Tedizolid Phosphate vs Linezolid for Treatment of Acute Bacterial Skin and Skin Structure Infections: The ESTABLISH-1 Randomized Trial

Prokocimer P, De Anda C, Fang E, et al (Trius Therapeutics Inc, San Diego, CA)
JAMA 309:559-569, 2013

Importance.—Acute bacterial skin and skin structure infections (ABSSSIs), including cellulitis or erysipelas, major cutaneous abscesses, and wound infections, can be life-threatening and may require surgery and hospitalization. Increasingly, ABSSSIs are associated with drug-resistant pathogens, and many antimicrobial agents have adverse effects restricting their use. Tedizolid phosphate is a novel oxazolidinone in development for the treatment of ABSSSIs.

Objectives.—To establish the noninferiority of tedizolid phosphate vs linezolid in treating ABSSSIs and compare the safety of the 2 agents.

Design, Setting, and Patients.—The Efficacy and Safety of 6-day Oral Tedizolid in Acute Bacterial Skin and Skin Structure Infections vs 10-day Oral Linezolid Therapy (ESTABLISH-1) was a phase 3, randomized, double-blind, noninferiority trial that was conducted from August 2010 through September 2011 at 81 study centers in North America, Latin America, and Europe. The intent-to-treat analysis set consisted of data from 667 adults aged 18 years or older with ABSSSIs treated with tedizolid phosphate (n = 332) or linezolid (n = 335).

Interventions.—A 200 mg once daily dose of oral tedizolid phosphate for 6 days or 600 mg of oral linezolid every 12 hours for 10 days.

Main Outcome Measures.—The primary efficacy outcome was early clinical response at the 48- to 72-hour assessment (no increase in lesion surface area from baseline and oral temperature of ≤37.6°C, confirmed by a second temperature measurement within 24 hours). A 10% noninferiority margin was predefined.

Results.—In the intent-to-treat analysis set, the early clinical treatment response rates were 79.5% (95% CI, 74.8% to 83.7%) of 332 patients in the tedizolid phosphate group and 79.4% (95% CI, 74.7% to 83.6%) of 335 patients in the linezolid group (a treatment difference of 0.1% [95% CI, −6.1% to 6.2%]). The sustained clinical treatment response rates at the end of treatment (day 11) were 69.3% (95% CI, 64.0% to 74.2%) in the tedizolid phosphate group and 71.9% (95% CI, 66.8% to 76.7%) in the linezolid group (a treatment difference of −2.6% [95%

CI, −9.6% to 4.2%]). Results of investigator-assessed clinical treatment success rates at a posttherapy evaluation visit (1-2 weeks after the end-of-treatment visit) were 85.5% (95% CI, 81.3% to 89.1%) in the tedizolid phosphate group and 86.0% (95% CI, 81.8% to 89.5%) in the linezolid group (a treatment difference of −0.5% [95% CI, −5.8% to 4.9%), and were similar for 178 patients with methicillin-resistant *Staphylococcus aureus* isolated from the primary lesion.

Conclusions and Relevance.—Tedizolid phosphate was a statistically noninferior treatment to linezolid in early clinical response at 48 to 72 hours after initiating therapy for an ABSSSI. Tedizolid phosphate may be a reasonable alternative to linezolid for treating ABSSSI.

Trial Registration.—clinicaltrials.gov Identifier: NCT01170221.

▶ It is important to include within this discussion the illustration of the types of studies used to obtain the antibiotics that are approved by the Food and Drug Administration (FDA) for surgical infections. The ESTABLISH-1 study is an industry-sponsored study performed and designed to meet new guidelines from the FDA for the purpose of drug registration. The new noninferiority criteria are rife with areas for bias. Although registration criteria were stated, where candidates were recruited and how was not mentioned. Additionally, the outcome efficacy was assessed in a nonblinded fashion by the investigator. Pharmaceutical companies must design studies that are consistent with FDA requirements. Although the study may show noninferiority in a study population, the application of the agent in clinical settings is left for the clinician to discern.

T. Pruett, MD

Effect of Eritoran, an Antagonist of MD2-TLR4, on Mortality in Patients With Severe Sepsis: The ACCESS Randomized Trial

Opal SM, for the ACCESS Study Group (Alpert Med School of Brown Univ, Providence, RI; et al)

JAMA 309:1154-1162, 2013

Importance.—Eritoran is a synthetic lipid A antagonist that blocks lipopolysaccharide (LPS) from binding at the cell surface MD2-TLR4 receptor. LPS is a major component of the outer membrane of gram-negative bacteria and is a potent activator of the acute inflammatory response.

Objective.—To determine if eritoran, a TLR4 antagonist, would significantly reduce sepsis-induced mortality.

Design, Setting, and Participants.—We performed a randomized, double-blind, placebo-controlled, multinational phase 3 trial in 197 intensive care units. Patients were enrolled from June 2006 to September 2010 and final follow-up was completed in September 2011.

Interventions.—Patients with severe sepsis (n = 1961) were randomized and treated within 12 hours of onset of first organ dysfunction in a 2:1 ratio with a 6-day course of either eritoran tetrasodium (105 mg total) or placebo, with n = 1304 and n = 657 patients, respectively.

Main Outcome Measures.—The primary end point was 28-day all-cause mortality. The secondary end points were all-cause mortality at 3, 6, and 12 months after beginning treatment.

Results.—Baseline characteristics of the 2 study groups were similar. In the modified intent-to-treat analysis (randomized patients who received at least 1 dose) there was no significant difference in the primary end point of 28-day all-cause mortality with 28.1% (366/1304) in the eritoran group vs 26.9% (177/657) in the placebo group (P=.59; hazard ratio, 1.05; 95% CI, 0.88-1.26; difference in mortality rate, −1.1; 95% CI, −5.3 to 3.1) or in the key secondary end point of 1-year all-cause mortality with 44.1% (290/657) in the eritoran group vs 43.3% (565/1304) in the placebo group, Kaplan-Meier analysis of time to death by 1 year, P=.79 (hazard ratio, 0.98; 0.85-1.13). No significant differences were observed in any of the prespecified subgroups. Adverse events, including secondary infection rates, did not differ between study groups.

Conclusions and Relevance.—Among patients with severe sepsis, the use of eritoran, compared with placebo, did not result in reduced 28-day mortality.

Trial Registration.—clinicaltrials.gov Identifier: NCT00334828.

► As technology progresses, efforts persist to improve outcomes. The role of supportive adjuncts in the management of surgical infections has been touted. The use of antiendotoxin agents and antibodies has been part of the surgical literature for decades. In animal models, such therapy provides therapeutic value. In the most recent iteration, eritoran (a synthetic lipid A antagonist) failed to modify outcomes in almost 2000 patients (with more than a quarter having surgical-related enrollment criteria). As with prior studies with antiendotoxin preparations, there was no clear benefit in survival for those receiving the active agent versus placebo. The issue remains as to most effective management of individuals with abdominal or soft tissue infections. Management of serious surgical infections is a combination of basic support and effective surgical manipulation of the primary source. The specific role of immune response modification has yet to be clarified.

T. Pruett, MD

Effect of an Investigational Vaccine for Preventing *Staphylococcus aureus* Infections After Cardiothoracic Surgery: A Randomized Trial

Fowler VG Jr, Allen KB, Moreira ED Jr, et al (Duke Univ Med Ctr and Duke Clinical Res Inst, Durham, NC; St Luke's Mid-America Heart and Vascular Inst, Kansas City, MO; McGill Univ, Montreal, Quebec, Canada; et al)

JAMA 309:1368-1378, 2013

Importance.—Infections due to *Staphylococcus aureus* are serious complications of cardiothoracic surgery. A novel vaccine candidate (V710) containing the highly conserved *S aureus* iron surface determinant B is immunogenic and generally well tolerated in volunteers.

Objective.—To evaluate the efficacy and safety of preoperative vaccination in preventing serious postoperative *S aureus* infection in patients undergoing cardiothoracic surgery.

Design, Setting, and Participants.—Double-blind, randomized, event-driven trial conducted between December 2007 and August 2011 among 8031 patients aged 18 years or older who were scheduled for full median sternotomy within 14 to 60 days of vaccination at 165 sites in 26 countries.

Intervention.—Participants were randomly assigned to receive a single 0.5-mL intramuscular injection of either V710 vaccine, 60 μg (n = 4015), or placebo (n = 4016).

Main Outcome Measures.—The primary efficacy end point was prevention of *S aureus* bacteremia and/or deep sternal wound infection (including mediastinitis) through postoperative day 90. Secondary end points included all *S aureus* surgical site and invasive infections through postoperative day 90.Three interim analyses with futility assessments were planned.

Results.—The independent data monitoring committee recommended termination of the study after the second interim analysis because of safety concerns and low efficacy. At the end of the study, the V710 vaccine was not significantly more efficacious than placebo in preventing either the primary end points (22/3528 V710 vaccine recipients [2.6 per 100 person-years] vs 27/3517 placebo recipients [3.2 per 100 person-years]; relative risk, 0.81; 95% CI, 0.44-1.48; $P = .58$) or secondary end points despite eliciting robust antibody responses. Compared with placebo, the V710 vaccine was associated with more adverse experiences during the first 14 days after vaccination (1219/3958 vaccine recipients [30.8%; 95% CI, 29.4%-32.3%] and 866/3967 placebo recipients [21.8%; 95% CI, 20.6%-23.1%], including 797 [20.1%; 95% CI, 18.9%-21.4%] and 378 [9.5%; 95% CI, 8.6%-10.5%] with injection site reactions and 66 [1.7%; 95% CI, 1.3%-2.1%] and 51 [1.3%; 95% CI, 1.0%-1.7%] with serious adverse events, respectively) and a significantly higher rate of multiorgan failure during the entire study (31 vs 17 events; 0.9 [95% CI, 0.6-1.2] vs 0.5 [95% CI, 0.3-0.8] events per 100 person-years; $P = .04$). Although the overall incidence of vaccine-related serious adverse events (1 in each group) and the all-cause mortality rate (201/3958 vs 177/3967; 5.7 [95% CI, 4.9-6.5] vs 5.0 [95% CI, 4.3-5.7] deaths per 100 person-years; $P = .20$) were not statistically different between groups, the mortality rate in patients with staphylococcal infections was significantly higher among V710 vaccine than placebo recipients (15/73 vs 4/96; 23.0 [95% CI, 12.9-37.9] vs 4.2 [95% CI, 1.2-10.8] per 100 person-years; difference, 18.8 [95% CI, 8.0-34.1] per 100 person-years).

Conclusions and Relevance.—Among patients undergoing cardiothoracic surgery with median sternotomy, the use of a vaccine against *S aureus* compared with placebo did not reduce the rate of serious postoperative *S aureus* infections and was associated with increased mortality among patients who developed *S aureus* infections. These findings do not support the use of the V710 vaccine for patients undergoing surgical interventions.

Trial Registration.—clinicaltrials.gov Identifier: NCT00518687.

▶ *Staphylococcus* continues to be the most common pathogen isolated from surgical site infection (SSI) after cardiac surgery. Animal models have shown a protective effect against *Staphylococcus* infections after vaccination. The possibility of reducing the incidence of deep SSI through immunologic means has resulted in development of clinical *Staphylococcus* vaccines. This report of a target of 8000 people enrolled into a double-blind, randomized, event-driven trial was established to answer the question of vaccine efficacy in cardiac surgery patients. The trial was terminated early because of concerns of poor outcomes in the vaccine group. This shows the importance of properly performed clinical trials. Although the number of overall deep infections/ *Staphylococcus* bacteremia was similar in the placebo and vaccine groups, the outcomes were worse in the vaccine group. This was a disappointing finding. Whether the worsened outcome after *Staphylococcus* infection seen in vaccine recipients is caused by the vaccine remains to be discerned. However, the finding must make one pause in the search for immunologic means to reduce clinical SSI.

T. Pruett, MD

Association Between Telomere Length and Experimentally Induced Upper Respiratory Viral Infection in Healthy Adults

Cohen S, Janicki-Deverts D, Turner RB, et al (Carnegie Mellon Univ, Pittsburgh, PA; Univ of Virginia Health Sciences Ctr, Charlottesville; et al)

JAMA 309:699-705, 2013

Importance.—Although leukocyte telomere length is associated with mortality and many chronic diseases thought to be manifestations of age-related functional decline, it is not known whether it relates to acute disease in younger healthy populations.

Objective.—To determine whether shorter telomeres in leukocytes, especially CD8CD28− T cells, are associated with decreased resistance to upper respiratory infection and clinical illness in young to midlife adults.

Design, Setting, and Participants.—Between 2008 and 2011, telomere length was assessed in peripheral blood mononuclear cells (PBMCs) and T-cell subsets (CD4, CD8CD28+, CD8CD28−) from 152 healthy 18- to 55-year-old residents of Pittsburgh, Pennsylvania. Participants were subsequently quarantined (single rooms), administered nasal drops containing a common cold virus (rhinovirus 39), and monitored for 5 days for development of infection and clinical illness.

Main Outcome Measures.—Infection (virus shedding or 4-fold increase in virus-specific antibody titer) and clinical illness (verified infection plus objective signs of illness).

Results.—Rates of infections and clinical illness were 69% (n = 105) and 22% (n = 33), respectively. Shorter telomeres were associated with greater odds of infection, independent of prechallenge virus-specific antibody, demographics, contraceptive use, season, and body mass index (PBMC: odds ratio [OR] per 1-SD decrease in telomere length, 1.71 [95% CI, 1.08-2.72]; n = 128 [shortest tertile 77% infected; middle, 66%; longest, 57%]; CD4: OR, 1.76 [95% CI, 1.15-2.70]; n = 146 [shortest tertile 80% infected; middle, 71%; longest, 54%]; CD8CD28+: OR, 1.93 [95% CI, 1.21-3.09], n = 132 [shortest tertile 84% infected; middle, 64%; longest, 58%]; CD8CD28−: OR, 2.02 [95% CI, 1.29-3.16]; n = 144 [shortest tertile 77% infected; middle, 75%; longest, 50%]). CD8CD28− was the only cell population in which shorter telomeres were associated with greater risk of clinical illness (OR, 1.69 [95% CI, 1.01-2.84]; n = 144 [shortest tertile, 26%; middle, 22%; longest, 13%]). The association between CD8CD28− telomere length and infection increased with age (CD8CD28− telomere length × age interaction, b = 0.09 [95% CI, 0.02-0.16], *P* = .01, n = 144).

Conclusion and Relevance.—In this preliminary study among a cohort of healthy 18- to 55-year-olds, shorter CD8CD28− T-cell telomere length was associated with increased risk for experimentally induced acute upper respiratory infection and clinical illness.

▶ The more one looks, the more one finds. Change in the end region of the chromosome, telomere length, is associated with immune modification that is found in aging individuals. However, telomere shortening can be seen in other conditions. The authors addressed telomere length and susceptibility to acute viral infection. It was found that shortening of the telomere was associated with an increased likelihood of acquisition of experimental infection. Additionally, telomeres were found to shorten with increasing body mass index and seasonality (shorter telomeres in the winter vs summer). This trial, in combination with the previous 2 studies relating to immunologic modulations affecting surgical patients, is another example of variables that may be extraordinarily influential in control of inocula within the surgical wound and the ability of the host to heal. The number of cellular variables required to control and eliminate pathogens contaminating the surgical wound is still undergoing study to increase our understanding. The literature on cytokine, innate immunity, and phagocytes will continue to be supplemented by factors influencing acquired and adaptive immunity and the reparative processes.

T. Pruett, MD

8 Endocrine

Can Established CT Attenuation and Washout Criteria for Adrenal Adenoma Accurately Exclude Pheochromocytoma?

Patel J, Davenport MS, Cohan RH, et al (Univ of Michigan Health System, Ann Arbor)
AJR Am J Roentgenol 201:122-127, 2013

Objective.—The purpose of this article is to determine the proportion of pheochromocytomas that mimic adrenal adenoma using established CT washout and attenuation criteria.

Materials and Methods.—The CT characteristics of pheochromocytomas confirmed by histologic analysis ($n = 46$) and ^{131}I-metaiodobenzylguanidine ($n = 1$) were compared with those of 98 adrenal adenomas (negative plasma and urinary metanephrines or catecholamines, and one or more of the following characteristics: unenhanced attenuation ≤ 10 HU, absolute washout ≥ 60%, and relative washout ≥ 40%). CT numbers were measured in all available phases (unenhanced [$n = 37$], 1-minute contrast enhanced [$n = 46$], and delayed contrast enhanced [$n = 43$]) using a region of interest that encompassed the majority of the mass. Absolute washout, relative washout, and degree of enhancement (1-minute minus unenhanced) were calculated. Mass size and heterogeneity were recorded and compared using the Student *t* test and a chi-square test, respectively.

Results.—Twenty-four of 47 (51%) pheochromocytomas were imaged with a triphasic examination using a 15-minute delay. Eight of 24 (33%) met relative (6/24 [25%]) or absolute (7/24 [29%]) washout criteria for the diagnosis of a lipid-poor adenoma. Four of these (50% [4/8]) were homogeneous on all three phases. None of the pheochromocytomas had an unenhanced attenuation of 10 HU or less. Pheochromocytomas were significantly larger than adrenal adenomas (mean diameter, 3.9 cm [range, 0.6–14 cm] vs 2.0 cm [range, 0.8–3.9 cm]; $p < 0.0001$) and were significantly less likely to be homogeneous (15/47 [32%] vs 95/98 [97%]; $p < 0.0001$), but there was overlap.

Conclusion.—A substantial minority of pheochromocytomas have absolute or relative washout characteristics that overlap with those of lipid-poor adenomas.

▶ Whether computed tomography (CT) findings alone are enough to exclude a diagnosis of pheochromocytoma (pheo) is often discussed. Here the authors examine a series of patients with proven pheos and compare them with patients with adrenal adenomas. The authors utilize an adrenal protocol for CT imaging of the adrenal glands that included imaging the adrenals 3 times: unenhanced, 1-minute contrast enhanced, and 15-minute contrast enhanced. Despite best current-day imaging criteria, the authors found that there is considerable overlap between pheos and lipid-poor adenomas in both the unenhanced and contrast-enhanced images as shown in Fig 1 of the original article. Even after calculating the washout characteristics of each nodule, there was still significant overlap between the pheos and the adenomas, again more evident for the lipid-poor adenomas. The authors conclude—and I wholeheartedly agree—that biochemical screening (plasma metanephrines is the test of choice) is necessary to exclude the possibility of a pheo, even if CT characteristics indicate a cortical adenoma.

T. J. Fahey, MD

Long-Term Cardio- and Cerebrovascular Events in Patients With Primary Aldosteronism

Mulatero P, Monticone S, Bertello C, et al (Univ of Torino, Italy)
J Clin Endocrinol Metab 98:4826-4833, 2013

Background.—Aldosterone plays a detrimental role on the cardiovascular system and PA patients display a higher risk of events compared with EH.

Objectives.—The objectives of the study were to compare cardio- and cerebrovascular events in patients with primary aldosteronism (PA) and matched essential hypertension (EH).

Methods.—We retrospectively compared the percentage of patients experiencing events at baseline and during a median follow-up of 12 years in 270 PA patients case-control matched 1:3 with EH patients and in PA subtypes [aldosterone-producing adenoma (n = 57); bilateral adrenal hyperplasia (n = 213)] vs matched EH.

Results.—A significantly higher number of PA patients experienced cardiovascular events over the entire period of the study (22.6% vs 12.7%, $P < .001$). At the diagnosis of PA, a higher number of patients had experienced total events (14.1% vs 8.4% EH, $P = .007$); furthermore, during the follow-up period, PA patients had a higher rate of events (8.5% vs 4.3% EH, $P = .008$). In particular, stroke and arrhythmias were more frequent in PA patients. During the follow-up, a higher percentage of PA patients developed type 2 diabetes. Parameters that were independently associated with the occurrence of all events were age, duration of hypertension, systolic blood pressure, presence of diabetes mellitus, and PA diagnosis. After division into PA subtypes, patients with either aldosterone-producing adenoma or bilateral adrenal hyperplasia displayed a higher rate of events compared with the matched EH patients.

Conclusions.—This study demonstrates in a large population of patients the pathogenetic role of aldosterone excess in the cardiovascular system

TABLE 2.—Events in PA and PA Subtypes and Matched EH Patients During the Study Period

Events	PA (n = 270)	EH (n = 810)	*P* Value	APA (n = 57)	EH (n = 171)	*P* Value	BAH (n = 213)	EH (n = 639)	*P* Value
CAD									
Patients with CAD at diagnosis, %	2.6	3.1	.6	5.3	2.3	.2	1.9	3.3	.3
Patients with CAD during follow-up, %	2.6	1.5	.2	1.7	1.8	.6	2.8	1.4	.2
Patients with CAD in total, %	5.2	4.6	.6	7	4.1	.4	4.7	4.7	1.00
Stroke									
Patients with stroke at diagnosis, %	7.4	3.5	.006	12.3	2.9	.01	6.1	3.6	.1
Patients with stroke during follow-up, %	3	1.4	.1	5.2	1.2	.1	2.4	1.6	.5
Patients with stroke in total, %	10.4	4.9	.002	17.5	4.1	.004	8.5	5.2	.1
Arrhythmias									
Patients with arrhythmias at diagnosis, %	4.8	2.2	.03	8.8	0.6	.03	3.8	2.7	.4
Patients with arrhythmias during follow-up, %	3	2.1	.4	1.7	1.7	.4	3.2	2.2	.4
Patients with arrhythmias in total, %	7.8	4.3	.02	10.5	2.3	.02	7	4.9	.2
HF									
Patients with HF at diagnosis, %	0.7	0.25	.2	1.7	0.6	.4	0.5	0.2	.4
Patients with HF during follow-up, %	3	0.12	.001	3.5	0	.06	2.8	0.1	.001
Patients with HF in total, %	3.7	0.37	.001	5.2	0.6	.051	3.3	0.3	.001

CAD category grouped patients with MI and unstable angina.

and thus the importance of early diagnosis and targeted PA treatment (Table 2).

▶ Primary hyperaldosteronism has slowly been increasingly recognized for its contribution to hypertension. This study very nicely examines the risk of cardiovascular events associated with primary hyperaldosteronism—both before and after treatment for the disease. Particularly interesting are the data in the report that separate events for patients with aldosterone-producing adenomas (APA) versus bilateral adrenal hyperplasia (BAH). Table 2 contains much of these data. It can be seen that patients with APA have a higher chance of presenting with stroke or an arrhythmia at diagnosis than patients with BAH, although there is no difference after treatment. The authors note in the text that patients who have adrenalectomy for an APA have a greater reduction in both systolic and diastolic blood pressure than patients treated pharmacologically for BAH. What is not addressed in the text in Table 2 is why there is a significantly greater incidence of heart failure in patients after being treated for primary hyperaldosteronism than in patients being treated for essential hypertension. This needs to be the focus of additional study, as it appears to be a significant source of long-term morbidity in those patients who have been treated. Finally, although not proven in the dataset here, the authors advocate for early recognition of primary hyperaldosteronism to prevent the excess morbidity seen before diagnosis in this study.

T. J. Fahey, MD

Comparative Outcomes of Laparoscopic and Open Adrenalectomy for Adrenocortical Carcinoma: Single, High-Volume Center Experience

Mir MC, Klink JC, Guillotreau J, et al (Cleveland Clinic, OH)
Ann Surg Oncol 20:1456-1461, 2013

Purpose.—Adrenocortical carcinoma (ACC) is a rare and clinically aggressive cancer. Previous studies reported increased recurrence rates associated with laparoscopic adrenalectomy (LA). We evaluated a single-center experience of LA versus open adrenalectomy (OA) for the management of ACC.

Methods.—Between 1993 and 2011, 44 consecutive patients with primary ACC were treated at our institution. Baseline patient characteristics and surgical and pathological outcomes were compared between OA and LA groups. Multivariable Cox proportional hazards analysis was used to estimate the association between OA versus LA with recurrence-free and overall survival.

Results.—Eighteen and 26 patients underwent LA and OA, respectively. Patients who underwent OA had larger tumors and more advanced clinical stage compared with LA group. During a median follow-up of 22 months, 22 recurrences and 26 deaths were observed. The 2-year, recurrence-free and overall survivals for OA and LA were 60 vs. 39 % ($P = 0.7$) and 54 vs. 58 % ($P = 0.6$), respectively. After adjusting for clinical stage, OA was associated with lower risk of recurrence (hazard ratio (HR) 0.4; 95 % confidence interval (CI) 0.2−1.2; $P = 0.099$) and improved overall survival (HR 0.5; 95 % CI 0.2−1.2; $P = 0.122$) compared with LA, although differences were not statistically significant.

Conclusions.—A nonstatistically significant increase in recurrence and death was observed among patients undergoing LA versus OA after adjusting for clinical stage. The rarity of this disease limits the ability to assess for significant differences in a single-institution series. Patients with suspected ACC should be considered for OA (Fig 1).

▶ The debate about whether adrenocortical carcinoma (ACC) should be resected by an open or laparoscopic approach continues, and this article does little to resolve the issue. The authors report on a reasonably large series of ACC over a nearly 20-year period. A total of 18 of 44 patients had a laparoscopic resection and 26 of 44 had an open resection. The strength of the study is that all operations were performed by a single group of surgeons (urologists) at a single institution (Cleveland Clinic). The authors conclude that open

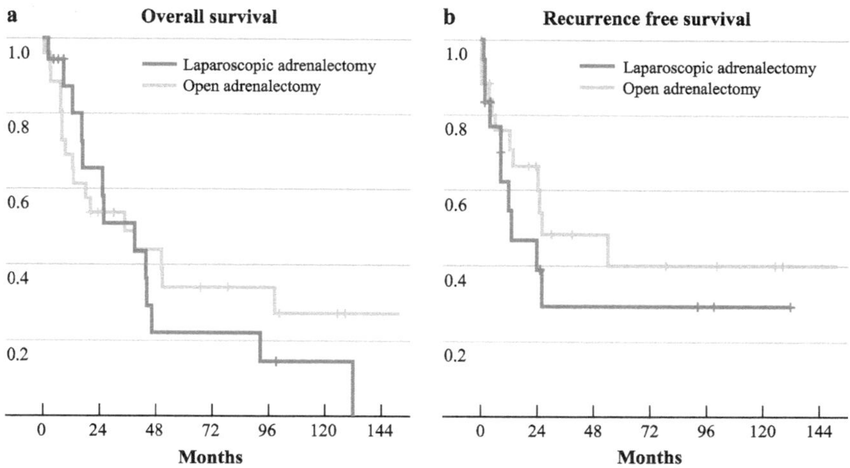

FIGURE 1.—Kaplan—Meier analysis of a overall and b recurrence-free survivals. (With kind permission from Springer Science+Business Media. Mir MC, Klink JC, Guillotreau J, et al. Comparative outcomes of laparoscopic and open adrenalectomy for adrenocortical carcinoma: single, high-volume center experience. *Ann Surg Oncol.* 2013;20:1456-1461, with permission from Society of Surgical Oncology.)

adrenalectomy should be the preferred approach based on their data—and this is the problem: The data do not support the conclusion at all. One wonders how the authors were able to keep their conclusions in the report. There is no statistical difference between the groups at all. The authors report that the recurrence-free survival is 60% for the open adrenalectomy group versus 39% for the laparoscopic adrenalectomy group at 2 years. But if one looks at Fig 1 from the report, the recurrence-free survival at 24 months appears to be virtually identical. And the recurrence-free survival at 5 years appears to be 40% and 30%, respectively, for open and laparoscopic procedures. Now, the groups were not even to start—the tumor size was smaller in the laparoscopic group (one of the few differences that was statistically different), although the authors account for this in their analysis. More important perhaps are some of the operative and pathologic details. The mean operating time in the laparoscopic group (with a mean tumor size of 7 cm) was 5 hours with a mean blood loss of 1500 mL. This is excessive, even for difficult much larger tumors. Furthermore, both the open and laparoscopic groups had a rate of positive margins of nearly 40%.

This article does little to convince me that all ACCs should be resected via an open approach. The implications for adopting such an approach are that all cortical tumors larger than 4 or 5 cm should be resected by an open approach to appropriately treat them if they prove to be cancer. Clearly, this is not necessary and definitely not proven in this report. Until a randomized, prospective trial is undertaken to address this issue, the decision as to whether to proceed via a laparoscopic approach or an open approach should depend on the technical skill and comfort level of the surgeon.

T. J. Fahey, MD

Molecular Screening for a Personalized Treatment Approach in Advanced Adrenocortical Cancer

De Martino MC, Al Ghuzlan A, Aubert S, et al (Institut Gustave Roussy, Villejuif, France; Centre Hospitalier Régional Universitaire, Lille, France; et al)

J Clin Endocrinol Metab 98:4080-4088, 2013

Context.—Adrenocortical cancer (ACC) is a rare cancer with poor prognosis and scant treatment options. In ACC, no personalized approach has emerged but no extensive molecular screening has been performed to date.

Objective.—The objective of the study was to evaluate the presence of a large number of potentially targetable molecular events in a large cohort of advanced ACC.

Design, Setting, and Participants.—We used hot spot gene sequencing (Ion Torrent, 40 patients) and comparative genomic hybridization (CGH; 28 patients; a subset of the entire cohort) in adult stage III-IV ACC samples to screen for mutations and copy number abnormalities of potential interest for therapeutic use in 46 and 130 genes, respectively.

Results.—At least one copy number alteration or mutation was found in 19 patients (47.5%). The most frequent mutations were detected on *TP53*, *ATM*, and *CTNNB1* [6 of 40 (15%), 5 of 40 (12.5%), and 4 of 40 (10%), respectively]. The most frequent copy number alterations identified were: amplification of the *CDK4* oncogene (5 of 28; 17.9%) and deletion of the *CDKN2A* (4 of 28; 14.3%) and *CDKN2B* (3 of 28; 10.7%) tumor suppressor genes. Amplifications of *FGFR1*, *FGF9*, or *FRS2* were discovered in three subjects (10.7%). Associated alterations were: deletions of *CDKN2A*, *CDKN2B* with *ATM* mutations, and *TP53* mutations with *CTNNB1* mutations.

Conclusions.—No simple targetable molecular event emerged. Drugs targeting the cell cycle could be the most relevant new therapeutic approach for patients with advanced ACC. Inhibitors of the fibroblast growth factor receptor pathway could also be a therapeutic option in a subset of patients, whereas other targeted therapies should be considered on a case-by-case basis.

▶ Adjuvant treatment for adrenocortical carcinoma (ACC) remains dismal—the primary treatment continues to rely on mitotane, an old drug with very limited efficacy and significant potential toxicity. Here the authors used targeted sequencing and comparative genomic hybridization to try to identify new targets, and the results are very disappointing. The results presented here, combined with those of previous reports, suggest that unlike gastrointestinal stromal tumors or melanoma, a single dominant mutation that drives or contributes to oncogenesis in most ACC is not going to be identified. Where does that leave us? Additional studies that more broadly characterize genomic abnormalities in ACC must be performed. It seems apparent that focused approaches looking at known genes are not going to lead to advances in the treatment of this deadly disease. Finally, treatment of ACC may require sequencing the entire tumor in each case to identify the underlying molecular aberrations and tailor adjuvant treatment in a truly personalized manner.

T. J. Fahey, MD

A Comprehensive Next Generation Sequencing–Based Genetic Testing Strategy To Improve Diagnosis of Inherited Pheochromocytoma and Paraganglioma

Rattenberry E, Vialard L, Yeung A, et al (Univ of Birmingham, Edgbaston, UK; Birmingham Women's Hosp NHS Trust, Edgbaston, UK; et al)

J Clin Endocrinol Metab 98:E1248-E1256, 2013

Context.—Pheochromocytomas and paragangliomas are notable for a high frequency of inherited cases, many of which present as apparently sporadic tumors.

Objective.—The objective of this study was to establish a comprehensive next generation sequencing (NGS)–based strategy for the diagnosis of patients with pheochromocytoma and paraganglioma by testing simultaneously for mutations in *MAX, RET, SDHA, SDHB, SDHC, SDHD, SDHAF2, TMEM127,* and *VHL.*

Design.—After the methodology for the assay was designed and established, it was validated on DNA samples with known genotype and then patients were studied prospectively.

Setting.—The study was performed in a diagnostic genetics laboratory.

Patients.—DNA samples from 205 individuals affected with adrenal or extraadrenal pheochromocytoma/head and neck paraganglioma (PPGL/HNPGL) were analyzed. A proof-of-principle study was performed using 85 samples known to contain a variant in 1 or more of the genes to be tested, followed by prospective analysis of an additional 120 samples.

Main Outcome Measures.—We assessed the ability to use an NGS-based method to perform comprehensive analysis of genes implicated in inherited PPGL/HNPGL.

Results.—The proof-of-principle study showed that the NGS assay and analysis gave a sensitivity of 98.7%. A pathogenic mutation was identified in 16.6% of the prospective analysis cohort of 120 patients.

Conclusions.—A comprehensive NGS-based strategy for the analysis of genes associated with predisposition to PPGL and HNPGL was established, validated, and introduced into diagnostic service. The new assay provides simultaneous analysis of 9 genes and allows more rapid and cost-effective mutation detection than the previously used conventional Sanger sequencing-based methodology.

▶ The number of genes that potentially harbor germline mutations in patients presenting with pheochromocytomas and paragangliomas has increased nearly 3-fold over the last decade. Several reports document the relatively high frequency of de novo germline mutations in patients presenting with pheochromocytomas and paragangliomas (PPGLs). Identifying these mutations is a labor-intensive and expensive task if it is to be done by traditional sequencing methods. However, the need to do so is compelling, as germline mutations have been identified approximately 20% of the time in patients without a family history of prior PPGLs. Here the authors outline a technique using Next-gen sequencing to identify mutations in 9 of the 10 genes currently known to be responsible for inherited PPGL. The advantage of Next-gen sequencing is that it is relatively inexpensive—excluding labor costs, a run costs less than $650 currently at our core facility—and it can also be easily adapted to identify additional mutations as they are discovered. The authors confirmed the utility of this technique in a large series of sporadic tumors, where they also found a germline mutation rate of 16.6%. The one patient with a germline mutation that was "missed" was a 6–base pair duplication that was detected but not in enough reads to be called a mutation. The discussion of the report highlights how important computational biologists are in establishing a program such as this and suggests that not every institution can or probably will be able to establish such a program independently. Nevertheless, the fact that the cost of genetic testing for these patients will be decreasing is encouraging for future generations.

T. J. Fahey, MD

Adrenalectomy for solid tumor metastases: Results of a multicenter European study

Moreno P, de la Quintana Basarrate A, Musholt TJ, et al (Hospital Universitari de Bellvitge, Barcelona, Spain; Hospital de Cruces, Barakaldo, Bizkaia, Spain; Univ Med Ctr of the Johannes Gutenberg Univ, Mainz, Germany; et al)
Surgery 154:1215-1223, 2013

Background.—We assessed the results of adrenalectomy for solid tumor metastases in 317 patients recruited from 30 European centers.

Methods.—Patients with histologically proven adrenal metastatic disease and undergoing complete removal(s) of the affected gland(s) were eligible.

Results.—Non-small cell lung cancer (NSCLC) was the most frequent tumor type followed by colorectal and renal cell carcinoma. Adrenal metastases were synchronous (≤6 months) in 73 (23%) patients and isolated in 213 (67%). The median disease-free interval was 18.5 months. Laparoscopic resection was used in 46% of patients. Surgery was limited to the adrenal gland in 73% of patients and R0 resection was achieved in 86% of cases. The median overall survival was 29 months (95% confidence interval, 24.69–33.30). The survival rates at 1, 2, 3, and 5 years were 80%, 61%, 42%, and 35%, respectively. Patients with renal cancer showed a median survival of 84 months, patients with NSCLC 26 months, and patients with colorectal cancer 29 months ($P = .017$). Differences in survival between metachronous and synchronous lesions were also significant (30 vs 23 months; $P = .038$).

Conclusion.—Surgical removal of adrenal metastasis is associated with long-term survival in selected patients.

▶ Adrenalectomy for metastatic disease is a relatively uncommon operation. The report by Moreno et al provides a nice follow-up of several patients from a large number of centers throughout Europe. The authors document that survival after adrenalectomy for metastatic disease remains reasonably good—35% at 5 years—and similar to survival after metastasectomy of other sites. It is interesting to note that only 46% of the operations were done laparoscopically, and it is not clear from the report or the talk at the American Association of Endocrine Surgeons meeting last year why the laparoscopic number was this low. Other studies have now convincingly shown the oncologic equivalence of a laparoscopic resection versus an open resection for metastatic lesions in the adrenal gland. Adrenalectomy for a metastasis can be a very difficult operation. I believe that this is related to response to adjuvant treatment (chemotherapy) that most of these patients have received. It is not uncommon to encounter significant scarring and inflammation in the peri-adrenal tissues when approaching metastatic lesions, so a laparoscopic approach for a metastatic lesion should be undertaken by surgeons experienced in laparoscopic adrenal surgery.

T. J. Fahey, MD

Outcome of Bilateral Adrenalectomy in Cushing's Syndrome: A Systematic Review

Ritzel K, Beuschlein F, Mickisch A, et al (Klinikum der Universität München, Germany)
J Clin Endocrinol Metab 98:3939-3948, 2013

Background.—The outcome of bilateral adrenalectomy (BADx) in patients with Cushing's syndrome (CS) is not well characterized.

Methods.—A literature search was performed with the search terms "bilateral adrenalectomy" or "total adrenalectomy" and "Cushing's" or "Cushing." Immediate and long-term outcomes after BADx in CS were analyzed using descriptive statistics (median [range]).

Results.—From 549 screened publications, 37 studies met inclusion criteria (1320 patients, 82% having Cushing's disease [CD], 13% having ectopic CS, and 5% having primary adrenal hyperplasia). Surgical morbidity and mortality of BADx (23 studies, 739 patients) were 18% (6–31) and 3% (0–15), respectively. In patients with CD, surgical mortality was below 1%. Although residual cortisol secretion due to accessory adrenal tissue or adrenal remnants was found in 3–34% (5 studies, 236 patients), less than 2% had a relapse of CS. Symptoms of hypercortisolism (eg, hypertension, obesity, or depression) improved in the majority of the patients after BADx (7 studies, 195 patients). The number of adrenal crises per 100 patient-years was 9.3 (6 studies, 203 patients). Nelson's syndrome occurred in 21% (0–47) of the patients (24 studies, 768 patients). Mortality (23 studies, 690 patients) was 17% (0–88) at a follow-up of 41 months (14–294). Remarkably, 46% of the patients died in the first year after surgery. The median ages at death were 62 years (CD) and 53 years (ectopic CS).

Conclusion.—BADx is relatively safe and provides adequate success. Excess mortality within the first year after surgery suggests that intensive clinical care for patients after BADx is warranted.

▶ The management of treatment-resistant Cushing syndrome remains a difficult clinical problem (Fig 1 in the original article). This report gives a nice representation of the indication for bilateral adrenalectomy at the author's institution, and this appears to be a good representation of the indication for bilateral adrenalectomy. The report highlights the fact that substantial morbidity and mortality exist after bilateral adrenalectomy, including an overall incidence of Nelson's syndrome of 21% and mortality after bilateral adrenalectomy of 17%. Unfortunately, the authors did not examine the data based on year of publication, and clearly many of the included studies were older (reports were included from 1980 through 2012). This is highlighted by the fact that 58% of the patients undergoing adrenalectomy in the group analyzed for surgical outcomes had open operations, a statistic that is surely heavily influenced by studies done even before the advent of laparoscopic surgery, although the authors do report that mortality rates were no different between the open and laparoscopic groups. Nevertheless, the authors rightfully conclude that particular attention should be given to these patients in the first year after surgery, as nearly 50% of the deaths occurred during the first postoperative year.

T. J. Fahey, MD

The Role of Proinsulin and Insulin in the Diagnosis of Insulinoma: A Critical Evaluation of the Endocrine Society Clinical Practice Guideline

Guettier J-M, Lungu A, Goodling A, et al (Natl Insts of Health, Bethesda, MD; et al)

J Clin Endocrinol Metab 98:4752-4758, 2013

Context.—An end of fast insulin ≥3 μIU/mL and a proinsulin concentration ≥5 pmol/L have been suggested as useful cutoffs for the diagnosis of insulinoma.

Objective.—The main objective was to evaluate the diagnostic performance of an end of fast insulin concentration ≥3 μIU/mL and an end of fast proinsulin concentration ≥5 pmol/L.

Design.—The design was a case-control series.

Setting.—The setting was a tertiary-care center.

Patients.—Fifty-six subjects with a positive 48-hour supervised fast had an insulinoma between June 2000 and April 2011. During this same time period, a diagnosis of insulinoma was excluded in 29 subjects who underwent a supervised fast.

Intervention.—48-hour supervised fast.

Main Outcome Measure.—The main outcome measures were serum insulin concentration and plasma proinsulin concentration.

Results.—Ninety-one percent of the patients with an insulinoma had a measured insulin concentration ≥5 μIU/mL at the end of fast. The sensitivity increased to 98% if the threshold to define inadequate insulin suppression was lowered to ≥3 μIU/mL. The median (interquartile range) end of fast proinsulin was 100 (53–270) pmol/L for cases and 6.8 (4.2–12.0) pmol/L for controls. An end of fast proinsulin value of ≥5 pmol/L could not distinguish cases from controls (59% false positive rate). All patients with an insulinoma (sensitivity 100%) and none of the control subject (specificity 100%) had end of fast proinsulin concentration ≥27 pmol/L.

Conclusions.—Using a current insulin assay 9% of insulinoma cases end the supervised fast with an insulin concentration below 5 μIU/mL. Inadequate insulin suppression defined using a threshold of ≥3 μIU/mL increases the sensitivity of the test. The value of the proinsulin test lies in its unique ability to distinguish cases from controls. A proinsulin concentration of ≥22 pmol/L best discriminates cases from controls. Reliance on an end of fast proinsulin cutoff value of 5 pmol/L does not augment sensitivity but greatly reduces specificity of the test.

▶ Making the diagnosis of an insulinoma can be a difficult problem. Here the authors analyze the current guidelines from the Endocrine Society using a retrospective cohort of patients seen at the National Institutes of Health over an 11-year period. The data indicate that the current guidelines—which suggest using an end-of-fast proinsulin level of greater than 5 pmol/L—provide for a highly sensitive test with a very low specificity. This is especially important in a disease like insulinoma because of the substantial difficulty in localizing small tumors. Localization usually requires invasive testing (endoscopic ultrasound scan), and if that is unsuccessful, even more invasive testing—either simultaneous arterial and portal vein catheterization—or surgery. Thus, the specificity of the biochemical testing is at least as important as the sensitivity of the test to avoid invasive testing—up to and including surgery. The authors demonstrate in this series that an end-of-fast proinsulin level of greater than 27 provides both 100% sensitivity and specificity. Furthermore, the data show that measuring proinsulin is significantly more sensitive and specific than measuring C-peptide. Although the series is relatively small, and it is virtually certain that a case of insulinoma will be identified that falls outside of these biochemical parameters, using a higher proinsulin level to establish the diagnosis makes sense here to avoid the potential morbidity of invasive testing with a false-positive test.

T. J. Fahey, MD

Circulating Tumor Cells As Prognostic Markers in Neuroendocrine Tumors

Khan MS, Kirkwood A, Tsigani T, et al (Univ College London (UCL) Cancer Inst; Cancer Res UK and UCL Cancer Trials Centre; et al)
J Clin Oncol 31:365-372, 2013

Purpose.—To determine the prognostic significance of circulating tumor cells (CTCs) in patients with neuroendocrine cancer.

Patients and Methods.—In this single-center prospective study, 176 patients with measurable metastatic neuroendocrine tumors (NETs) were recruited. CTCs were measured using a semiautomated technique based on immunomagnetic separation of epithelial cell adhesion molecule–expressing cells

Results.—Overall, 49% patients had ≥ one CTC, 42% had ≥ two CTCs, and 30% had ≥ five CTCs in 7.5 mL blood. Presence of CTCs was associated with increased burden, increased tumor grade, and elevated serum chromogranin A (CgA). Using a 90-patient training set and 85-patient validation set, we defined a cutoff of < one or ≥ one as the optimal prognostic threshold with respect to progression-free survival (PFS). Applying this threshold, the presence of ≥ one CTC was associated with worse PFS and overall survival (OS; hazard ratios [HRs], 6.6 and 8.0, respectively; both $P < .001$). In multivariate analysis, CTCs remained significant when other prognostic markers, grade, tumor burden, and CgA were included. Within grades, presence of CTCs was able to define a poor prognostic subgroup. For grade 1, HRs were 5.0 for PFS ($P = .017$) and 7.2 for OS ($P = .023$); for grade 2, HRs were 3.5 for PFS ($P = .018$) and 5.2 for OS ($P = .036$)

Conclusion.—CTCs are a promising prognostic marker for patients with NETs and should be assessed in the context of clinical trials with defined tumor subtypes and therapy.

▶ Clinically available determinants of prognosis are generally lacking for neuroendocrine tumors (NETs). Chromogranin A and Ki-67 index have been used to assess prognosis in NETs. Ki-67 is particularly useful for identifying more aggressive tumors, but it fails to provide much prognostic input for most gastrointestinal NETs—the low-grade tumors. This report introduces circulating tumor cells (CTCs) as a potential new biomarker for prognosis for NETs that appears to be helpful in stratifying patients in the low and moderately differentiated groups as scored by Ki-67 index. However, the graphs shown in Fig 1 in the original article suggest that Ki-67 index is at least as good as the presence or absence of CTCs in predicting both progression-free and overall survival. Thus, although new biomarkers are desperately needed in NETs, whether CTCs will hold up as a biomarker in future studies remains to be seen. Nevertheless, future studies looking at response to treatment may benefit from inclusion of CTC determination in the analysis.

T. J. Fahey, MD

Presentation, Management, and Outcomes of Hyperparathyroidism in Octogenarians and Nonagenarians

Oltmann SC, Schneider DF, Sippel RS, et al (Univ of Wisconsin-Madison)
Ann Surg Oncol 20:4195-4199, 2013

Background.—Various elective surgical procedures are routinely performed on patients ≥80 years of age. With primary hyperparathyroidism (PHPT), surgical management is the only treatment. The goal of this study was to compare presentation and outcome of patients ≥80 to that of those <80 years of age.

Methods.—Retrospective review of a prospectively collected database of all parathyroidectomies for PHPT performed at a university hospital. Patients ≥80 years at the time of surgery compared with patients <80 years.

Results.—Over 13 years, 1,826 patients underwent parathyroidectomy for PHPT. A total of 154 patients were ≥80 years at the time of surgery (8.4 %), ranging from 80 to 91 years. Patients ≥80 years had higher serum PTH, creatinine and vitamin D levels and lower T scores. Calcium levels were similar. Patients ≥80 years had a greater history of hypertension, coronary artery disease, congestive heart failure, and stroke. Psychiatric disease was less common. Patients ≥80 years had the procedure under local anesthesia only more often. Use of a unilateral approach was equivalent. Rates of adenoma, double adenoma, and hyperplasia were comparable. Patients ≥80 years were observed overnight more frequently. Stays >24 h and disease recurrence and persistence, as well as morbidity rates, were all equivalent.

Conclusion.—Disease presentation of PHPT in patients ≥80 is similar to <80. Despite increased comorbidities, parathyroidectomy is a safe procedure in this patient population with a noted equivalent complication rate to younger patients. Operative management remains the only treatment. Patient age should not be a deterrent to offer curative surgical intervention.

► As the population ages, surgeons are frequently challenged to make decisions regarding suitability for surgery in the elderly and very elderly. This report from the group at the University of Wisconsin shows very nicely that parathyroidectomy is a safe operation even in the very elderly, and although the authors don't state this, when performed by high-volume, expert endocrine surgeons. As might be expected, these patients did have a higher incidence of comorbidities than the younger comparison group. However, they had a similar (low) incidence of complications. Whether these results can be reproduced in the community setting with less-experienced surgeons is not clear. What the study does not tell us is: Who did the authors not operate on? Were there patients who were deemed to be too risky for surgery? To really confidently conclude that surgery is safe in octogenarians with primary hyperparathyroidism, it would have been nice to know if there were some patients who did not undergo operation. The fact that patients 80 or older were less likely to be considered as having mild disease than the younger group (15% vs 24%) suggests that perhaps some older patients with milder disease may not have undergone surgery. Most of the older patients still had general anesthesia in this study, but a higher percentage did have local anesthesia only (15%) than in the younger group (8%). It is possible that the use of local anesthesia in more of the cohort could have allowed earlier (same day) discharge for more of the older group (bringing it back into balance with the younger group). Nevertheless, this study serves as an excellent demonstration that parathyroidectomy can be safely carried out, even in a population with advanced age, when the surgery is performed by experienced surgeons.

T. J. Fahey, MD

Bone Mineral Density Evolution After Successful Parathyroidectomy in Patients With Normocalcemic Primary Hyperparathyroidism

Koumakis E, Souberbielle J-C, Sarfati E, et al (Hôpital Cochin, Paris, France; Centre de Recherche "Croissance et Signalisation," Paris, France; et al)
J Clin Endocrinol Metab 98:3213-3220, 2013

Context.—It is unclear whether bone mineral density (BMD) improves in patients with normocalcemic primary hyperparathyroidism (PHPT) after parathyroidectomy (PTX).

Objective.—The objective of the study was to evaluate and compare the impact of PTX on BMD change at 1 year in normocalcemic vs hypercalcemic PHPT.

Design.—This was a longitudinal cohort study.

Setting.—The study took place at a referral center.

Patients.—We included 60 PHPT patients (mean age 64.0 ± 10.1 years), successfully treated by PTX by the same surgeon. Two groups were individualized according to baseline serum total (albumin corrected) calcium: 39 patients with normal baseline serum total calcium (normocalcemic group) and 21 patients with hypercalcemia at baseline (hypercalcemic group).

Main Outcome Measure.—BMD changes 1 year after PTX were measured.

Results.—In the normocalcemic group, BMD increased significantly by +2.3 ± 5.0% at the spine ($P = .016$) and +1.9 ± 5.7% at the hip ($P = .048$). In the hypercalcemic group, BMD increased significantly by +4.0 ± 3.8% at the spine ($P = .0003$) and +3.2 ± 4.2% at the hip ($P = .003$). There was no difference in these BMD gains between both groups ($P > .1$). The presence of multiple adenomas or hyperplasia was more frequent in the normocalcemic group than in the hypercalcemic group ($P = .04$).

Conclusion.—Our results indicate for the first time that successful PTX in normocalcemic PHPT patients with osteoporosis is followed with mild but significant BMD improvement at the spine and hip at 1 year, comparable with that observed in hypercalcemic PHPT, suggesting that PTX may be beneficial in normocalcemic PHPT.

▶ Eucalcemic hyperparathyroidism is increasingly being recognized as a real clinical entity. How to treat these patients remains a dilemma for endocrinologists and endocrine surgeons alike. Should they have surgery? This report provides evidence that those patients with osteoporosis and eucalcemic hyperparathyroidism will benefit from parathyroidectomy. Whether these findings can be extended to all patients with diminished bone density will require further study. Of note, the increases in bone density occurred at both the spine and femoral neck—but not at the distal radius. The authors note this and discuss it briefly, only to say that increases in bone density at the distal radius are variable in other studies of bone density after parathyroidectomy for primary hyperparathyroidism. Finally, the authors note that multigland disease is more common in patients undergoing parathyroidectomy for eucalcemic hyperparathyroidism. This mirrors my experience with these patients, and a 4-gland exploration is necessary in most of these cases.

T. J. Fahey, MD

Cardiovascular dysfunction in symptomatic primary hyperparathyroidism and its reversal after curative parathyroidectomy: Results of a prospective case control study

Agarwal G, Nanda G, Kapoor A, et al (Sanjay Gandhi Postgraduate Inst of Med Sciences, Lucknow, India)

Surgery 154:1394-1404, 2013

Background.—Cardiovascular mortality in primary hyperparathyroidism (PHPT) is attributed to myocardial and endothelial dysfunction. In this prospective, case-control study we assessed cardiovascular dysfunction in patients with symptomatic PHPT and its reversal after successful parathyroidectomy.

Methods.—Fifty-six patients with symptomatic PHPT underwent two-dimensional echocardiography, tissue Doppler (diastolic function assessment), serum N-terminal pro-brain natriuretic peptide (s-NTproBNP, a myocardial damage marker), and endothelial- and smooth muscle–dependent vasodilatory response (vascular dysfunction) studies before, 3, and 6 months after parathyroidectomy; 25 age-matched controls were studied similarly.

Results.—Patients had greater left ventricular mass (192 ± 70 vs 149 ± 44 g; $P = .006$), interventricular septal thickness (10.8 ± 2.5 vs 9.0 ± 1.6 mm; $P = .001$), posterior wall thickness (9.9 ± 2.0 vs 8.6 ± 2.2 mm; $P = .004$), and diastolic dysfunction (lower E/A transmitral flow velocity ratio [1.0 ± 0.4 vs 1.3 ± 0.4; $P = .01$). Patients had greater s-NTproBNP (4,625 ± 1,130 vs 58 ± 49 pg/mL; $P = .002$) and lower endothelial-mediated vasodilation (9.3 ± 8.6 vs 11.7 ± 6.3%; $P = .03$) and smooth muscle–mediated vasodilation (20.1 ± 17.9 vs

23.8 ± 11.2%; $P = .01$). Improvements in left ventricular mass, systolic and diastolic function, and smooth muscle–mediated vasodilation were noted from 3 to 6 months after parathyroidectomy. Endothelial-mediated vasodilation did not improve significantly. S-NTproBNP levels mirrored echocardiographic changes with a substantial, sustained decrease. Results were similar in hypertensive and normotensive patients.

Conclusion.—Symptomatic PHPT patients have substantial cardiac and vascular dysfunction, which improve by 6 months after parathyroidectomy. Objective cardiovascular evaluation may improve outcomes in symptomatic PHPT patients.

▶ This report from Dr Agarwal in Lucknow, India is a nicely done study looking at cardiovascular changes before and after parathyroidectomy. The authors document that there are quantifiable differences in patients with primary hyperparathyroidism and controls in a number of parameters but, perhaps most importantly, left ventricular mass. Fortunately, these detrimental changes reverse themselves in most cases after 3 to 6 months. It is important to note that the patients in this study had symptomatic hyperparathyroidism, and the mean calcium level was 11.5 with a mean parathyroid hormone level of 338—not the average patient who presents with hyperparathyroidism in the United States. So whether these findings can be extrapolated to much less severe hyperparathyroidism that we see in most of our patients here in the United States is unclear. Nevertheless, this report corroborates and to some extent provides a mechanism to explain older data that document an improvement in cardiovascular morbidity with correction of hyperparathyroidism.

T. J. Fahey, MD

The Clinical Course of Treated Hyperparathyroidism Among Patients Receiving Hemodialysis and the Effect of Cinacalcet: The EVOLVE Trial

Parfrey PS, Chertow GM, Block GA, et al (Health Sciences Ctr, St John's, Newfoundland, Canada; Stanford Univ School of Medicine, Palo Alto, CA; Denver Nephrology, CO; et al)

J Clin Endocrinol Metab 98:4834-4844, 2013

Context.—The clinical course of secondary hyperparathyroidism (sHPT) in patients on hemodialysis is not well described, and the effect of the calcimimetic cinacalcet on disease progression is uncertain.

Objective.—Our objective was to describe 1) the clinical course of sHPT in patients treated with phosphate binders and/or vitamin D sterols and 2) the impact of cinacalcet on the occurrence of severe unremitting HPT, defined by the persistence of markedly elevated PTH concentrations together with hypercalcemia or parathyroidectomy (PTX).

Design and Setting.—This was a randomized, double-blind, placebo-controlled, global, multicenter clinical trial.

Patients.—Of 5755 patients screened with moderate to severe sHPT, 3883 patients on hemodialysis were included in the trial.

Main Outcome Measures.—Outcomes included PTX; severe, unremitting HPT; and use of commercial cinacalcet (a protocol violation).

Intervention.—Intervention was cinacalcet (30–180 mg daily) or placebo for up to 64 months.

Results.—In the 1935 patients randomized to placebo, 278 patients (14%) underwent PTX (median PTH 1872 pg/mL within the previous 12 weeks from surgery). Age, sex, geographic region, co-morbidity, calcium-containing phosphate binder use, and baseline serum calcium, phosphorus, and PTH concentrations were associated with PTX. Commercial cinacalcet was started in 443 (23%) patients (median PTH 1108 pg/mL before treatment began). Severe unremitting HPT developed in 470 patients (24%). In a multivariable Cox model, the relative hazard (comparing patients randomized to cinacalcet versus placebo) of severe unremitting HPT was 0.31 (95% confidence interval = 0.26–0.37). The relative hazard differed little when adjusted by baseline clinical characteristics.

Conclusions.—Severe unremitting HPT develops frequently in patients on hemodialysis despite conventional therapy, and cinacalcet substantially reduces its occurrence.

▶ Last year the EVOLVE trial reported that cinacalcet did not appreciably reduce the incidence of major cardiovascular events or death in patients with moderate to severe secondary hyperparathyroidism who were on dialysis.[1] Here the trial reports that cinacalcet does reduce the occurrence of severe secondary hyperparathyroidism, despite current best medical therapy. This finding is not a surprise and justifies why patients on dialysis are routinely started on cinacalcet. Fig 1 in the original article clearly delineates the drop in the number of patients undergoing parathyroidectomy in the 6 regions around the world in patients on cinacalcet vs placebo. However, it is interesting that patients appear to have been referred for surgery earlier in the placebo group (median PTH 1872) compared with the cinacalcet group (median PTH 2143), as reported in Table 3 in the original article. There are no statistics provided to allow comparison of these 2 groups, and how this might affect the rate of parathyroid surgery in the 2 groups if it were equal cannot be analyzed from the data provided. It would be interesting to analyze the data to see if earlier referral for parathyroidectomy resulted in reduced cardiovascular events.

T. J. Fahey, MD

Reference

1. EVOLVE Trial Investigators, Chertow GM, Block GA, Correa-Rotter R, et al. Effect of cinacalcet on cardiovascular disease in patients undergoing dialysis. *N Engl J Med.* 2012;367:2482-2494.

Preoperative BRAF(V600E) Mutation Screening Is Unlikely to Alter Initial Surgical Treatment of Patients With Indeterminate Thyroid Nodules: A Prospective Case Series of 960 Patients

Kleiman DA, Sporn MJ, Beninato T, et al (New York Presbyterian Hosp—Weill Cornell Med College)

Cancer 119:1495-1502, 2013

Background.—Preoperative B-type Raf kinase Val600Glu mutation, or BRAF(V600E), analysis has been proposed as a tool to guide initial surgery for indeterminate thyroid nodules. This study sought to determine if cytologic markers of malignancy are associated with the BRAF(V600E) mutation and if preoperative BRAF(V600E) testing would alter the initial management of patients with indeterminate nodules.

Methods.—Patients who underwent surgery for a thyroid nodule between 2003 and 2012 at a tertiary care center were prospectively enrolled. Stored nodule samples were retrospectively genotyped for the BRAF(V600E) mutation. BRAF(V600E) status, demographics, cytologic and histopathologic findings, and choice of initial surgery were examined.

Results.—A total of 960 patients were enrolled, of which 310 (32%) had an indeterminate nodule. The BRAF(V600E) mutation was identified in 13 patients (4%), 12 of whom had either cytologic atypia or were Bethesda category V. Three percent of Bethesda category III or IV nodules that were malignant harbored the mutation compared with 42% of Bethesda category V malignancies. Nuclear grooves ($P = .030$), pseudoinclusions ($P < .001$), and oval nuclei ($P = .022$) were all more common among BRAF(V600E) mutants. The sensitivities of using BRAF testing alone, cytologic atypia/Bethesda category V classification, or both, were 15%, 73%, and 76%, respectively. Twelve of the 13 BRAF(V600E) mutants had total thyroidectomies initially due to worrisome cytologic features, and therefore the initial management of only one patient would have been altered if BRAF(V600E) testing had been performed preoperatively.

Conclusions.—Preoperative mutation screening for BRAF(V600E) does not meaningfully improve risk stratification and is unlikely to alter the initial management of patients with indeterminate nodules (Table 4).

▶ BRAF mutation testing has been proposed to be an adjunct to routine fine-need aspiration and cytology to aid in the discrimination of benign and malignant thyroid nodules. This report by Kleiman shows that, at least by itself, it has limited utility as a molecular diagnostic test. In the 2 Bethesda categories that generate the most uncertainty for patients and physicians about how to proceed (Bethesda III and IV), BRAF mutations were found in only 3% of the cancers (Table 4). Even for Bethesda V lesions, the sensitivity for BRAF mutations detecting malignancy was only 42%, which is less than the sensitivity of the cytology itself. If you recommend that a patient with a Bethesda V lesion proceed with a total thyroidectomy, the added benefit of determining BRAF mutation status is very limited. As a side note, and perhaps even more importantly, BRAF mutation testing can be used as a method to identify patients who do not need surgery. Whether

TABLE 4.—Correlation Between BRAF(V600E) Status and Outcome Among Various Subgroups of the Study Population

Subgroup		Malignant (n = 89)	Benign (n = 221)	
All indeterminate nodules (Bethesda III, IV or V)	BRAF(V600E)	13 (15%)	0 (0%)	Sensitivity: 15% Specificity: 100%
	Wild-type	76 (85%)	221 (100%)	PPV: 100% NPV: 74%
		Malignant (n = 63)	Benign (n = 211)	
Bethesda III or IV (FLUS/AUS or follicular neoplasm)	BRAF(V600E)	2 (3%)	0 (0%)	Sensitivity: 3% Specificity: 100%
	Wild-type	61 (97%)	211 (100%)	PPV: 100% NPV: 78%
		Malignant (n = 26)	Benign (n = 10)	
Bethesda V (suspicious for PTC)	BRAF(V600E)	11 (42%)	0 (0%)	Sensitivity: 42% Specificity: 100%
	Wild-type	15 (58%)	10 (100%)	PPV: 100% NPV: 40%
		Malignant (n = 61)	Benign (n = 84)	
Any atypia	BRAF(V600E)	11 (18%)	0 (0%)	Sensitivity 18% Specificity 100%
	Wild-type	50 (82%)	84 (100%)	PPV 100% NPV 63%
		Malignant (n = 23)	Benign (n = 135)	
Bethesda III or IV without atypia	BRAF(V600E)	1 (4%)	0 (0%)	Sensitivity 4% Specificity 100%
	Wild-type	22 (96%)	135 (100%)	PPV 100% NPV 86%

Abbreviations: AUS, atypia of undetermined significance; BRAF(V600E), B-type Raf kinase Val600Glu mutation; FLUS, follicular lesion of undetermined significance; NPV, negative predictive value; PPV, positive predictive value.

BRAF mutation testing can ultimately be used to tailor the extent of surgery—specifically whether to include central neck dissection as part of the surgical management—is still uncertain, as noted in the report by Zeiger et al.[1]

T. J. Fahey, MD

Reference

1. Zeiger MA, Li C, Aragon Han P, et al. Does BRAF V600E mutation predict aggressive features in papillary thyroid cancer? Results from four endocrine surgery centers. *J Clin Endocrinol Metab*. 2013;98:3702-3712.

Targeted Next-Generation Sequencing Panel (ThyroSeq) for Detection of Mutations in Thyroid Cancer

Nikiforova MN, Wald AI, Roy S, et al (Univ of Pittsburgh Med Ctr, PA)
J Clin Endocrinol Metab 98:E1852-E1860, 2013

Objectives.—Next-generation sequencing (NGS) allows for high-throughput sequencing analysis of large regions of the human genome. We explored the use of targeted NGS for simultaneous testing for multiple mutations in thyroid cancer.

Design.—A custom panel (ThyroSeq) was designed to target 12 cancer genes with 284 mutational hot spots. Sequencing was performed to analyze DNA from 228 thyroid neoplastic and nonneoplastic samples including 105 frozen, 72 formalin-fixed, and 51 fine-needle aspiration samples representing all major types of thyroid cancer.

Results.—Only 5–10 ng of input DNA was sufficient for successful analysis of 99.6% of samples. The analytical accuracy for mutation detection was 100% with the sensitivity of 3%–5% of mutant allele. ThyroSeq DNA assay identified mutations in 19 of 27 of classic papillary thyroid carcinomas (PTCs) (70%), 25 of 30 follicular variant PTCs (83%), 14 of 18 conventional (78%) and 7 of 18 oncocytic follicular carcinomas (39%), 3 of 10 poorly differentiated carcinomas (30%), 20 of 27 anaplastic (ATCs) (74%), and 11 of 15 medullary thyroid carcinomas (73%). In contrast, 5 of 83 benign nodules (6%) were positive for mutations. Most tumors had a single mutation, whereas several ATCs and PTCs demonstrated two or three mutations. The most common mutations detected were *BRAF* and *RAS* followed by *PIK3CA, TP53, TSHR, PTEN, GNAS, CTNNB1*, and *RET.* The *BRAF* mutant allele frequency was 18%–48% in PTCs and was lower in ATCs.

Conclusions.—The ThyroSeq NGS panel allows simultaneous testing for multiple mutations with high accuracy and sensitivity, requires a small amount of DNA and can be performed in a variety of thyroid tissue and fine-needle aspiration samples, and provides quantitative assessment of mutant alleles. Using this approach, the point mutations were detected in 30%–83% of specific types of thyroid cancer and in only 6% of benign thyroid nodules and were shown to be present in the majority of cells within the cancer nodule.

▶ This report by Nikiforova is another in a series from the Pittsburgh group leading the way in the molecular diagnosis of thyroid nodules and thyroid cancer. The authors have created a very nice platform using next-generation sequencing to analyze a panel of genes that are potentially mutated in thyroid cancer. The technique appears to show great promise, although there are a couple of points that need further explanation and future study. First, the source of the fine-needle aspiration (FNA) samples is not clear in the report. Were these FNA samples obtained ex vivo after the specimen was removed? If so, this will require additional study to prove that FNA samples obtained by standard technique will still have such an excellent yield and success at going through next-generation sequencing. Another concern going forward will be the cost of such an approach. Although the cost of next-generation sequencing has been coming down, it still costs at least $600 to $650 per sample, not including labor costs to prepare the sample. So, although ThyroSeq appears to hold great promise going forward, additional study is needed before applying the test clinically.

T. J. Fahey, MD

Is Potassium Iodide Solution Necessary Before Total Thyroidectomy for Graves Disease?

Shinall MC Jr, Broome JT, Baker A, et al (Vanderbilt Univ Med Ctr, Nashville, TN)

Ann Surg Oncol 20:2964-2967, 2013

Background.—Potassium iodide (KI) has traditionally been used to reduce gland vascularity and diminish blood loss in patients undergoing thyroidectomy for Graves disease (GD). Current American Thyroid Association (ATA) guidelines (Recommendation 22) call for its routine administration in GD but avoidance in toxic multinodular goiter (TMNG).

Methods.—A retrospective review (July 2008—May 2012) of perioperative data was performed on 162 patients undergoing total thyroidectomy without preoperative KI and compared to 102 patients with TMNG. Statistical analysis included Student's t test, χ^2 test, and multivariate linear regression.

Results.—Compared to TMNG patients, GD patients had a lower mean age (42.7 vs. 49.6 years, $p < 0.001$) and were less likely to be obese (37 vs. 54%, $p = 0.047$). No patients were provided KI in preparation. GD patients did not differ significantly from TMNG patients with respect to mean estimated blood loss (55.4 vs. 51.5 mL, $p = 0.773$) or mean operative time (131.5 vs. 122.6 min, $p = 0.084$). GD patients had a lower rate of transient hypocalcemia (31 vs. 49%, $p = 0.004$), but the two groups did not statistically differ in rates of prolonged hypocalcemia, temporary recurrent laryngeal nerve (RLN) palsy, prolonged RLN paralysis, or hematoma formation.

Conclusions.—Although current ATA recommendations for the management of GD call for routine use of KI before thyroidectomy, this large series demonstrates no appreciable detriment to patient outcomes when this goal is not met.

▶ This is a large, single-center review of the authors' experience with the surgical management of Graves disease. The authors are to be commended for excellent outcomes in what is typically one of the most challenging groups of patients for thyroid surgery. They conclude that potassium iodide (KI) does not reduce blood loss at surgery for Graves disease. The major flaw in the article is that the authors do not have a comparison group that did receive KI. Instead, they used patients undergoing surgery for toxic multinodular goiter who also did not receive KI. Overlooking this, the authors recorded a mean blood loss of only 55 mL in this series, which is remarkably low, even for nontoxic goiter. It must be pointed out once again that the authors are experienced endocrine surgeons practicing in a referral center where they see a substantial number of patients for surgical treatment of Graves disease. Whether these results can be extrapolated to the practicing surgeon who performs only a handful of thyroid operations a year is doubtful. However, it is not clear that KI will help in that situation either. The authors have provided evidence that the guidelines from the American Thyroid Association, which recommend the use of KI in the preoperative management of Graves disease, may not be based on solid ground. Through my experience, I believe that the authors are correct, although a better study is needed to prove this.

T. J. Fahey, MD

Anaesthesia for massive retrosternal thyroidectomy in a tertiary referral centre

Dempsey GA, Snell JA, Coathup R, et al (Univ Hosp Aintree NHS Foundation Trust, Liverpool, UK)

Br J Anaesth 111:594-599, 2013

Background.—Retrosternal goitre (RSG) is an uncommon problem encountered rarely by anaesthetists working outside specialized head and neck (H&N) surgical units. Traditional anaesthetic teaching warns of difficult airway management in these patients. The incidence and extent of these problems is unclear.

Methods.—We have performed a retrospective review of the anaesthetic management all patients with massive RSG (extending to the aortic arch or beyond) presenting for thyroidectomy at University Hospital Aintree from January 2007 to May 2012.

Results.—Five hundred and seventy-three patients underwent a thyroidectomy procedure at Aintree University Hospitals NHS Foundation Trust (AUH) between January 2007 and May 2012. Of these, 34 cases were documented as having a RSG. Review of each patient's preoperative computerized tomography imaging identified 19 patients with massive RSG. There was one case of failed intubation. All other patients underwent uneventful tracheal intubation via direct laryngoscopy. All glands were removed through the neck with no requirement to proceed to sternotomy. There were no instances of postoperative respiratory problems or tracheomalacia. Three patients suffered recurrent laryngeal nerve (RLN) injuries.

Conclusion.—When managed within a dedicated H&N operating theatre we have found a low incidence of difficult tracheal intubation, difficult mechanical ventilation nor postoperative respiratory difficulties in patients with massive RSG and mid-tracheal compression because of benign multinodular goitre. Surgical complications, however, are more frequent than those associated with cervical thyroidectomy with RLN injury and postoperative bleeding more likely.

► Substernal goiters typically produce consternation among the anesthesiologists—and rightfully so—as intubation can sometimes be difficult. This series from a busy head and neck center in England shows that intubation in patients with substernal goiter is associated with a low incidence of difficult intubation. At first glance it would seem that the authors did not really examine their own data, as 1 of 19 patients had a failed intubation and required emergency tracheostomy, an unacceptably high number. However, the authors go on to delineate that this case was initially attempted in an operating room (and presumably with surgeons and anesthesiologists) not dedicated to head and neck (or endocrine) surgery and anesthesia. In fact, the patient was the only one in the series who had an attempt at induction with inhalation anesthetics only. The remaining 18 cases had intubation by direct laryngoscopy (only one by fiber optic), and in none of these cases was there difficulty in passing the tube. To me, this makes sense. In virtually all cases of substernal goiter, the tracheal compression and deviation occur below the level of the vocal cords, thus, bringing into question the need for awake fiberoptic intubation. Probably the most important lesson that can be learned from this series is that an experienced anesthesia team and an experienced surgical team are necessary to safely conduct these operations.

T. J. Fahey, MD

A multi-institutional international study of risk factors for hematoma after thyroidectomy

Campbell MJ, McCoy KL, Shen WT, et al (Univ of California, San Francisco; The Univ of Pittsburgh Med Ctr, PA; et al)
Surgery 154:1283-1291, 2013

Background.—Cervical hematoma can be a potentially fatal complication after thyroidectomy, but its risk factors and timing remain poorly understood.

Methods.—We conducted a retrospective, case-control study identifying 207 patients from 15 institutions in 3 countries who developed a hematoma requiring return to the operating room (OR) after thyroidectomy.

Results.—Forty-seven percent of hematoma patients returned to the OR within 6 hours and 79% within 24 hours of their thyroidectomy. On univariate analysis, hematoma patients were older, more likely to be male, smokers, on active antiplatelet/anticoagulation medications, have Graves' disease, a bilateral thyroidectomy, a drain placed, a concurrent parathyroidectomy, and benign pathology. Hematoma patients also had more blood loss, larger thyroids, lower temperatures, and higher blood pressures postoperatively. On multivariate analysis, independent associations with hematoma were use of a drain (odds ratio, 2.79), Graves' disease (odds ratio, 2.43), benign pathology (odds ratio, 2.22), antiplatelet/anticoagulation medications (odds ratio, 2.12), use of a hemostatic agent (odds ratio, 1.97), and increased thyroid mass (odds ratio, 1.01).

Conclusion.—A significant number of patients with a postoperative hematoma present >6 hours after thyroidectomy. Hematoma is associated with patients who have a drain or hemostatic agent, have Graves' disease, are actively using antiplatelet/anticoagulation medications or have large thyroids. Surgeons should consider these factors when individualizing patient disposition after thyroidectomy.

▶ This large multi-institutional study raises some concerns regarding the widespread trend toward outpatient thyroidectomy in the United States. It is now customary for insurance companies to deny approval for admission after thyroid surgery, although of course a patient can be kept overnight if deemed appropriate by the surgeon (but with no guarantee of payment by the insurance companies). In this study, only 47% of the patients who required re-exploration for hematoma underwent re-exploration within the standard 6-hour timeframe allotted for patient recovery after thyroidectomy as an outpatient. The authors were able to identify factors that were more highly associated with bleeding; however, clearly that did not account for all or even most of the cases of hematoma. Additionally, it is not clear what percentage of these cases were emergent as opposed to semi-elective. So the question is—does this study provide enough information to support or counter using a 6-hour timeframe as an adequate time for observation after thyroidectomy? The answer is—not really. What really needs to be understood from a cohort of patients like this is what happened to the patients between 6 and 24 hours that required re-exploration? Were these admitted patients that were emergently taken back to the operating room? Or did these patients have enough time to get back to the hospital if they were already discharged? Thus, the data are very useful in suggesting that there are some classes of patients who have higher risk for postoperative hematoma, and these should be watched more diligently or for longer. But it does not help to resolve the dilemma of how long to keep the standard postoperative patient. More in-depth analysis is needed to sort out this question.

T. J. Fahey, MD

Ten percent tall cells confer the aggressive features of the tall cell variant of papillary thyroid carcinoma

Beninato T, Scognamiglio T, Kleiman DA, et al (New York Presbyterian Hosp - Weill Cornell Med College)

Surgery 154:1331-1336, 2013

Background.—The tall cell (TC) variant of papillary thyroid carcinoma (PTC) is more aggressive than classic PTC, but the percentage of TC necessary to diagnose this variant has been debated. We aimed to better determine what percentage of TC correlates with a more aggressive phenotype.

Methods.—Cases from 2005 to 2010 that were the TC variant of PTC or PTC with TC features were identified and compared with classic PTCs. All cases were reviewed to determine what percent, if any, of the tumors consisted of TC.

Results.—One hundred forty-one cases of PTC were reviewed. Eighty-three cases had some TC component, and 58 cases had none. There were no differences in patient demographics. Tumors with ≥10% TC had more extrathyroidal extension, angiolymphatic invasion, positive surgical margin, and lymph node involvement than classic PTC. There were more recurrences in patients with ≥10% TC, but this was not significant. Similar findings were also observed with increasing percentages of TC.

Conclusion.—The aggressive features conferred by the presence of TC in PTCs occur with as little as 10% TC and are maintained with increasing percentages. Therefore, TC in a PTC should be reported if they comprise at least 10% of the tumor.

▶ The importance that is assigned to the histology of papillary thyroid cancer (PTC) is considerable, as it often influences postoperative treatment and subsequent follow-up. Tall cell histology has become one of the most frequently identified histologic factors associated with more aggressive behavior, yet the percentage of the tumor cells deemed tall cells that are necessary to label a tumor tall cell is variable. Here Beninato et al suggest that the threshold for labeling a tumor as tall cell might be considered as low as 10%. The authors show that compared with classic PTC without tall cells, using a 10% threshold of tall cells is still associated with other histologic features that signal potentially more aggressive tumors, such as extrathyroidal extension and the presence of lymph node metastases. It is interesting to note that with careful pathologic examination of these cases, the presence of some tall cells was identified in 46% of cases that had been signed out as classic PTC—a very high percentage and much higher than previous reports in the literature. This could be completely explained by the very stringent criteria that were used to reclassify tumors—any tall cells seen in the specimen. If the criteria for reclassifying the tumor were set at 30%, 50%, or 70%, the percentage of tumors reclassified would have been much lower—11%, 5%, and 0%—numbers that are completely consistent with those reported in the literature.

It is not surprising that a smaller percentage of presumably more aggressive cells drives the ultimate behavior of the tumor, as this is seen in multiple other carcinomas, including poorly differentiated and anaplastic carcinomas of the thyroid.

T. J. Fahey, MD

Stimulated Thyroglobulin at Recombinant Human TSH-Aided Ablation Predicts Disease-free Status One Year Later

Melo M, Costa G, Ribeiro C, et al (Univ and Hosp Ctr of Coimbra, Portugal; et al)
J Clin Endocrinol Metab 98:4364-4372, 2013

Context.—Thyroglobulin (Tg) levels measured at the time of remnant ablation after thyroid hormone withdrawal (THW) were shown to have prognostic value in predicting disease-free status.

Objectives.—Our objectives were to determine whether stimulated Tg levels, measured at the time of remnant ablation performed under recombinant human TSH (rhTSH) stimulation, has value in predicting absence of detectable disease 1 year after radioiodine therapy and to compare the results obtained with this approach with a cohort of patients submitted to ablation after THW.

Design.—This was a prospective observational study.

Setting and Patients.—The study included 293 consecutive patients treated for a differentiated thyroid carcinoma with no initial evidence of distant metastasis. All patients were submitted to a total or near-total thyroidectomy, followed by ablation either under rhTSH (n = 151) or endogenous TSH stimulation (n = 142). Patients with positive Tg antibodies were excluded.

Main Outcome Measures.—The predictive value of Tg at ablation was assessed by receiver operating characteristic curve analysis.

Results.—In the rhTSH group, 96 patients (73.3%) were considered disease-free at 1 year. Stimulated Tg at ablation after rhTSH was found to be an independent prognostic indicator of disease persistence 12 months later. The highest-accuracy cutoff value for absence of detectable disease was defined as 7.2 ng/mL, with a negative predictive value of 90%. In the THW group, Tg at ablation also proved to have independent predictive value. Using the same threshold (7.2 ng/mL), the negative predictive value of Tg was 95% in the THW group.

Conclusions.—When rhTSH was used, stimulated Tg at ablation had independent predictive value for disease-free status 1 year later. A low stimulated Tg at rhTSH-aided ablation may be considered a favorable prognosis factor.

▶ This report examines the utility of using the stimulated thyroglobulin (Tg) at the time of postoperative radioactive iodine (RAI) administration to predict the presence of disease recurrence 1 year after treatment and compares that with the use of thyroid hormone withdrawal. Recombinant human thyroid-stimulating hormone (rhTSH)-stimulated Tg has been shown to be essentially equivalent to thyroid hormone withdrawal for the preparation of patients for RAI administration with equivalent outcomes using the 2 techniques. The advantages of using rhTSH stimulation are the avoidance of significant hypothyroid symptoms using thyroid hormone withdrawal and a significant reduction in exposure to radiation from the excess radioactive iodine (approximately 35%). This study documents that a low Tg at the time of RAI administration is useful in predicting a disease-free status at 1 year. Ultimately, with larger cohorts of patients and longer follow-up, it may be possible to identify patients treated with total thyroidectomy and postoperative RAI who can be declared disease free after completing treatment and forego follow-up testing completely. One note of concern about the study—a study like this is highly dependent on the ability to accurately determine Tg, and Tg levels are directly influenced by the presence of Tg antibodies. The assay used for antibody detection in this study was not a sensitive assay as far as I can tell. It had a sensitivity of 10 IU/mL, and reference value was less than 40 IU/mL. By comparison, the better Tg antibody tests have reference values of less than 1 IU/mL. This may explain the fact that 1 of 13 patients in the rhTSH-stimulated group who had an undetectable Tg at the time of treatment had a recurrence at 1 year.

T. J. Fahey, MD

Does *BRAF* V600E Mutation Predict Aggressive Features in Papillary Thyroid Cancer? Results From Four Endocrine Surgery Centers

Li C, Aragon Han P, Lee KC, et al (The Johns Hopkins Univ School of Medicine, Baltimore, MD; et al)

J Clin Endocrinol Metab 98:3702-3712, 2013

Background.—Existing evidence is controversial regarding the association between *BRAF* mutation status and aggressive features of papillary thyroid cancer (PTC). Specifically, no study has incorporated multiple surgical practices performing routine central lymph node dissection (CLND) and thus has patients who are truly evaluable for the presence or absence of central lymph node metastases (CLNMs).

Methods.—Consecutive patients who underwent total thyroidectomy and routine CLND at 4 tertiary endocrine surgery centers were retrospectively reviewed. Descriptive and bivariable analyses examined demographic, patient, and tumor-related factors. Multivariable analyses examined the odds of CLNM associated with positive *BRAF* status.

Results.—In patients with classical variant PTC, bivariate analysis found no significant associations between *BRAF* mutation and aggressive clinicopathologic features; multivariate analysis demonstrated that *BRAF* status was not an independent predictor of CLNM. When all patients with PTC were analyzed, including those with aggressive or follicular subtypes, bivariate analysis showed *BRAF* mutation to be associated with LNM, advanced American Joint Committee on Cancer (AJCC) stage, and histologic subtype. Multivariable analyses showed *BRAF*, age, size, and extrathyroidal extension to be associated with CLNM.

Conclusion.—Although *BRAF* mutation was found to be an independent predictor of central LNM in the overall cohort of patients with PTC, this relationship lost significance when only classical variant PTC was included in the analysis. The usefulness of *BRAF* in predicting the presence of LNM remains questionable. Prospective studies are needed before *BRAF* mutation can be considered a reliable factor to guide the treatment of patients with PTC, specifically whether to perform prophylactic CLND (Table 2).

▶ This nicely coordinated study addresses the important question of whether *BRAF* status should be used as a preoperative variable to direct treatment of patients presenting with papillary thyroid cancer (PTC). The study shows nicely that if you look at all patients with PTC—including classical and follicular variants—that *BRAF* mutation is associated with the presence of lymph node metastases. However, this association is almost entirely driven by the relationship between *BRAF* mutation and the classic variant PTC. If one examines the relationship between *BRAF* mutation and lymph node metastases in just classic variant PTC, there is no difference in the presence of lymph node metastases in *BRAF*+ or *BRAF*− tumors. The implications are several. First, preoperative determination of *BRAF* mutation status should not determine whether a prophylactic central neck dissection should be done, as the rate of central neck lymph

TABLE 2.—Bivariate Analyses of Associations Between *BRAF* Mutation Status and Clinicopathologic Features in Patients With CVPTC Only

Clinicopathologic Features	*BRAF* Mutation-Positive, n (%)	*BRAF* Mutation-Negative, n (%)	*P*
Gender			
Female	193 (76.3)	52 (83.9)	.198
Male	60 (23.7)	10 (16.1)	
Age, y			
<45	116 (45.9)	32 (51.6)	.415
≥45	137 (54.1)	30 (48.4)	
Tumor size, cm			
≤2	167 (66.0)	45 (72.6)	.323
>2	86 (34.0)	17 (27.4)	
Multifocality			
No	133 (52.6)	35 (56.5)	.583
Yes	120 (47.4)	27 (43.6)	
LVI			
Absent	226 (89.3)	54 (87.1)	.616
Present	27 (10.7)	8 (12.9)	
Surgical margins			
Negative	221 (87.4)	55 (88.7)	.771
Positive	32 (12.6)	7 (11.3)	
LNM			
Absent	103 (40.7)	30 (48.4)	.273
Present	150 (59.3)	32 (51.6)	
ETE			
Absent	193 (76.3)	45 (72.6)	.543
Present	60 (23.7)	17 (27.4)	
AJCC stage			
I	157 (62.1)	46 (74.2)	.233
II	13 (5.1)	3 (4.8)	
III	68 (26.9)	9 (14.5)	
IV	15 (5.9)	4 (6.5)	

node metastases in these groups of patients is essentially identical (Table 2). Second, the study brings into question the conclusions of numerous previous studies that argue that *BRAF* mutation is a marker for more aggressive tumors. Really, it is a best marker for classical variant PTC. The distinction between classical variant and follicular variant PTC needs to be made in future studies considering the implications of *BRAF* mutation in PTC.

T. J. Fahey, MD

Is Thyroid Cancer Recurrence Risk Increased After Transplantation?

Tisset H, the TUTHYREF network (Université Lyon 1, France; et al)
J Clin Endocrinol Metab 98:3981-3988, 2013

Context.—An increased cancer mortality is reported in transplanted patients.

Objective.—This multicentric study aimed to investigate the rate of thyroid cancer recurrence after transplantation.

Results.—Sixty-eight patients (35 male/33 female) with a history of both thyroid cancer and organ transplantation were recruited via two nationwide French networks. Histological analysis identified 58 papillary (88%), 5 follicular (7.5%), and 3 poorly differentiated cancer cases (4.5 %). Thirty-one patients (52%) presented high recurrence risk tumors. In the 36 patients with thyroid cancer diagnosed after transplantation, the 5-year disease-free survival (DFS) was 74.7% (SE: 7.3%). One patient died after progression of a poorly differentiated cancer. Persistent disease was observed in six high-risk patients. One of them underwent a second transplantation and disease remained stable after 5 years of follow-up. Thyroid cancer had been diagnosed before transplantation in 32 patients. One patient with cystic fibrosis and thyroid lung metastases at the time of lung transplantation underwent a 4-year remission. For the 31 patients in remission at the time of transplantation, the 5-year DFS was 93.1% (SE: 4.8%). Two patients with local recurrence presented subsequent remission. For the entire study population, the 5-year and 9-year DFS were 81.9% (SE: 5.5%) and 75.6% (SE: 7.9%), respectively. Recurrence or persistent disease occurred in patients with high-risk tumors.

Conclusions.—The prognosis of thyroid cancer does not seem to be altered by transplantation. This suggests that a history of thyroid cancer should not be considered a contraindication.

▶ The evaluation of patients with end-stage renal disease (ESRD) before listing on a transplant list is comprehensive. In recent years, we have seen an increase in the number of patients with ESRD referred for evaluation of both thyroid nodules and thyroid cancer when being evaluated for possible transplantation. After surgery, for those who do have thyroid cancer, we are asked to clear the patient as cancer free before listing, which in many cases is like looking into the crystal ball. Waiting a year and then doing a thyrogen-stimulated thyroglobulin test is clearly one option, but these patients are anxious to be listed, and another year—before even being listed—is a long time for a patient on dialysis. This article provides some level of confidence that it is safe to list patients for transplant after their initial treatment is completed. The study, although the largest of its kind to date, still has small numbers (only 32 patients diagnosed with thyroid cancer before transplantation and 36 diagnosed after transplantation), and patients were accrued over 40 years (from 1970 to 2010). Still, the study provides evidence that patients who are treated for thyroid cancer remain at low risk for recurrence and that recurrences, when they do occur, are manageable, similar to patients in the general population. Discovery of thyroid cancer in the pretransplant screening process should not prevent listing for transplant.

T. J. Fahey, MD

Selumetinib-Enhanced Radioiodine Uptake in Advanced Thyroid Cancer

Ho AL, Grewal RK, Leboeuf R, et al (Memorial Sloan-Kettering Cancer Ctr and Weill Cornell Med College, NY)

N Engl J Med 368:623-632, 2013

Background.—Metastatic thyroid cancers that are refractory to radioiodine (iodine-131) are associated with a poor prognosis. In mouse models of thyroid cancer, selective mitogen-activated protein kinase (MAPK) pathway antagonists increase the expression of the sodium–iodide symporter and uptake of iodine. Their effects in humans are not known.

Methods.—We conducted a study to determine whether the MAPK kinase (MEK) 1 and MEK2 inhibitor selumetinib (AZD6244, ARRY-142886) could reverse refractoriness to radioiodine in patients with metastatic thyroid cancer. After stimulation with thyrotropin alfa, dosimetry with iodine-124 positron-emission tomography (PET) was performed before and 4 weeks after treatment with selumetinib (75 mg twice daily). If the second iodine-124 PET study indicated that a dose of iodine-131 of 2000 cGy or more could be delivered to the metastatic lesion or lesions, therapeutic radioiodine was administered while the patient was receiving selumetinib.

Results.—Of 24 patients screened for the study, 20 could be evaluated. The median age was 61 years (range, 44 to 77), and 11 patients were men. Nine patients had tumors with BRAF mutations, and 5 patients had tumors with mutations of *NRAS*. Selumetinib increased the uptake of iodine-124 in 12 of the 20 patients (4 of 9 patients with BRAF mutations and 5 of 5 patients with *NRAS* mutations). Eight of these 12 patients reached the dosimetry threshold for radioiodine therapy, including all 5 patients with *NRAS* mutations. Of the 8 patients treated with radioiodine, 5 had confirmed partial responses and 3 had stable disease; all patients had decreases in serum thyroglobulin levels (mean reduction, 89%). No toxic effects of grade 3 or higher attributable by the investigators to selumetinib were observed. One patient received a diagnosis of myelodysplastic syndrome more than 51 weeks after radioiodine treatment, with progression to acute leukemia.

Conclusions.—Selumetinib produces clinically meaningful increases in iodine uptake and retention in a subgroup of patients with thyroid cancer that is refractory to radioiodine; the effectiveness may be greater in patients with *RAS*-mutant disease. (Funded by the American Thyroid Association and others; ClinicalTrials.gov number, NCT00970359.).

► The management of radioiodine (RAI)-refractory metastatic thyroid cancer remains a challenging problem. Most deaths from follicular cell-derived thyroid cancer are secondary to this group of tumors, and the 10-year survival of patients with RAI-refractory metastatic differentiated thyroid cancer is only 10%. This study is a landmark study showing a substantial advance in the treatment of these patients. The biologic basis for optimism that this treatment strategy would work stems from the observation that inhibition of BRAF mutations can lead to re-expression of the sodium-iodine symporter (NIS). However, as seen in Fig 1 of the original article, this is not yet a cure-all. Only 8 of 20 patients had enough of an increase in iodine uptake to qualify for repeat treatment with RAI. This appeared to vary based on the type of mutation, and, somewhat surprisingly, this was most common in patients who had tumors that harbored NRAS mutations. Unfortunately, only 1 of the 9 patients with BRAF mutant tumors (by far the most common mutation in papillary thyroid cancers) had an increase in iodine uptake sufficient to allow for repeat treatment. Whether this is caused by inadequate selectivity of the mitogen-activated protein kinase inhibitor to induce re-expression of NIS in BRAF-mutant tumors will require additional study with more selective BRAF inhibitors going forward.

T. J. Fahey, MD

The Clinical and Economic Burden of a Sustained Increase in Thyroid Cancer Incidence

Aschebrook-Kilfoy B, Schechter RB, Shih Y-CT, et al (Univ of Chicago, IL)
Cancer Epidemiol Biomarkers Prev 22:1252-1259, 2013

Background.—Thyroid cancer incidence is increasing worldwide at an alarming rate, yet little is known of the impact this increase will have on society. We sought to determine the clinical and economic burden of a sustained increase in thyroid cancer incidence in the United States and to understand how these burdens correlate with the National Cancer Institute's (NCI) prioritization of thyroid cancer research funding.

Methods.—We used the NCI's SEER 13 database (1992—2009) and Joinpoint regression software to identify the current clinical burden of thyroid cancer and to project future incidence through 2019. We combined Medicare reimbursement rates with American Thyroid Association guidelines, and our clinical practice to create an economic model of thyroid cancer. We obtained research-funding data from the NCI's Office of Budget and Finance.

Results.—By 2019, papillary thyroid cancer will double in incidence and become the third most common cancer in women of all ages at a cost of $18 to $21 billion dollars in the United States. Despite these substantial clinical and economic burdens, thyroid cancer research remains significantly underfunded by comparison, and in 2009 received only $14.7 million (ranked 30th) from the NCI.

Conclusion.—The impact of thyroid cancer on society has been significantly underappreciated, as is evidenced by its low priority in national research funding levels.

Impact.—Increased awareness in the medical community and the general public of the societal burden of thyroid cancer, and substantial increases in research on thyroid cancer etiology, prevention, and treatment are needed to offset these growing concerns.

▶ The authors of this report have outlined some neglected facts about the clinical and economic burdens of the increase in thyroid cancer. The economic impact is potentially huge—21 trillion dollars in costs over the 10-year period from 2010 to 2019. They go on to note that thyroid cancer research is grossly underfunded by the National Cancer Institute compared with other significant cancers. As an individual who is familiar with the struggles trying to get federal funding for thyroid cancer research, additional funding for thyroid cancer research would be welcome. However, the authors should note that the incidence of death secondary to thyroid cancer has essentially remained stable, even while incidence rates have skyrocketed. Although it is unclear if the death rate from thyroid cancer will remain flat as time goes on, one can expect that it will not increase substantially. Thus, the argument could be made that current funding levels are adequate. On the other hand, research into the epidemiology of the increase is badly needed and should be funded by the government given the substantial economic burden facing the health care system as a result of the increased number of cases of thyroid cancer identified. Large, prospective studies should be undertaken to answer the questions: what subcentimeter nodules should undergo fine-needle aspiration, what patients can simply be observed, does the introduction of molecular testing ultimately reduce costs if included as part of the algorithm for all indeterminate nodules, and who really needs or benefits from radioactive iodine administration as a postoperative adjuvant treatment? Although it does not appear that there will soon be an increase in deaths due to differentiated thyroid cancers, the economic burden of caring for these patients could be suffocating.

T. J. Fahey, MD

9 Nutrition

Clinical and Immunological Impact of Early Postoperative Enteral Immunonutrition After Total Gastrectomy in Gastric Cancer Patients: A Prospective Randomized Study

Marano L, Porfidia R, Pezzella M, et al (Second Univ of Naples, Italy)

Ann Surg Oncol 20:3912-3918, 2013

Background.—Enteral immunodiet has been gaining increasing attention, but experimental data of its clinical effects in patients with gastric cancer are inconsistent, contradictory, and poorly investigated. The aim of this study was to assess the impact of early postoperative enteral immunonutrition on clinical and immunological outcomes in a homogeneous group of gastric cancer patients submitted to total gastrectomy.

Methods.—A total of 109 patients with gastric cancer were randomized to receive early postoperative enteral immunonutrition (formula supplemented with arginine, omega-3 fatty acids and ribonucleic acid [RNA]), or an isocaloric-isonitrogenous control. The postoperative outcome was evaluated based on clinical variables, including postoperative infectious complications, anastomotic leak rate, and length of hospitalization. In addition, state of cellular immunity was evaluated and compared between the 2 groups.

Results.—The incidence of postoperative infectious complications in the immunodiet group (7.4%) was significantly ($p < .05$) lower than that of the control group (20%), as well as the anastomotic leak rate (3.7% in immunodiet group vs 7.3% in standard nutrition group, $p < .05$). Mortality rate did not show any significant differences; patients of the immunodiet group were found to have a significantly reduced length of hospitalization (12.7 ± 2.3 days) when compared with standard diet group (15.9 ± 3.4 days, $p = .029$). The data on cellular immunity showed that the postoperative $CD4^+$ T-cell counts decreased in both groups, but the reduction in the IED group was significantly higher ($p = .032$) compared with the SND group.

Conclusions.—Early postoperative enteral immunonutrition significantly improves clinical and immunological outcomes in patients undergoing gastrectomy for gastric cancer.

► Several clinical trials have addressed the question as to whether certain nutrients such as arginine, Ω-3 fatty acids, and RNA in pharmacologic dosages would enhance the patient's immune status and ultimately lead to improved outcomes. Our own trial in patients with upper gastrointestinal (GI) malignances compared standard enteral feeding with an experimental diet containing these additional nutrients. In that trial, there was a significant reduction in postoperative infectious complications. Several prospective clinical studies replicated these results. Other trials, however, did not find significant differences in patient outcomes, yet a more recent meta-analysis found improved outcomes in malnourished GI cancer patients that received immunonutrition perioperatively.

The strength of the prospective clinical trial reported by Marano et al is that it focused only on gastric cancer patients undergoing surgery. Mean infectious complications, postoperative anastomotic leaks, and postoperative length of stay were markedly reduced in the immunonutrition group compared with the control group.

These findings coupled with earlier reports suggest that enteral immunonutrition can be significantly beneficial to the GI cancer patient undergoing major surgery.

J. M. Daly, MD

Plasma Arginine Levels and Blood Glucose Control in Very Preterm Infants Receiving 2 Different Parenteral Nutrition Regimens

Burgess L, Morgan C, Mayes K, et al (Liverpool Women's Hosp, UK; Alder Hey Children's Hosp, Liverpool, UK)

JPEN J Parenter Enteral Nutr 38:243-253, 2014

Background.—Improving parenteral nutrition (PN) amino acid (AA) intake in very preterm infants is associated with less hyperglycemia. AAs stimulate newborn insulin secretion with arginine, demonstrating a specific effect. We hypothesized that low arginine levels would be associated with increased insulin-treated hyperglycemia and higher mean daily blood glucose levels in very preterm infants.

Methods.—We performed a secondary analysis on previous study data comparing high-protein/calorie PN (HPC-PN) and control groups in infants <29 weeks' gestation. Infants were substratified (within original groups) according to high (highARG) and low (lowARG) plasma arginine levels on days 8–10 using a reference population-derived threshold for high/low arginine (57 μmol/L). Daily protein, arginine, carbohydrate intake, mean daily blood glucose, and insulin treatment data from the first 15 days of life were collected.

Results.—Control group infants (n = 60) were stratified into lowARG (n = 41) and highARG (n = 19) groups. There were no differences in basic demographic data or carbohydrate intake. LowARG infants had higher mean daily blood glucose levels ($P < .05$) and a trend to more insulin treatment on days 6–10. HPC-PN group infants (n = 55) were stratified into lowARG (n = 33) and highARG (n = 22) groups. LowARG infants had lower gestation and birth weight and were sicker than highARG infants. There were no differences in carbohydrate intake. LowARG infants had higher mean daily blood glucose levels ($P < .01$) and more insulin treatment ($P < .01$) on days 1–5 and 6–10. Insulin-treated hyperglycemia was also associated with low plasma glutamine levels.

Conclusion.—Low plasma arginine levels (≤57 μmol/L) in very preterm infants are associated with poorer blood glucose control.

▶ It is well known that the administration of arginine increases plasma insulin levels, which leads to anabolism. It is less clear what a deficit in circulating arginine levels actually means physiologically to glucose metabolism. This study evaluated the relationship between plasma arginine levels and blood glucose levels and the need for insulin intervention in very low birth weight infants.

As pointed out by the authors, infants that had low plasma arginine levels also had higher plasma glucose levels and required more interventions with insulin administrations. This study suggests but does not prove that administration of greater amounts of arginine to low birth weight infants may be beneficial to plasma glucose control. Because arginine also stimulates human growth hormone, it may also be beneficial to the growth and development of these infants.

J. M. Daly, MD

Clinical Effects of Probiotic *Bifidobacterium longum* BB536 on Immune Function and Intestinal Microbiota in Elderly Patients Receiving Enteral Tube Feeding

Akatsu H, Iwabuchi N, Xiao J-Z, et al (Choju Med Inst, Toyohashi, Aichi, Japan; Morinaga Milk Industry Co, Ltd., Zama, Kanagawa, Japan; et al)
JPEN J Parenter Enteral Nutr 37:631-640, 2013

Background.—Immune system function declines with age. We evaluated the effects of supplementation with the probiotic *Bifidobacterium longum* BB536 on immune function and intestinal microbiota in the elderly.

Materials and Methods.—In a double-blind study, 45 elderly patients fed by enteral tube feeding (mean [SD] age 81.7 [8.7] years) were given BB536 (n = 23) or a placebo powder (n = 22) for 12 weeks and were observed for an additional 4 weeks posttreatment. At week 4, all patients received an influenza vaccination (A/H1N1, A/H3N2, and B). Clinical data were assessed, including body temperature, bowel movements, fecal microbiota, and immunological biomarkers in blood.

Results.—BB536 intake significantly increased cell numbers of bifidobacteria in fecal microbiota. There was a tendency toward an increase ($P = .085$ at week 4 and $P = .070$ at week 16) of serum IgA in the BB536 group compared with the placebo group. BB536 intake did not significantly affect hemagglutination inhibition (HI) titers in response to the influenza vaccine. Natural killer (NK) cell activity decreased significantly in the placebo group during the intervention but not in the BB536 group. Among those subjects with low NK cell activity (<55%, n = 10 for each group), a significant intergroup difference ($P < .05$) was observed in the changed values from baseline of NK cell activity at weeks 8 and 12.

Conclusions.—These results shed new light on the potential of long-term ingestion of BB536 in increasing the cell number of bifidobacteria in intestinal microbiota and modulating immune function in the elderly.

▶ Multiple approaches have been used to enhance the immune systems of individuals who are chronically immune-suppressed by factors such as age. In the elderly, it is critical to obtain the maximum response to administration of the influenza vaccine. In other studies, the use of the probiotic *Bifidobacterium longum* has been shown to enhance immune function. This randomized, controlled study of 45 elderly patients receiving tube feeding was done to evaluate the response to influenza vaccination after specific bacterial administration. Clearly, intestinal bacterial flora was changed in the experimental group, and immune responses to the vaccination seemed better. However, the numbers of patients were too small to obtain statistical significance between the 2 groups except for responses such as natural killer activity (questionable significance). Further work is necessary to determine if the authors' hypothesis is correct regarding administration of probiotics along with enteral feedings.

J. M. Daly, MD

A Protocol of Early Aggressive Acceleration of Tube Feeding Increases Ileus Without Perceptible Benefit in Severely Burned Patients

Kesey J, Dissanaike S (Univ Med Ctr, Lubbock, TX; Texas Tech Univ Health Sciences Ctr, Lubbock)

J Burn Care Res 34:515-520, 2013

Optimal nutrition is essential to the recovery of burned patients. The authors evaluated the efficacy of an aggressive nutrition delivery protocol. The following protocol was implemented: initiation of tube feeds within 4 hours, acceleration to goal rate within 8 hours, and tolerance of gastric residual volumes of 400 ml. Patients on the protocol formed the study group whereas patients admitted immediately before implementation served as controls for a study period of 7 days after admission. Outcome variables included ileus, prokinetic medication use, intensive care unit and overall length of stay, ventilator days and mortality. Variables were compared using bivariate analysis. The 42 study subjects and 34 controls were similar at baseline. Time to initiation was similar (6.8 vs 9.4 hours; $P = .226$), however, goal rate was achieved much sooner in the study group (11.2 vs 20.9 hours; $P < .001$). Number of hours spent at goal was different on days 1 and 2 (6.62 vs 2.74, $P = .003$ and 17.24 vs 13.18, $P = .032$) with no difference thereafter. Residual volumes in the study group were higher from day 2 onward, and remained increased throughout the study period (401 vs 234 ml average; $P = .449$). Clinical ileus was much more common in the study group (8 cases vs 1, $P = .037$). There was no difference in length of stay or mortality. The protocol was successfully implemented and resulted in early achievement of goal tube feed rates. However, this resulted in tube feed intolerance as manifested by more cases of clinical ileus.

► Patients with major burn injuries have significant catabolic issues, which last usually until their burn wounds are covered by skin and healed. Prior studies have found that early initiation of enteral tube feeding compared with later onset of feeding significantly improves the clinical outcomes of these patients. Unfortunately, often gastrointestinal intolerance occurs that limits the ability of caregivers to provide adequate nutrition early after injury. Intestinal ileus, gastric dyskinesia, and tracheal aspiration are major complications of aggressive enteral feeding attempts.

In this retrospective, cohort study, the authors found that aggressive initiation and progression of feeding led to improved administration of nutrients but also to increased gastric residual volumes. Because there were no differences in clinical outcomes comparing the 2 groups, use of the more aggressive nutrition protocol may not be worth the potential increased risk of gastric aspiration. It is apparent from this study that a multidisciplinary nutrition support team should manage enteral nutrition support in patients after major burn injury.

J. M. Daly, MD

A Disease-Specific Enteral Nutrition Formula Improves Nutritional Status and Functional Performance in Patients With Head and Neck and Esophageal Cancer Undergoing Chemoradiotherapy: Results of a Randomized, Controlled, Multicenter Trial

Fietkau R, Lewitzki V, Kuhnt T, et al (Erlangen Univ Hosp, Germany; Univ Hosp, Rostock, Germany; et al)

Cancer 119:3343-3353, 2013

Background.—In patients with head and neck and esophageal tumors, nutritional status may deteriorate during concurrent chemoradiotherapy (CRT). The aim of this study was to investigate the influence of enteral nutrition enriched with eicosapentaenoic acid (EPA) and docosahexaenoic acid (DHA) on body composition and nutritional and functional status.

Methods.—In a controlled, randomized, prospective, double-blind, multicenter study, 111 patients with head and neck and esophageal cancer undergoing concurrent CRT received either an enteral standard nutrition (control group) or disease-specific enteral nutrition Supportan®-containing EPA + DHA (experimental group) via percutaneous endoscopic gastrostomy. The primary endpoint was the change of body cell mass (BCM) following CRT at weeks 7 and 14 compared with the baseline value. Secondary endpoints were additional parameters of body composition, anthropometric parameters, and nutritional and functional status.

Results.—The primary endpoint of the study, improvement in BCM, reached borderline statistical significance. Following CRT, patients with experimental nutrition lost only 0.82 ± 0.64 kg of BCM compared with 2.82 ± 0.77 kg in the control group ($P = .055$). The objectively measured nutritional parameters, such as body weight and fat-free mass, showed a tendency toward improvement, but the differences were not significant. The subjective parameters, in particular the Kondrup score (P =.0165) and the subjective global assessment score (P =.0065) after follow-up improved significantly in the experimental group, compared with the control group. Both enteral regimens were safe and well tolerated.

Conclusion.—Enteral nutrition with EPA and DHA may be advantageous in patients with head and neck or esophageal cancer by improving parameters of nutritional and functional status during CRT.

▶ It has long been hypothesized that disease-specific nutritional formulae could be utilized to better improve nutritional outcomes in different groups of patients. Some nutritional formulae contain ingredients such as arginine to improve cell-mediated immunity in surgical patients. Other compositions use omega-3 fatty acids as supplements to alter the inflammatory responses to injury. In this randomized, controlled study, the authors used a formula supplemented with omega-3 fatty acids in patients undergoing radiation therapy for head and neck and esophageal cancers. They noted less weight loss (nearly statistically significant) in the supplemented group compared with the standard enteral nutrition group and significant differences in subjective measures (Kondrup and Subjective Global Assessment scores). It is important to note that nutritional therapy was administered by tube feeding in all patients. Sadly, to fully power the prospective study, 138 more patients would have been required for the second phase. Prospective, randomized studies such as these are very difficult and expensive to carry out, and the sponsor did not want to continue the trial. Nevertheless, there is interesting evidence now from several sources that disease-specific nutrition may be of benefit compared with standard enteral feeding. If the cost of nutritional intervention is similar, then there is little to argue with regarding its use in head and neck and esophageal cancer patients undergoing radiation treatment.

J. M. Daly, MD

Parenteral Fish Oil Lipid Emulsions in the Critically Ill: A Systematic Review and Meta-Analysis

Manzanares W, Dhaliwal R, Jurewitsch B, et al (Universidad de la República (UDELAR), Montevideo, Uruguay; Kingston General Hosp, Ontario, Canada; St Michael's Hosp and Univ of Toronto, Ontario, Canada; et al)
JPEN J Parenter Enteral Nutr 38:20-28, 2014

Introduction.—ω-3 Polyunsaturated fatty acids contained in fish oils (FO) possess major anti-inflammatory, antioxidant, and immunologic properties that could be beneficial during critical illness. We hypothesized that parenteral FO-containing emulsions may improve clinical outcomes in the critically ill.

Methods.—We searched computerized databases from 1980–2012. We included randomized controlled trials (RCTs) conducted in critically ill adult patients that evaluated FO-containing emulsions, either in the context of parenteral nutrition (PN) or enteral nutrition (EN).

Results.—A total of 6 RCTs (n = 390 patients) were included; the mean methodological score of all trials was 10 (range, 6–13). When the results of these studies were aggregated, FO-containing emulsions were associated with a trend toward a reduction in mortality (risk ratio [RR], 0.71; 95% confidence interval [CI], 0.49–1.04; $P = .08$; heterogeneity $I^2 = 0\%$) and a reduction in the duration of mechanical ventilation (weighted mean difference in days [WMD], −1.41; 95% CI, −3.43 to 0.61; $P = .17$). However, this strategy had no effect on infections (RR, 0.76; 95% CI, 0.42–1.36; $P = .35$) and intensive care unit length of stay (WMD, −0.46; 95% CI, −4.87 to 3.95; $P = .84$, heterogeneity $I^2 = 75\%$).

Conclusion.—FO-containing lipid emulsions may be able to decrease mortality and ventilation days in the critically ill. However, because of the paucity of clinical data, there is inadequate evidence to recommend the routine use of parenteral FO. Large, rigorously designed RCTs are required to elucidate the efficacy of parenteral FO in the critically ill.

▶ Use of ω-3 fatty acids in vitro changes cell lipid membrane composition, resulting in the production of less inflammatory cytokines in the case of macrophages and neutrophils. In vivo, diets high in fish oils have also been linked to a more suppressed inflammatory reactive state perhaps because of the same in vitro effects on inflammatory cells. Improved cardiovascular outcomes caused by anticoagulant and anti-inflammatory effects have been shown using diets high in fish oils. These diets as well as dietary fish oil supplements have been recommended in recent years for these reasons.

The authors evaluated 10 randomized, controlled, trials that sought to evaluate the effects of fish oil supplemented nutrition compared with nonsupplemented nutrition in critically ill patients. There were few significant differences between groups. This may be because of the duration of the feeding, the critical nature of the underlying illnesses, the amount of the ω-3 fatty acids given, and the fact that critical illness supersedes nutritional supplements. Nevertheless, further studies are needed before the routine use of fish oil–supplemented nutrition is recommended for hospitalized, critically ill patients.

J. M. Daly, MD

Use of Exclusive Enteral Nutrition Is Just as Effective as Corticosteroids in Newly Diagnosed Pediatric Crohn's Disease

Soo J, Malik BA, Turner JM, et al (Stollery Children's Hosp, Edmonton, Alberta, Canada)

Dig Dis Sci 58:3584-3591, 2013

Background.—The efficacy of exclusive enteral nutrition (EEN) in induction of remission in pediatric Crohn's disease (CD) is reported to be equivalent to that of corticosteroids (CS).

Aims.—Our objective was to compare the efficacy of EEN and CS in inducing remission in pediatric onset CD and the effects of the treatment on nutritional status and bone mineral density (BMD).

Methods.—Medical charts were retrospectively studied for patients diagnosed with CD between 2000 and 2010 at the Stollery children's hospital in Edmonton, Alberta. Anthropometric and dual-energy X-ray absorptiometry (DXA) data were collected to assess effects of therapy; clinical remission, relapse, and severity were defined on the basis of the pediatric Crohn's disease activity index.

Results.—To induce remission at first presentation, 36 patients (mean age 12.9 years) received EEN and 69 (mean age 11.2 years) received CS. Remission (88.9% in the EEN group versus 91.3% in the CS group ($p = 0.73$) at 3 months) and relapse (40.6 vs. 28.6%, respectively ($p = 0.12$) over 12 months) were similar in both treatment groups. Thirty-four patients had paired DXA scans at the time of diagnosis and one year later: 16 given EEN and 18 given CS. Change in BMD spine z-scores based on bone age adjusted for height and chronological age was greater for EEN patients but not statistically significant (Δz-score 0.30 vs. 0.03, $p = 0.28$).

Conclusions.—EEN has similar efficacy to corticosteroids; however, EEN may lead to better BMD accrual. EEN should be preferred to corticosteroids as first-line therapy for induction of remission in pediatric CD.

▶ Treatment of Crohn disease in children is problematic. Standard therapies include corticosteroids. However, starting in the 1970s, total parenteral nutrition was initiated in an effort to promote bowel rest. Early reports suggested benefit in terms of nutritional status of the children and avoidance of corticosteroids.

Later, enteral nutritional formulas (elemental vs special diets) were used in children to promote anabolism and growth while potentially reducing the dosage or use of steroids. In this article, Soo et al retrospectively reviewed 105 children with Crohn disease that were treated over a 10-year period. As noted, the rates of remission and relapse were similar between those given early enteral feeding compared with those given steroids.

One must view this as a possible association, as this was purely a retrospective review. Nevertheless, the article raises the question regarding the avoidance of steroids in the treatment of children with Crohn disease.

J. M. Daly, MD

Tolerability and Safety of Enteral Nutrition in Critically Ill Patients Receiving Intravenous Vasopressor Therapy

Mancl EE, Muzevich KM (Virginia Commonwealth Univ Health System, Richmond)

JPEN J Parenter Enteral Nutr 37:641-651, 2013

Background.—Enteral nutrition (EN) is recommended within the first 24-48 hours following admission to an intensive care unit (ICU) once resuscitation and hemodynamic stability have been achieved; however, hemodynamic stability is not well defined.

Objective.—To evaluate the tolerability and safety of EN in critically ill patients receiving intravenous (IV) vasopressor therapy.

Methods.—A retrospective medical record review was conducted in an urban academic medical center and included adult ICU patients from 2011 who received concomitant EN and IV vasopressor therapy for ≥1 hour. EN tolerance was defined as an absence of gastric residuals ≥300 mL, emesis, positive finding on abdominal imaging, and evidence of bowel ischemia/perforation.

Results.—Two hundred fifty-nine patients received 346 episodes of concomitant EN and IV vasopressor therapy. Overall EN tolerability was 74.9%. Adverse events included rising serum lactate (30.6%), elevated gastric residuals (14.5%), emesis (9.0%), positive finding on kidney/ureter/bladder radiograph (4.3%), and bowel ischemia/perforation (0.9%). An inverse relationship was found between maximum norepinephrine equivalent dose and EN tolerability (12.5 mcg/min for patients who tolerated EN vs 19.4 mcg/min, $P = .0009$). This relationship remained statistically significant after controlling for other variables ($P = .019$). Patients who tolerated EN were less likely to have received dopamine (63.8% vs 77.6%, $P = .018$) or vasopressin (58.9% vs 77.9%, $P = .0027$). These patients received concomitant therapy for less time and received more nutrition.

Conclusions.—Most patients receiving IV vasopressor therapy tolerate EN. Tolerability was related to the maximum cumulative vasopressor dose and may be related to the specific vasopressor administered.

▶ Use of enteral nutrition is an important adjunct in critically ill patients in the intensive care unit (ICU). It is often difficult to properly feed these patients because of diet tolerability. These patients are often receiving multiple medications, they may be in shock for at least a portion of their time in the ICU, and they require hemodynamic support pharmacologically. This retrospective report by Mancl et al is important because it focused on those 259 patients requiring vasopressin during their ICU stay and when the patients were receiving enteral feeding. Importantly, 75% of patients tolerated the feeding despite requiring vasopressin to support them hemodynamically. The most devastating complication, bowel ischemia and perforation, occurred in only 0.9% of patients in their series. Because of the size of their series, the authors were able to determine the average maximum tolerated norepinephrine equivalent dose (12.5 μg/min).

Despite its retrospective nature, the study provides important insights. It demonstrates that enteral feeding can continue in critically ill ICU patients with careful attention to detail despite administration of vasopressin. However, as the required dosage increases to provide better hemodynamic support, intolerability to tube feeding begins to occur.

J. M. Daly, MD

Impact of Early Parenteral Nutrition on Muscle and Adipose Tissue Compartments During Critical Illness

Casaer MP, Langouche L, Coudyzer W, et al (Univ Hosps Leuven, Belgium)
Crit Care Med 41:2298-2309, 2013

Objective.—The goal of enhanced nutrition in critically ill patients is to improve outcome by reducing lean tissue wasting. However, such effect has not been proven. This study aimed to assess the effect of early administration of parenteral nutrition on muscle volume and composition by repeated quantitative CT.

Design.—A preplanned substudy of a randomized controlled trial (Early Parenteral Nutrition Completing Enteral Nutrition in Adult Critically Ill Patients [EPaNIC]), which compared early initiation of parenteral nutrition when enteral nutrition was insufficient (*early parenteral nutrition*) with tolerating a pronounced nutritional deficit for 1 week in ICU (*late parenteral nutrition*). Late parenteral nutrition prevented infections and accelerated recovery.

Setting.—University hospital.

Patients.—Fifteen EPaNIC study neurosurgical patients requiring prescheduled repeated follow-up CT scans and six healthy volunteers matched for age, gender, and body mass index.

Intervention.—Repeated abdominal and femoral quantitative CT images were obtained in a standardized manner on median ICU day 2 (interquartile range, 2–3) and day 9 (interquartile range, 8–10). Intramuscular, subcutaneous, and visceral fat compartments were delineated manually. Muscle and adipose tissue volume and composition were quantified using standard Hounsfield Unit ranges.

Measurements and Main Results.—Critical illness evoked substantial loss of femoral muscle volume in 1 week's time, irrespective of the nutritional regimen. Early parenteral nutrition reduced the quality of the muscle tissue, as reflected by the attenuation, revealing increased intramuscular water/lipid content. Early parenteral nutrition also increased the volume of adipose tissue islets within the femoral muscle compartment. These changes in skeletal muscle quality correlated with caloric intake. In the abdominal muscle compartments, changes were similar, albeit smaller. Femoral and abdominal subcutaneous adipose tissue compartments were unaffected by disease and nutritional strategy.

Conclusions.—Early parenteral nutrition did not prevent the pronounced wasting of skeletal muscle observed over the first week of critical illness. Furthermore, early parenteral nutrition increased the amount of adipose tissue within the muscle compartments.

▶ Many studies have sought to evaluate the role of early parenteral nutrition in critically ill patients. Those patients in the intensive care unit suffering trauma or sepsis develop severe muscle wasting, and the theory has been that early initiation of parenteral nutrition might prevent much of this muscle wasting. Early studies have noted that early initiation of enteral nutrition has reduced the complications and mortality rates of burn patients compared with late initiation of enteral nutrition. Additional studies in different subsets of critically ill patients have supported this concept.

In this metabolic study, small numbers of patients were given early total parenteral nutrition (TPN) and were compared with those receiving late initiation of TPN. Normal volunteers acted as controls for the computed tomography scan determination of normal muscle composition. Results show that TPN alone does not improve muscle composition but does increase muscle accumulation of fat and water. These results are to be expected because although many have shown improved nitrogen balance in patients given TPN vs no feeding, it is unclear where the nitrogen is being used to maximum efficiency.

J. M. Daly, MD

Effect of Hyperalimentation and Insulin-Treated Hyperglycemia on Tyrosine Levels in Very Preterm Infants Receiving Parenteral Nutrition

Mayes K, Tan M, Morgan C (Alder Hey Childrens' Hosp, Liverpool, UK; Liverpool Women's Hosp, UK)

JPEN J Parenter Enteral Nutr 38:92-98, 2014

Background.—Hyperalimentation describes the increase in glucose, amino acids (AAs), and lipid intake designed to overcome postnatal growth failure in preterm infants. Preterm infants are dependent on phenylalanine metabolism to maintain tyrosine levels because of tyrosine concentration limits in parenteral nutrition (PN). We hypothesized that hyperalimentation would increase individual AA levels when compared with the control group but avoid high phenylalanine/tyrosine levels.

Aim.—To compare the plasma AA profiles on days 8–10 of life in preterm infants receiving a hyperalimentation vs a control regimen.

Methods.—Infants <29 weeks' gestation were randomized to receive hyperalimentation (30% more PN macronutrients) or a control regimen. Data were collected to measure macronutrient (including protein) intake and PN intolerance, including hyperglycemia, insulin use, urea, and AA profile. Plasma profiles of 23 individual AA levels were measured on days 8–10 using ion exchange chromatography.

Results.—One hundred forty-two infants were randomized with 118 AA profiles obtained on days 8–10. There were no differences in birth weight or gestation between groups. There was an increase ($P < .05$) in 8 of 23 median individual plasma AA levels when comparing hyperalimentation ($n = 57$) with controls ($n = 61$). Only tyrosine levels (median; interquartile range) were lower with hyperalimentation: 27 (15–52) μmol/L vs 43 (24–69) μmol/L ($P < .01$). Hyperalimentation resulted in more insulin-treated hyperglycemia. No difference between the groups was apparent in tyrosine levels when substratified for insulin-treated hyperglycemia. All insulin vs no insulin comparisons showed lower tyrosine levels with insulin treatment ($P < .01$).

Conclusion.—Hyperalimentation can result in paradoxically low plasma tyrosine levels associated with an increase in insulin-treated hyperglycemia.

▶ It has been more than 45 years since total parenteral nutrition was first used for the growth and development of infants, yet the best formulations of nutrients still elude investigators. Preterm infants are at risk for a variety of medical problems and, with so little reserve, require precise nutrient formulations to improve outcomes, reduce the incidence of fatty liver, and maximize growth potential. The authors evaluated hyperalimentation versus standard care in an attempt to determine whether amino acid supplementation would improve phenylalanine and tyrosine levels, which are critical to infants but not adults.

The authors noted that plasma tyrosine levels actually declined regardless of whether insulin was required to maintain euglycemia. The results of this clinical trial emphasize again the need for prospective randomized studies to obtain definitive results, leading to appropriate biological conclusions.

J. M. Daly, MD

Arginine appearance and nitric oxide synthesis in critically ill infants can be increased with a protein-energy–enriched enteral formula

de Betue CTI, Joosten KFM, Deutz NEP, et al (Maastricht Univ Med Ctr, Netherlands; Erasmus MC – Sophia Children's Hosp, Rotterdam, Netherlands; Texas A and M Univ, College Station)

Am J Clin Nutr 98:907-916, 2013

Background.—Arginine is considered an essential amino acid during critical illness in children, and supplementation of arginine has been proposed to improve arginine availability to facilitate nitric oxide (NO) synthesis. Protein-energy–enriched enteral formulas (PE-formulas) can improve nutrient intake and promote anabolism in critically ill infants. However, the effect of increased protein and energy intake on arginine metabolism is not known.

Objective.—We investigated the effect of a PE-formula compared with that of a standard infant formula (S-formula) on arginine kinetics in critically ill infants.

Design.—A 2-h stable-isotope tracer protocol was conducted in 2 groups of critically ill infants with respiratory failure because of viral bronchiolitis, who received either a PE-formula ($n = 8$) or S-formula ($n = 10$) in a randomized, blinded, controlled setting. Data were reported as means ± SDs.

Results.—The intake of a PE-formula in critically ill infants (aged 0.23 ± 0.14 y) resulted in an increased arginine appearance (PE-formula: 248 ± 114 μmol · kg^{-1} · h^{-1}; S-formula: 130 ± 53 μmol · kg^{-1} · h^{-1}; $P = 0.012$) and NO synthesis (PE-formula: 1.92 ± 0.99 μmol · kg^{-1} · h^{-1}; S-formula: 0.84 ± 0.36 μmol · kg^{-1} · h^{-1}; $P = 0.003$), whereas citrulline production and plasma arginine concentrations were unaffected.

Conclusion.—In critically ill infants with respiratory failure because of viral bronchiolitis, the intake of a PE-formula increases arginine availability by increasing arginine appearance, which leads to increased NO synthesis, independent of plasma arginine concentrations. This trial was registered at www.trialregister.nl as NTR515.

▶ The relationship of parenteral nutrients and their multiple biologic and pharmacologic effects is often unclear. For example, arginine is a nonessential amino acid but has been thought of as conditionally essential in children and adults during periods of critical illness. Its immunologic effects are to enhance the T-cell immune cascade, but it is also a precursor to nitrous/nitric oxide, a potent vasodilator and bronchodilator. This randomized, controlled study in critically ill children with viral bronchiolitis showed that increasing nutritional intake of protein and energy led to increasing arginine and nitric oxide appearance. It will be extremely valuable to understand if this increase actually had a beneficial effect on ventilatory patterns and oxygenation as well as on outcomes in these critically ill children. Finally, it will be important to understand the duration of this pharmacologic response to increased protein and energy in this population of critically ill children.

J. M. Daly, MD

Early Enteral Nutrition Prevents Intra-abdominal Hypertension and Reduces the Severity of Severe Acute Pancreatitis Compared with Delayed Enteral Nutrition: A Prospective Pilot Study

Sun J-K, Li W-Q, Ke L, et al (Nanjing Univ School of Medicine, Jiangsu Province, China)

World J Surg 37:2053-2060, 2013

Background.—To investigate the effects of early enteral nutrition (EEN) on intra-abdominal pressure (IAP) and disease severity in patients with severe acute pancreatitis (SAP).

Methods.—Enteral nutrition (EN) was started within 48 h after admission in the EEN group and from the 8th day in the delayed enteral nutrition (DEN) group. The IAP and intra-abdominal hypertension (IAH) incidence were recorded for 2 weeks. The caloric intake and feeding intolerance (FI) incidence were recorded daily after EN was started. The severity markers and clinical outcome variables were also recorded.

Results.—Sixty patients were enrolled to this study. No difference about IAP was found. The IAH incidence of the EEN group was significantly lower than that of the DEN group from the 9th day (8/30 versus 18/30; $P = 0.009$) after admission. The FI incidence of the EEN group was higher than that of the DEN group during the initial 3 days of feeding (25/30 versus 12/30; $P = 0.001$; 22/30 versus 9/30; $P = 0.001$; 15/30 versus 4/30; $P = 0.002$). Patients with an IAP < 15 mm Hg had lower FI incidence than those with an IAP ≥ 15 mmHg on the 1st day (20/22 versus 17/38; $P < 0.001$), the 3rd day (11/13 versus 8/47; $P < 0.001$), and the 7th day

(3/5 versus 3/55; $P = 0.005$) of feeding. The severity markers and clinical outcome variables of the EEN group were significantly improved.

Conclusions.—Early enteral nutrition did not increase IAP. In contrast, it might prevent the development of IAH. In addition, EEN might be not appropriate during the initial 3–4 days of SAP onset. Moreover, EN might be of benefit to patients with an IAP <15 mmHg. Early enteral nutrition could improve disease severity and clinical outcome, but did not decrease mortality of SAP.

▶ Since Alexander's groundbreaking work using early enteral nutrition in burn patients, many studies have attempted to replicate the beneficial effects of early enteral nutrition. This randomized, controlled study used early enteral nutrition compared with delayed enteral nutrition in 60 very ill patients with severe acute pancreatitis. Appropriately, they sought to evaluate physiologic effects such as intra-abdominal pressures (IAP), intra-abdominal hypertension (IAH), and tolerance. Intuition would have suggested that early enteral nutrition would increase IAP and IAH, yet the authors found just the opposite. However, tolerance was better in the group that received delayed enteral nutrition. Unfortunately, this methodology did not improve mortality rates. Clearly, further work is needed, perhaps in a multicenter trial with hundreds of patients, to determine the potential outcome benefits of this modified approach to enteral feeding.

J. M. Daly, MD

Enhanced Protein-Energy Provision via the Enteral Route Feeding Protocol in Critically Ill Patients: Results of a Cluster Randomized Trial

Heyland DK, Murch L, Cahill N, et al (Kingston General Hosp, Ontario, Canada; et al)

Crit Care Med 41:2743-2753, 2013

Objectives.—To determine the effect of the enhanced protein-energy provision via the enteral route feeding protocol, combined with a nursing educational intervention on nutritional intake, compared to usual care.

Design.—Prospective, cluster randomized trial.

Setting.—Eighteen ICUs from United States and Canada with low baseline nutritional adequacy.

Patients.—One thousand fifty-nine mechanically ventilated, critically ill patients.

Interventions.—A novel feeding protocol combined with a nursing educational intervention.

Measurements and Main Results.—The two primary efficacy outcomes were the proportion of the protein and energy prescriptions received by study patients via the enteral route over the first 12 days in the ICU. Safety outcomes were the prevalence of vomiting, witnessed aspiration, and ICU-acquired pneumonia. The proportion of prescribed protein and energy delivered by enteral nutrition was greater in the intervention sites compared to the control sites. Adjusted absolute mean difference between groups in the protein and energy increases were 14% (95% CI, 5–23%; $p = 0.005$) and 12% (95% CI, 5–20%; $p = 0.004$), respectively. The intervention sites had a similar improvement in protein and calories when appropriate parenteral nutrition was added to enteral sources. Use of the enhanced protein-energy provision via the enteral route feeding protocol was associated with a decrease in the average time from ICU admission to start of enteral nutrition compared to the control group (40.7–29.7 hr vs 33.6–35.2 hr, $p = 0.10$). Complication rates were no different between the two groups.

Conclusions.—In ICUs with low baseline nutritional adequacy, use of the enhanced protein-energy provision via the enteral route feeding protocol is safe and results in modest but statistically significant increases in protein and calorie intake.

▶ Appropriate use of parenteral nutrition in surgical and medical intensive care units (ICUs) is absolutely necessary to prevent complications and to maximize the efficacy of such feeding. This is important because many studies have looked at the adverse consequences of hyperglycemia and the benefits and problems of early nutritional intervention in critically ill patients. In addition to evaluating nutrient formulations, it is important to understand the team of health care providers in the ICU with regard to their knowledge and diligence in the provision of total parenteral nutrition.

This interesting study used a cluster design in 18 ICUs gathering data for more than 1000 patients. The authors concluded that patient safety was improved and that earlier initiation of parenteral nutrition could be achieved.

Overall outcomes were similar between groups. The lack of differences in overall outcomes is not surprising given that the nutritional support is meant to "support" the patient and not specifically to treat the critical illness. A knowledgeable (nutrition support) team of health care providers is important to improve the safety of parenteral nutrition administration in critically ill patients.

J. M. Daly, MD

Clinical and Immunological Impact of Early Postoperative Enteral Immunonutrition After Total Gastrectomy in Gastric Cancer Patients: A Prospective Randomized Study

Marano L, Porfidia R, Pezzella M, et al (Second Univ of Naples, Italy)

Ann Surg Oncol 20:3912-3918, 2013

Background.—Enteral immunodiet has been gaining increasing attention, but experimental data of its clinical effects in patients with gastric cancer are inconsistent, contradictory, and poorly investigated. The aim of this study was to assess the impact of early postoperative enteral immunonutrition on clinical and immunological outcomes in a homogeneous group of gastric cancer patients submitted to total gastrectomy.

Methods.—A total of 109 patients with gastric cancer were randomized to receive early postoperative enteral immunonutrition (formula supplemented with arginine, omega-3 fatty acids and ribonucleic acid [RNA]), or an isocaloric–isonitrogenous control. The postoperative outcome was evaluated based on clinical variables, including postoperative infectious complications, anastomotic leak rate, and length of hospitalization. In addition, state of cellular immunity was evaluated and compared between the 2 groups.

Results.—The incidence of postoperative infectious complications in the immunodiet group (7.4%) was significantly ($p < .05$) lower than that of the control group (20%), as well as the anastomotic leak rate (3.7% in immunodiet group vs 7.3% in standard nutrition group, $p < .05$). Mortality rate did not show any significant differences; patients of the immunodiet group were found to have a significantly reduced length of hospitalization (12.7 ± 2.3 days) when compared with standard diet group (15.9 ± 3.4 days, $p = .029$). The data on cellular immunity showed that the postoperative $CD4^+$ T-cell counts decreased in both groups, but the reduction in the IED group was significantly higher ($p = .032$) compared with the SND group.

Conclusions.—Early postoperative enteral immunonutrition significantly improves clinical and immunological outcomes in patients undergoing gastrectomy for gastric cancer.

▶ In the last 20 years, there has been a marked shift in concepts of nutritional support from providing nutrition with standard formulations to controlled clinical trials evaluating the pharmacologic effects of individual nutrients and their biologic and clinical outcomes. Nutrients such as arginine, glutamine, omega-3 fatty acids, RNA, and others have been studied. *Immunonutrition* is a term coined by Alexander and refers to nutrients administered in larger-than-normal amounts in an effort to improve clinical outcomes. He showed that such nutrition could improve outcomes in burn patients. Daly[1] and others also showed an improvement in clinical outcomes in patients with upper gastrointestinal cancers that underwent operative resection. This study showed similar benefits to an arginine-enriched diet in a homogenous group of gastric cancer patients. At this time, the evidence of multiple trials recommends the use of immunonutrition in these elective surgery patients.

J. M. Daly, MD

Reference

1. Daly JM, Lieberman MD, Goldfine J, et al. Enteral nutrition with supplemental arginine RNA and Omega-3 fatty acids in postoperative patients: Immunologic, metabolic and clinical outcome. *Surgery.* 1992;112:56-67.

Enteral L-Arginine Supplementation for Prevention of Necrotizing Enterocolitis in Very Low Birth Weight Neonates: A Double-Blind Randomized Pilot Study of Efficacy and Safety

Polycarpou E, Zachaki S, Tsolia M, et al (General District Hosp Athens "Alexandra," Greece; Athens Univ, Greece)

JPEN J Parenter Enteral Nutr 37:617-622, 2013

Background.—Necrotizing enterocolitis (NEC) is the most common acquired gastrointestinal disease in premature infants and has high mortality and morbidity. Endothelial nitric oxide is an important regulator of vascular perfusion and is synthetized from the amino acid L-arginine. Hypoargininemia is frequently observed in preterm neonates and may predispose them to NEC. Our objective was to determine the effect of enteral L-arginine supplementation on the incidence and severity of NEC in very low birth weight (VLBW) neonates.

Materials and Methods.—We conducted a parallel blind randomized pilot study, comprising VLBW neonates with birth weight ≤1500 g and gestational age ≤34 weeks. VLBW neonates were randomly assigned to receive enteral L-arginine supplementation (1.5 mmol/kg/d bid) between the 3rd and 28th day of life or placebo. Diagnosis and classification of NEC were done according to modified Bell's criteria.

Results.—Eighty-three neonates were randomized to the arginine ($n = 40$) or placebo ($n = 43$) group. No adverse effects were observed in neonates receiving L-arginine supplementation. The incidence of NEC stage III was significantly lower in the arginine-supplemented group (2.5% vs 18.6%, $P = .030$).

Conclusions.—Enteral L-arginine supplementation of 1.5 mmol/kg/d bid can be safely administered in VLBW neonates from the 3rd to the 28th day of life. Enteral L-arginine supplementation appears to reduce the incidence of stage III NEC in VLBW infants. Larger studies are needed to further evaluate the effect of L-arginine supplementation in preventing NEC in VLBW infants.

► Arginine supplementation is thought to have major biological effects on wound healing, t-cell immune function, macrophage functions, and increased nitric oxide production with consequent vasodilation. As pointed out by the authors, necrotizing enterocolitis (NEC) is a common and terrible illness in preterm infants, leading to high mortality rates.

They hypothesized that use of L-arginine supplementation would increase nitric oxide production and improve the vascular supply to the colon, perhaps reducing the incidence of NEC.

This randomized, prospective trial engaged 83 preterm infants with or without L-arginine supplementation at 1.5 mmol/kg/d twice a day. Importantly, the incidence of NEC decreased from 19% to 2.5%, a significant reduction in these infants.

If these results are borne out by further studies, a new standard of care for preterm infants will have been developed that should markedly improve the outcomes for these often very ill infants. Prevention of enterocolitis is a major step forward in neonatology.

J. M. Daly, MD

Early Enteral Fat Supplement and Fish Oil Increases Fat Absorption in the Premature Infant with an Enterostomy

Yang Q, Ayers K, Chen Y, et al (Wake Forest Univ Health Science, Winston-Salem, NC)

J Pediatr 163:429-434, 2013

Objective.—To test the hypothesis that in the premature infant with an enterostomy, early enteral supplementation with Microlipid (fat supplement) and fish oil increases enteral fat absorption and decreases the requirement for Intralipid (intravenous fat emulsion).

Study Design.—Premature infants (<2 months old) with an enterostomy after surgical treatment for necrotizing enterocolitis or spontaneous intestinal perforation and tolerating enteral feeding at 20 mL/kg/day were randomized to usual care (control 18 infants) or early supplementing enteral fat and fish oil (treatment 18 infants). Intravenous fat emulsion was decreased as enteral fat intake was increased. Daily weight, ostomy output, and nutrition data were recorded. Weekly 24-hour ostomy effluent was collected until bowel reanastomosis, and fecal fat, fecal liquid, and dry feces were measured. Fat absorption (g/kg/d) was calculated by subtracting fecal fat from dietary fat. The fecal liquid and dry feces were reported as mg/g wet stool. Date were analyzed by using ANOVA and mixed-effects model.

Results.—The interval from initial postoperative feeding to bowel reanastomosis varied from 2 to 10 weeks. The treatment group received more dietary fat and less intravenous fat emulsion and had higher enteral fat absorption, less fecal liquid, and drier feces than the control group. These effects were greater among infants with a high ostomy compared with those with a low ostomy. Enteral fat intake was significantly correlated with fat absorption.

Conclusion.—Early enteral fat supplement and fish oil increases fat absorption and decreases the requirement for intravenous fat emulsion. This approach could be used to promote bowel adaptation and reduce the use of intravenous fat emulsion in the premature infant with an enterostomy.

► It has been assumed that oral administration of fatty acid supplements would dramatically increase fecal fat levels and result in fecal losses of water and electrolytes. The authors tested these assumptions in a prospective randomized trial in infants requiring parenteral nutrition. These infants had enterostomies that allowed for enteral feeding as well. Those infants randomized to enteral fat supplements had their intravenous lipid emulsions reduced as the enteral fat intake was increased.

Interestingly, as the enteral fat supplements were increased, the infants had less fecal liquid and drier feces compared with controls. Those infants with a high ostomy had a greater chance of better fat absorption and better outcomes in terms of enteral intake. These results should lead to a greater use of enteral fat supplements and perhaps less steatohepatitis in such infants. Further studies are necessary to prove this theory, however.

J. M. Daly, MD

Minimizing unnecessary parenteral nutrition after appendectomy in children

Bell R, Betts J, Idowu O, et al (Children's Hosp and Res Ctr at Oakland, CA)
J Surg Res 184:164-168, 2013

Background.—Consensus guidelines have indicated that postoperative parenteral nutrition (PN) might provide benefit when patients are expected to be nil per os (NPO) ≥7 d and when PN is administered ≥5 d. We hypothesized that most children receiving PN after appendectomy do not satisfy these criteria.

Methods.—The medical records of the patients who had undergone appendectomy for perforated appendicitis from 2006-2011 were analyzed, and the proportion meeting the criteria for beneficial PN was determined. The clinical parameters independently associated with the criteria for beneficial PN (PN therapy ≥5 d, ileus ≥5 d, NPO ≥7 d) were identified using multiple regression analysis.

Results.—A total of 1612 patients were treated for appendicitis. Of these, 587 met the inclusion criteria (age < 16 y, perforated appendicitis, appendectomy within 24 h, no previous indication for PN). Of the 587 patients, 12.1% received PN; 43.8% of these received PN for ≥5 d. The predictors of PN duration of ≥5 d included preoperative symptoms for ≥3 d ($P < 0.01$) and initiation of PN by postoperative day 3 ($P = 0.047$). Preoperative symptoms for ≥3 d, imaging showing a discrete abscess or bowel obstruction, and operative findings of diffuse peritonitis predicted ileus of ≥5 d and NPO of ≥7 d ($P < 0.01$ for all). Major complications were more common in patients with ileus lasting ≥5 d.

Conclusions.—Fewer than one-half of patients receiving PN in the present cohort met the consensus-based guidelines for postoperative PN. The preoperative symptom duration, preoperative imaging findings demonstrating abscess and/or bowel obstruction, and intraoperative findings of diffuse peritonitis might predict prolonged ileus and longer recovery periods for children undergoing surgery for perforated appendicitis.

► Generally, nutritional support is thought to be beneficial after 5 days of inadequate nutritional intake. Children have less of a safety net than adults, however. This retrospective study sought to understand the use of parenteral nutrition in children undergoing appendectomy. As expected, those children suffering from intestinal ileus after 5 days postoperatively had more severe illness with intra-abdominal abscesses, peritonitis, and perforated appendicitis. They also had greater postoperative complications.

Because of the retrospective nature of the study, it is impossible to understand the true benefits of parenteral nutrition, but there appeared to be few complications of this intervention. If one uses generally accepted indications for initiation of parenteral nutrition, then at least 50% of the children did not meet these criteria, suggesting that parenteral nutrition was overused. The results of this study further emphasize that nutritional protocols can be very useful to more properly allocate resources when it comes to nutritional support.

J. M. Daly, MD

Multiple Micronutrient Deficiencies among Patients with Intestinal Failure during and after Transition to Enteral Nutrition

Ubesie AC, Kocoshis SA, Mezoff AG, et al (Cincinnati Children's Hosp Med Ctr, OH)

J Pediatr 163:1692-1696, 2013

Objectives.—To determine the prevalence of deficiencies of specific micronutrients (iron, zinc, magnesium, phosphorus, selenium, copper, folate, and vitamins A, D, E, and B12) in children with intestinal failure (IF), and to identify risk factors associated with developing these deficiencies.

Study Design.—This study was a retrospective review of prospectively collected data from 178 children with IF managed by the Intestinal Care Center of Cincinnati Children's Hospital Medical Center between August 1, 2007, and July 31, 2012. Transition to full enteral nutrition (FEN) was defined as the period during which the patient received between 20% and 100% of estimated required nutrition enterally. FEN was defined as the patient's ability to tolerate 100% estimated required nutrition enterally for >2 weeks.

Results.—Necrotizing enterocolitis was the most common cause of IF (27.5%). Iron was the most common micronutrient deficiency identified both during (83.9%) and after (61%) successful transition to FEN, with a significant reduction in the percentage of patients with iron deficiency between these 2 periods ($P = .003$). Predictors of micronutrient deficiency after successful transition to FEN included birth weight ($P = .03$), weight percentile ($P = .02$), height percentile ($P = .04$), and duration of parenteral nutrition (PN) ($P = .013$). After multivariate adjustments, only duration of PN remained statistically significant ($P = .03$).

Conclusion.—Micronutrient deficiencies persist in patients with IF during and after transition to FEN. These data support the need for routine monitoring and supplementation of these patients, especially those on prolonged PN.

▶ The requirements for protein, fat, and carbohydrate in the composition of total parenteral nutrition (TPN) of adults and children are quite clear. The exact requirements for micronutrients are somewhat controversial. This is an excellent study in that the data were collected prospectively and then retrospectively reviewed to determine the effect of long-term TPN in children with intestinal failure on micronutrient deficiencies. As noted by the authors, iron deficiency was the most common problem in these children as they transitioned to full enteral nutrition, but other deficiencies were also identified. The duration of TPN was the most significant factor associated with micronutrient deficiency.

Thus, it appears that not only should children be more closely monitored for micronutrient deficiencies, but that transition to enteral nutrition should occur at the earliest time.

J. M. Daly, MD

Body composition in paediatric intestinal failure patients receiving long-term parenteral nutrition

Pichler J, Chomtho S, Fewtrell M, et al (Med Univ Vienna, Austria; UCL Inst of Child Health, UK; et al)

Arch Dis Child 99:147-153, 2014

Objective.—Outcome of children with intestinal failure (IF) has improved on treatment with parenteral nutrition (PN). The effects of PN and IF on body composition (BC) are unknown. The aim was to review BC in PN-treated children and those weaned off and to compare with reference data.

Design.—Children on long-term/home PN underwent measurement of regional fat mass (FM) and lean mass (LM) using dual energy X-ray absorptiometry. Underlying diseases were intestinal enteropathy, n = 15, short bowel syndrome (SBS), n = 8 and intestinal dysmotility, n = 11. PN duration was median 10 years. Fat Mass Index (FMI) and Lean Mass Index (LMI) were compared in children with and without intestinal inflammation, steroid treatment and according to PN dependency.

Results.—34 children aged 5–20 years were studied. They were short, mean height SD score (SDS) −1.8 ($p < 0.001$) and light (mean weight SDS −0.86, $p < 0.001$) with high body mass index (BMI) SDS: mean 0.4 ($p = 0.04$) and low Limb LMI SDS −0.9 ($p < 0.001$). Children with SBS had low FMI SDS −0.8 ($p = 0.01$). BC did not significantly differ between diagnostic groups or with steroid treatment. Patients with intestinal inflammation (n = 20) had higher BMI SDS than those without, $p = 0.007$. Totally, PN-dependent children, n = 11 had higher BMI SDS, $p = 0.004$, total body FMI SDS, $p = 0.008$ and trunk FMI SDS, $p = 0.001$ compared with patients partially dependent and off PN.

Conclusions.—Significantly low limb LM was seen in all patient groups with high FM in children on total PN. Children with IF requiring PN treatment > 27 days may benefit from BC monitoring and PN adjustment according to results in order to maximise linear growth and health in later life.

▶ It is extremely important to monitor growth rates in children and particularly to measure body compositional changes in children receiving home parenteral nutrition. Unfortunately, to date, there have been little long-term data to evaluate the nutritional effectiveness of long-term nutritional support. This study by Pichler et al provides the opportunity to compare growth rates and body compositional changes over a median duration of 10 years. As noted by the authors, complete dependence on home total parenteral nutrition led to increased regional fat mass and lower lean limb muscle mass. However, it must be remembered that those requiring complete dependence on home total parenteral nutrition because of intestinal failure generally have more advanced disease. They may not have as much physical exercise because of their primary disease processes, which would then influence their body composition by decreasing lean body mass and increasing fat mass, as caloric intake remains elevated. One wonders if a physical therapy program tailored to each child's abilities should be a major part of their home parenteral nutrition program. It is unclear that simply changing the nutritional regimen would alter these compositional changes. This study provides an important benchmark for future reference for home TPN in children.

J. M. Daly, MD

Protocol-Driven Enteral Nutrition in Critically Ill Children: A Systematic Review

Wong JJ-M, Ong C, Han WM, et al (KK Women's and Children's Hosp, Singapore)

JPEN J Parenter Enteral Nutr 38:29-39, 2014

Enteral nutrition (EN) protocols are thought to improve clinical outcomes in the pediatric intensive care unit (PICU); however, critical evaluation of their efficacy is limited. We conducted a systematic review with the aim of assessing the effect of EN protocols on important clinical outcomes in these children. We searched MEDLINE, Cochrane Database for Reviews, Embase, and CINAHL using predetermined keywords and MESH terms. We included randomized controlled trials (RCTs) and observational studies that involved EN protocols in children admitted to the PICU for >24 hours. We included studies that reported at least 1 of our outcomes of interest. Studies that exclusively studied premature neonates or adults were excluded. Primary outcomes were PICU or hospital mortality, PICU or hospital length of stay (LOS), duration of mechanical ventilation, gastrointestinal (GI) complications, and infective complications. Secondary outcomes were time to initiate feeds and time to achieve goal feeds. In total, we included 9 studies (total 1564 children) in our systematic review (1 RCT, 4 before-and-after studies, 1 single-arm cohort study, 1 prospective descriptive study, and 2 audits). There is low-level evidence that the use of EN protocols is associated with a reduction in GI and infective complications and improved timeliness of feed initiation and achievement of goal feeds. Current medical literature does not have compelling data on the effects of an EN protocol on clinical outcomes among critically ill children. Future clinical trials should look into using standardized interventions and outcome measures to strengthen the existing evidence.

▶ It seems clear that the use of standardized protocols improves the outcomes of patients with a variety of diseases and medical interventions. The use of total parenteral nutrition (TPN) is no exception. In this meta-analysis of 9 studies in more than 1500 pediatric patients, the use of standardized protocols was associated with significant reductions in infectious and gastrointestinal complications. Because the adequate provision of nutrients is the goal of TPN, it was valuable to see that protocols improved the initiation of TPN and advancement to goal feedings. TPN should be used whenever adequate enteral nutrition cannot be done. In general, the children that receive TPN are ill, and it is critical to avoid any complications with its use.

Thus, it is important to incorporate the results of this study into our daily practices and develop and use standardized protocols for the use of TPN, improving the quality of our care for these patients.

J. M. Daly, MD

Lack of Preoperative Enteral Nutrition Reduces Gut-Associated Lymphoid Cell Numbers in Colon Cancer Patients: A Possible Mechanism Underlying Increased Postoperative Infectious Complications During Parenteral Nutrition

Okamoto K, Fukatsu K, Hashiguchi Y, et al (Natl Defense Med College, Saitama, Japan; Univ of Tokyo, Japan; Teikyo Univ School of Medicine, Tokyo, Japan; et al)

Ann Surg 258:1059-1064, 2013

Objective.—To examine preoperative dietary influences on gut-associated lymphoid tissue (GALT) cell number in the context of postoperative infectious complications.

Background.—There is little clinical evidence regarding whether nutritional routes affect GALT size and/or phenotype. The influence of GALT atrophy on clinical outcomes is also unclear.

Method.—Patients with complete obstruction of the colon due to a tumor were excluded from this study. Study 1. Resected terminal ileum specimens, from 62 patients [preoperative parenteral nutrition (PN): n = 15, preoperative oral feeding (OF): n = 47] who underwent right colectomy during the period from 1997 to 2004 at our department, were immunohistochemically stained for counting numbers of T, IgA-producing, and mature and immature dendritic cells (DCs) in the lamina propria (LP) and intraepithelial space.

Study 2. We reviewed 341 patients (PN: n = 99, OF: n = 242) with colon cancer who underwent colectomy during this period for postoperative complications.

Results.—Study 1. T cell numbers in the LP and intraepithelial space and IgA-producing cell number in the LP were significantly lower in the PN than in the OF group. Mature DC number in the LP was significantly lower in the PN than in the OF group, whereas total DC numbers (both mature and immature DC) were similar in the 2 groups.

Study 2. The PN group had significantly higher rates of total infectious complications, surgical site infection, pneumonia, infectious colitis, and central venous catheter infection.

Conclusions.—Lack of enteral delivery of nutrients reduces numbers of T and IgA-producing cells, as well as mature DCs, in GALT of colon cancer patients, as it does in animal models. A close association between GALT changes and infectious complication morbidity was confirmed.

▶ The importance of the gut-associated lymphoid tissue system within the small intestine (predominantly the terminal ileum) to the postoperative infectious outcomes in surgical patients is unclear. This retrospective study evaluated 15 patients that received preoperative parenteral nutrition compared with 42 patients that had received oral nutrition before operation. Samples of terminal ileum were evaluated histologically. The parenteral nutrition group had lower T-cell and dendritic cell numbers than the orally fed group. The authors then retrospectively studied 341 patients and found greater infectious complications compared with the orally fed group.

This study suffers from its retrospective nature and the lack of truly comparable controls (why did patients receive TPN in the preoperative period?). However, as many have stated previously, it is important to maintain the intestine structure (gross and histologic) and function by oral feeding if possible before operation.

J. M. Daly, MD

Serial Transverse Enteroplasty Allows Children with Short Bowel to Wean from Parenteral Nutrition

Mercer DF, Hobson BD, Gerhardt BK, et al (Univ of Nebraska Med Ctr, Omaha)
J Pediatr 164:93-98, 2014

Objective.—To analyze the effects of serial transverse enteroplasty (STEP) on parenteral and enteral calories in children with short bowel syndrome, and examine short- and long-term complications.

Study Design.—A retrospective analysis of prospectively-collected data from a large single center cohort of patients undergoing STEP procedure was analyzed. Baseline demographic and clinical information, operative data, and short- and long-term complications were recorded. Detailed growth and nutritional data were obtained for 6 months prior and 12 months following STEP procedure.

Results.—Sixty-eight procedures were performed in 51 patients over a 68-month period. Median bowel length at first STEP was 51 cm with a median length gain of 54%. Repeat STEP patients had longer initial length (77 cm) and reduced length gain (20%). Operative times and blood loss were low, with few complications. Parenteral calorie requirement was stable or rising for 6 months prior to STEP, but decreased to median <20 kCal/kg/d at 1 year postop. Longer length gains were associated with higher risk of stricture formation. Seven children were transplanted, and 60% of nontransplanted children were enterally independent, with the remainder making ongoing progress; 48/51 children are alive at a median of 39 months follow-up.

Conclusions.—STEP is shown to be safe, well tolerated, and to have definitive benefit in reducing parenteral calorie requirements over the first year following the procedure. It has an important role in achieving enteral independence in children with short bowel syndrome.

▶ We have seen previously how important it is to wean children suffering from short bowel syndrome and intestinal failure from long-term total parenteral nutrition support. Otherwise, patients totally dependent on parenteral nutrition suffer from both metabolic and infectious complications of long-term intravenous catheterization. In this retrospective study, a surgical intervention (serial transverse enteroplasty [STEP]) was evaluated as to its ability to help lengthen the small intestine, allowing for better enteral nutrition. It is clear that the first STEP procedure has the best chance of creating greater lengthening of the bowel compared with a repeat STEP procedure, but problems of stricture formation occurred. Importantly, however, the procedure decreased the need for total parenteral nutrition, leading to a greater chance of enteral nutritional independence.

Long-term evaluation of these children is critical to determine the most effective timing and completeness of surgical interventions such as STEP procedures.

J. M. Daly, MD

Effect of intravenous lipid emulsion in patients with acute glyphosate intoxication

Gil H-W, Park J-S, Park S-H, et al (Soonchunhyang Univ Cheonan Hosp, Republic of Korea)

Clin Toxicol 51:767-771, 2013

Background.—Although glyphosate intoxication has been considered minimally toxic in animals, severe toxicity has been observed in humans due to surfactant. We aimed to examine the potential therapeutic effects of intravenous lipid emulsion (ILE) on the patients with acute glyphosate intoxication.

Methods.—This study enrolled 64 glyphosate-intoxicated patients with allocation to two groups: those treated with ILE (ILE group, $n = 22$), and control patients treated with only supportive (conservative) care. Control patients were selected by matching for the amount ingested and time since ingestion. Twenty-two control patients were separately selected from the 42 patients receiving supportive care only. In ILE group, 20% lipid emulsion product was injected intravenously at the rate of 20 mL/h for the patients who ingested less than 100 ml of glyphosate. In the patients who ingested more than 100 ml of glyphosate, the loading dose was 500 ml for 2–3 h according to the status of the patients, followed by a maintenance dose of 1000 ml for the next 24 h.

Results.—Thirteen patients received high dose of ILE because the ingestion amount was more than 100 ml. None of the ILE group suffered from the complication of hypotension, while approximately 41% of the control group developed the complication. Additionally, arrhythmia was not observed in the ILE group. The incidence of mental change, respiratory failure, and acute kidney injury was similar between the two groups.

Conclusions.—ILE administration was associated with lower incidence of hypotension and arrhythmia in patients with acute glyphosate intoxication. ILE administration seems to be an effective treatment modality in patients who ingested sufficient amount of glyphosate herbicide that is expected to bring about significant toxicity.

▶ Glyphosate is the most common herbicide used worldwide. Apparently, glyphosate intoxication occurs with some frequency, and the results can be devastating with hypotension, renal and respiratory failure, metabolic acidosis, and other adverse effects, which may lead to death. Case reports have suggested that intravenous lipid infusions may be of benefit acutely because of the lipid interactions with glyphosate and surfactant. This prospective study evaluated 64 patients who ingested glyphosate in an effort to commit suicide. After gastric lavage and resuscitation, which was done in all patients, 22 individuals received intravenous lipid emulsion infusions (ILE). Importantly, those treated with the ILE showed less hypotension and fewer arrhythmias but did not appreciably improve the other adverse effects of the glyphosate.

Treatment with intravenous lipid emulsions appears to be an important modality along with immediate gastric lavage, physiologic support, and intensive monitoring. It appears most useful in those individuals that ingested more than 100 mL of glyphosate.

J. M. Daly, MD

Physical and Cognitive Performance of Patients with Acute Lung Injury 1 Year after Initial Trophic versus Full Enteral Feeding: EDEN Trial Follow-up

Needham DM, for the NIH NHLBI ARDS Network (Johns Hopkins Univ, Baltimore, MD; et al)

Am J Respir Crit Care Med 188:567-576, 2013

Rationale.—We hypothesized that providing patients with acute lung injury two different protein/calorie nutritional strategies in the intensive care unit may affect longer-term physical and cognitive performance.

Objectives.—To assess physical and cognitive performance 6 and 12 months after acute lung injury, and to evaluate the effect of trophic versus full enteral feeding, provided for the first 6 days of mechanical ventilation, on 6-minute-walk distance, cognitive impairment, and secondary outcomes.

Methods.—A prospective, longitudinal ancillary study of the ARDS Network EDEN trial evaluating 174 consecutive survivors from 5 of 12 centers. Blinded assessments of patients' arm anthropometrics, strength, pulmonary function, 6-minute-walk distance, and cognitive status (executive function, language, memory, verbal reasoning/concept formation, and attention) were performed.

Measurements and Main Results.—At 6 and 12 months, respectively, the mean (SD) percent predicted for 6-minute-walk distance was 64% (22%) and 66% (25%) ($P = 0.011$ for difference between assessments), and 36 and 25% of survivors had cognitive impairment ($P = 0.001$). Patients performed below predicted values for secondary physical tests with small improvement from 6 to 12 months. There was no significant effect of initial trophic versus full feeding for the first 6 days after randomization on survivors' percent predicted for 6-minutewalk distance, cognitive impairment status, and all secondary outcomes.

Conclusions.—EDEN trial survivors performed below predicted values for physical and cognitive performance at 6 and 12 months, with some improvement over time. Initial trophic versus full enteral feeding for the first 6 days after randomization did not affect physical and cognitive performance.

▶ This interesting prospective longitudinal study evaluated the effects of trophic feeding (400 kcal/d) versus full feeding (1300 kcal/d) for the first 6 days or until extubation, whichever came first in 174 consecutive survivors of acute lung injury. After this period, those receiving 400 kcal/d were switched to full feeding of 1300 kcal/d. Survivors had physical and cognitive studies performed at later time periods. As noted, there were few differences between the groups at the time periods measured in either cognitive or physical attributes.

I applaud the authors for the long-term evaluation of survivors in terms of the physical and cognitive consequences of hospital treatment of acute lung injury because these results provide benchmarks for all who treat these very ill patients. However, it would be very unlikely that an average difference of 5400 kcal administered over 6 days would change the physical and cognitive outcomes of survivors 6 and 12 months after injury.

J. M. Daly, MD

Variation in Feeding Practices following the Norwood Procedure

Lambert LM, for the Pediatric Heart Network Investigators (Primary Children's Med Ctr, Salt Lake City, UT; et al)

J Pediatr 164:237-242.e1, 2014

Objectives.—To assess variation in feeding practice at hospital discharge after the Norwood procedure, factors associated with tube feeding, and associations among site, feeding mode, and growth before stage II.

Study Design.—From May 2005 to July 2008, 555 subjects from 15 centers were enrolled in the Pediatric Heart Network Single Ventricle Reconstruction Trial; 432 survivors with feeding data at hospital discharge after the Norwood procedure were analyzed.

Results.—Demographic and clinical variables were compared among 4 feeding modes: oral only (n = 140), oral/tube (n = 195), nasogastric tube (N-tube) only (n = 40), and gastrostomy tube (G-tube) only (n = 57). There was significant variation in feeding mode among sites (oral only 0%-81% and G-tube only 0%-56%, $P < .01$). After adjusting for site, multivariable modeling showed G-tube feeding at discharge was associated with longer hospitalization, and N-tube feeding was associated with greater number of discharge medications ($R^2 = 0.65$, $P < .01$). After adjusting for site, mean pre–stage II weight-for-age *z*-score was significantly higher in the oral-only group (−1.4) vs the N-tube–only (−2.2) and G-tube-only (−2.1) groups ($P = .04$ and.02, respectively).

Conclusions.—Feeding mode at hospital discharge after the Norwood procedure varied among sites. Prolonged hospitalization and greater number of medications at the time of discharge were associated with tube feeding. Infants exclusively fed orally had a higher weight-for-age *z* score pre–stage II than those fed exclusively by tube. Exploring strategies to prevent morbidities and promote oral feeding in this highest risk population is warranted.

▶ It is often valuable to review practices in an attempt to define best practices—those that are associated with the highest quality of care. In this instance, the authors reviewed feeding practices in 432 children discharged from the hospital after major cardiac surgery (Norwood procedure). As expected, those children that were healthiest at discharge were able to eat and sustain themselves. Their average body weight for age was the best, and they required fewer medications. The sickest children who were going to require long-term enteral nutritional support required placement of a gastrostomy tube for support. They required a longer length of hospital stay. What this study underlines is that there is no single method for nutritionally supporting children at the time of discharge from the hospital. One chooses the best method calibrated to the anticipated duration needed for artificial feeding.

J. M. Daly, MD

The Association Between Home Parenteral Nutrition and Patients With FAP-Associated Intra-Abdominal Desmoids: A Retrospective Study

Shatnawei A, Habib M, Hamilton C, et al (The Cleveland Clinic, OH)

JPEN J Parenter Enteral Nutr 37:683-688, 2013

Background.—Intra-abdominal desmoid tumors (IADTs) are a common complication of familial adenomatous polyposis (FAP). Treatment is not standardized for advanced disease. Medical and surgical treatments may be ineffective in preventing complications, which can cause intestinal failure. Home parenteral nutrition (HPN) can be a life-saving treatment in these patients. The aim of this study was to investigate the association with HPN in FAP-IADTs.

Methods.—A retrospective review of FAP patients with IADTs at the Cleveland Clinic (CC) between 1980 and 2009 was performed. Patients and tumor characteristics were retrieved from the CC Jagelman Registry for Inherited Neoplasms and CC HPN database. Inclusion criteria were FAP-IADTs and 6-month follow up at CC. Exclusion criteria were <6-month follow-up, lack of 3-dimensional lesion or sheet desmoid, and/or incomplete medical records. Kaplan-Meier curves were analyzed for HPN and non-HPN groups.

Results.—One hundred fifty-four patients were included and divided into 2 groups: HPN (n = 41, 26.6%) and non-HPN (n = 113, 73.4%). The HPN group was more likely to have advanced-stage disease and significantly higher incidence of chronic abdominal pain, narcotic dependency, bowel obstruction, ureteral obstruction, deep vein thrombosis, pulmonary embolism, fistulae, and sepsis ($P < .05$). The need for HPN represented a strong predictor of mortality (5-year survival HPN = 72% vs non-HPN = 95%), but duration of HPN did not affect mortality.

Conclusion.—HPN, although a life-saving treatment, is an independent poor prognostic factor associated with high morbidity and mortality.

▶ It was in the 1970s that the first patient with short gut syndrome caused by a complete resection of an abdominal mesenteric desmoid tumor was reported. She required home total parenteral nutrition (TPN) and was never able to live independent of her home TPN. Ultimately, she died of sepsis secondary to multiple central venous catheterizations and inability to continue her home TPN. In this report from an institution with perhaps the largest series of patients having intra-abdominal desmoid tumors, home TPN was required in 41 of 154 patients. As expected, there were greater complications in the group requiring home TPN compared with those on oral diets primarily because of the extent of their disease and the complications associated with their lack of small intestine.

Previous work has shown the efficacy of administering growth hormone, glutamine, and other substances in an effort to enhance the adaptability of the small intestine after major resection and diminish the continued requirement of home TPN.

Thus, home TPN is life saving, but further work is required to enable these patients to ultimately support themselves independent of home TPN.

J. M. Daly, MD

Alternative lipid emulsions in the critically ill: a systematic review of the evidence

Manzanares W, Dhaliwal R, Jurewitsch B, et al (Universidad de la República (UDELAR), Montevideo, Uruguay; Kingston General Hosp, Ontario, Canada; St Michael's Hosp and Univ of Toronto, Ontario, Canada; et al)
Intensive Care Med 39:1683-1694, 2013

Purpose.—Parenteral lipid emulsions (LEs) are commonly rich in long-chain triglycerides derived from soybean oil (SO). SO-containing emulsions may promote systemic inflammation and therefore may adversely affect clinical outcomes. We hypothesized that alternative oil-based LEs (SO-sparing strategies) may improve clinical outcomes in critically ill adult patients compared to products containing SO emulsion only. The purpose of this systematic review was to evaluate the effect of parenteral SO-sparing strategies on clinical outcomes in intensive care unit (ICU) patients.

Methods.—We searched computerized databases from 1980 to 2013. We included randomized controlled trials (RCTs) conducted in critically ill adult patients that evaluated SO-sparing strategies versus SO-based LEs in the context of parenteral nutrition.

Results.—A total of 12 RCTs met the inclusion criteria. When the results of these RCTs were statistically aggregated, SO-sparing strategies were associated with clinically important reductions in mortality (risk ratio, RR 0.83; 95 % confidence intervals, CI 0.62, 1.11; $P = 0.20$), in duration of ventilation (weighted mean difference, WMD −2.57; 95 % CI −5.51, 0.37; $P = 0.09$), and in ICU length of stay (LOS) (WMD −2.31; 95 % CI −5.28, 0.66; $P = 0.13$) but none of these differences were statistically significant. SO-sparing strategies had no effect on infectious complications (RR 1.13; 95 % CI 0.87, 1.46; $P = 0.35$).

Conclusion.—Alternative oil-based LEs may be associated with clinically important reductions in mortality, duration of ventilation, and ICU LOS but lack of statistical precision precludes any clinical recommendations at this time. Further research is warranted to confirm these potential positive treatment effects.

▶ Since 1967 when Stanley Dudrick and colleagues reported the use of total parenteral nutrition in humans providing nutrients for growth and development during bowel rest, many types of solutions have been studied in an attempt to maximize nutritional and metabolic benefits, enhance the immune system, and decrease the inflammatory response to autoimmune diseases, trauma, and systemic infection. This report depicts a meta-analysis of 12 randomized, controlled human studies evaluating the type of lipid emulsion infused in an effort to decrease the inflammatory response. Others have used omega-3 fatty acid–enriched solutions to diminish the inflammatory response to the omega-6 fatty acids commonly in use. This report, evaluating many randomized studies, notes a significant reduction in mortality and duration in ventilation requirements with the use of nonsoybean lipid emulsion solutions.

I agree with the authors that further studies are indicated in critically ill intensive care unit patients to improve their outcomes.

J. M. Daly, MD

Postoperative Enteral Nutrition Improves Survival After Orthotopic Small Bowel Transplantation in Mice

Wang J, Li Y, Li J (Nanjing Univ School of Medicine, China)
Transplant Proc 45:2543-2545, 2013

Background.—The aim of this study was to assess the effect postoperative enteral nutrition support on the survival after orthotopic small bowel transplantation in mice.

Methods.—A model of orthotopic small bowel transplantation used C57BL/6 mice as both donors and recipients.

Results.—We demonstrated that postoperative ileus was the deciding complication after transplantation. Postoperative enteral nutritional support resolved this problem and significantly improved survival and growth rates after transplantation.

Conclusion.—These data suggest the importance of routine nutritional support after orthotopic small bowel transplantation in mice.

► Small bowel transplantation has come a long way in the treatment of those with short bowel syndrome and intestinal failure. There is some trepidation in providing early enteral nutritional support in these patients because of potential infectious and motility complications after transplant. Thus, it can be valuable to evaluate an animal model to determine the potential benefits or harm that might ensue with this approach. Because of denervation, small intestinal ileus is a common problem in patients and also in this mouse model. Interestingly, in this mouse model, ileus was reduced, and weight gain was promoted when enteral nutrition was supplied after small bowel transplantation. It is as though the provision of liquid nutrition within the small bowel not only did not stress the bowel but promoted proper peristaltic activity. Studies such as these provide some value, but the concepts must be tested carefully in humans before we can be sure of these results.

J. M. Daly, MD

Circadian Rhythm of Energy Expenditure and Oxygen Consumption

Leuck M, Levandovski R, Harb A, et al (Laboratiório de Cronobiologia Hospital de Clinicas de Porto Alegre (HCPA)/Universidade Federal do Rio Grande do Sul (UFRGS), Porto Alegre, Brazil)

JPEN J Parenter Enteral Nutr 38:263-268, 2014

Background.—This study aimed to evaluate the effect of continuous and intermittent methods of enteral nutrition (EN) administration on circadian rhythm.

Materials and Methods.—Thirty-four individuals, aged between 52 and 80 years, were fed through a nasoenteric tube. Fifteen individuals received a continuous infusion for 24 hours/d, and 19 received an intermittent infusion in comparable quantities, every 4 hours from 8:00 to 20:00. In each patient, 4 indirect calorimetric measurements were carried out over 24 hours (A: 7:30, B: 10:30, C: 14:30, and D: 21:30) for 3 days.

Results.—Energy expenditure and oxygen consumption were significantly higher in the intermittent group than in the continuous group (1782 ± 862 vs 1478 ± 817 kcal/24 hours, $P = .05$; 257 ± 125 vs 212 ± 117 mL/min, $P = .048$, respectively). The intermittent group had higher levels of energy expenditure and oxygen consumption at all the measured time points compared with the continuous group. Energy expenditure and oxygen consumption in both groups were significantly different throughout the day for 3 days.

Conclusion.—There is circadian rhythm variation of energy expenditure and oxygen consumption with continuous and intermittent infusion for EN. This suggests that only one indirect daily calorimetric measurement is not able to show the patient's true needs. Energy expenditure is higher at night with both food administration methods. Moreover, energy expenditure and oxygen consumption are higher with the intermittent administration method at all times.

▶ The role of feeding in daily energy expenditure is unclear. Standard regular diets are given 3 to 4 times per day. Enteral feeding given via tubes can be administered either continuously or intermittently. This prospective, randomized trial in 34 subjects sought to understand the differences in energy expenditure comparing these 2 methods of feeding. As noted previously, energy expenditure was greater at night than during the day. In addition, average energy expenditure was greater with intermittent feeding compared with continuous feeding. Part of the explanation may be in the hormonal milieu that continuous feeding creates compared with intermittent feeding. This hormonal milieu is not limited simply to insulin and glucagon but includes cortisol and the epinephrine metabolites, which may be elevated by intermittent feeding compared with continuous feeding. Thus, it would be valuable to test this hypothesis by measuring those hormones that can be affected by the type, method, and duration of enteral feeding.

J. M. Daly, MD

Tube Feeding Increases the Gastric-Emptying Rate Determined by Gastroesophageal Scintigraphy

Chen W, Codreanu I, Yang J, et al (Univ of Pennsylvania School of Medicine, Philadelphia)

Clin Nucl Med 38:962-965, 2013

Objective.—The aim of this study was to determine whether tube feeding affects the rate of gastric emptying determined by gastroesophageal reflux scintigraphy in pediatric patients.

Methods.—Gastroesophageal reflux scintigraphy studies of 700 pediatric patients aged 1 week to 16 years were retrospectively analyzed. From these, 350 subjects received their study meal via a feeding tube, and 350 subjects received their meal as oral feeding. Gastric-emptying rate at 60 minutes was calculated, and the results compared. Stratification analysis for age, sex, and type and volume of administered meal was also performed.

Results.—The average rate of the gastric emptying was higher in the tube feeding compared with oral feeding group (52.9% ± 17.9% vs 44.2% ± 15.1% gastric emptying at 1 hour, $P < 0.01$). The prevalence of fast gastric emptying, defined as greater than 50% emptying at 60 minutes, was also higher in the tube feeding group, being registered in 59.7% (209/350 cases) versus only 31.4% (110/350 cases) in the oral feeding group, $P < 0.01$. The difference persisted following stratification analysis for sex, age, and type and volume of ingested meal.

Conclusions.—Our findings show that tube feeding increases the rate of gastric emptying determined by gastroesophageal reflux scintigraphy in pediatric patients. The effect proved independent on such factors as sex, age, and type or volume of ingested meal.

▶ It is important to understand the physiologic responses to oral and tube feeding to determine whether such responses in individual patients are abnormal. In this study, Chen et al evaluated 700 pediatric patients who had undergone a gastric scintigraphy study evaluating gastric emptying. As noted, tube feeding was associated with faster emptying times compared with oral feeding.

It is uncertain why this difference in gastric emptying occurred, as several other factors were stratified and analyzed and did not provide answers. Was it because tube feeding is usually continuous and oral feeding is intermittent? Thus, the stomach is used to having liquid diets in the former and more solid diets in the latter, which require more gastric peristalsis to break up the food to pass onward to the duodenum. The answers are unclear from this report, but the study does provide important benchmarks on average gastric emptying times for children fed orally or by tube.

J. M. Daly, MD

10 Gastrointestinal

Patient perspectives on postoperative visits after common general operative procedures

Wright GP, Wolf AM, Ambrosi G, et al (Grand Rapids Med Education Partners/ Michigan State Univ General Surgery Residency Program; Michigan State Univ College of Human Medicine, Grand Rapids; et al)

Surgery 154:934-940, 2013

Background.—Many postoperative concerns after common general operative procedures may be addressed over the phone, thereby saving time and resources for both the patient and surgeon.

Methods.—Over a 6-month time period, patients who underwent laparoscopic cholecystectomy, appendectomy for uncomplicated appendicitis, and inguinal or umbilical hernia repair were mailed an anonymous survey. The primary outcome measure was whether or not patients felt their concerns could have been addressed adequately over the phone in place of an office visit.

Results.—A total of 1,406 surveys were mailed with 339 responses (24%: 174 laparoscopic cholecystectomy, 83 inguinal hernia, 41 appendectomy, and 41 umbilical hernia). One hundred twelve (33%) felt their concerns could have been addressed adequately over the phone without an office visit. Patients who spent less time with their doctor at the appointment favored telephone follow-up ($P < .001$). Patients undergoing inguinal hernia were less interested in telephone follow-up compared with laparoscopic cholecystectomy (15% vs 41%; $P < .001$), appendectomy (15% vs 34%; $P = .018$), and umbilical hernia (15% vs 37%; $P = .010$). Of 66 patients (20%) with self-reported complications, 44% sought care from a healthcare provider other than their primary surgeon.

Conclusion.—These observations are important for healthcare organizations seeking to maximize surgeon efficiency while improving patient satisfaction.

► Resources for the treatment of our patients are limited, and we have moved toward physician extenders providing significant portions of care. General surgeons perform a fair number of low-risk, high-volume procedures that may be amenable to alternate care models. As part of our postoperative management and obligation, we have always and traditionally seen our patients in the clinic 1 to 3 weeks after the procedure or discharge. This group investigated the concept of a phone call postoperative check rather than an actual visit in the clinic. About one-third of patients felt this was acceptable, and many of these actually preferred this. Types of operations included in this study were laparoscopic cholecystectomy, appendectomy, and inguinal/umbilical hernia repair. Inguinal hernia repair patients largely resisted the concept of the phone postoperative visit, but the others were amenable to this. The fear of this approach is that complications may be missed with just a simple phone call. But it is likely that appropriate and validated scripts could be developed to mitigate this risk. If one-third of your patients could simply have a phone call from a nurse that was trained in this approach and agreed to this care model, significant time would open in your clinic schedule and in your week. This concept may save health care dollars and may become a necessity as more patients come into the system with the roll out of the Affordable Care Act.

J. Hines, MD

A Trial of Intraoperative Low-Tidal-Volume Ventilation in Abdominal Surgery

Futier E, for the IMPROVE Study Group (Hôpital Estaing, Clermont-Ferrand, France; et al)

N Engl J Med 369:428-437, 2013

Background.—Lung-protective ventilation with the use of low tidal volumes and positive end-expiratory pressure is considered best practice in the care of many critically ill patients. However, its role in anesthetized patients undergoing major surgery is not known.

Methods.—In this multicenter, double-blind, parallel-group trial, we randomly assigned 400 adults at intermediate to high risk of pulmonary complications after major abdominal surgery to either nonprotective mechanical ventilation or a strategy of lung-protective ventilation. The primary outcome was a composite of major pulmonary and extrapulmonary complications occurring within the first 7 days after surgery.

Results.—The two intervention groups had similar characteristics at baseline. In the intention-to-treat analysis, the primary outcome occurred in 21 of 200 patients (10.5%) assigned to lung-protective ventilation, as compared with 55 of 200 (27.5%) assigned to nonprotective ventilation (relative risk, 0.40; 95% confidence interval [CI], 0.24 to 0.68; $P = 0.001$). Over the 7-day postoperative period, 10 patients (5.0%) assigned to lung-protective ventilation required noninvasive ventilation or intubation for acute respiratory failure, as compared with 34 (17.0%) assigned to nonprotective ventilation (relative risk, 0.29; 95% CI, 0.14 to 0.61; $P = 0.001$). The length of the hospital stay was shorter among patients receiving lung-protective ventilation than among those receiving nonprotective ventilation (mean difference, −2.45 days; 95% CI, −4.17 to −0.72; $P = 0.006$).

Conclusions.—As compared with a practice of nonprotective mechanical ventilation, the use of a lung-protective ventilation strategy in intermediate-risk and high-risk patients undergoing major abdominal surgery was associated with improved clinical outcomes and reduced health

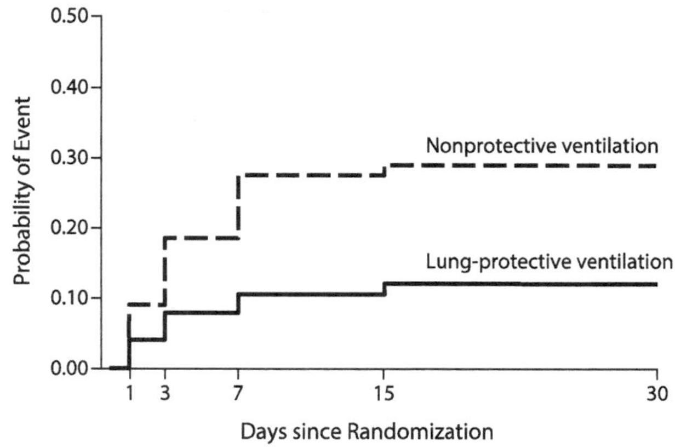

No. at Risk						
Nonprotective ventilation	200	182	163	145	142	142
Lung-protective ventilation	200	192	184	179	176	175

FIGURE 2.—Kaplan–Meier Estimates of the Probability of the Composite Primary Outcome. Data for the Kaplan–Meier estimates of the probability of the composite primary outcome of major pulmonary or extrapulmonary complications were censored at 30 days after surgery. Major pulmonary complications included pneumonia or the need for invasive or noninvasive ventilation for acute respiratory failure. Major extrapulmonary complications were sepsis, severe sepsis, septic shock, and death. $P < 0.001$ by the log-rank test for the between-group difference in the probability of the primary outcome. (Reprinted from Futier E, for the IMPROVE Study Group. A trial of intraoperative low-tidal-volume ventilation in abdominal surgery. *N Engl J Med.* 2013;369:428-437, Copyright 2013, with permission from Massachusetts Medical Society.)

care utilization. (IMPROVE ClinicalTrials.gov number, NCT01282996) (Fig 2).

▶ A team approach to patient care has been embraced across the country,[1] and this study may be a good way for us to build our quality improvement efforts with our anesthesia colleagues. The Intraoperative Protective Ventilation (IMPROVE) trial from France randomly assigned patients undergoing abdominal surgery to traditional high-tidal volume ventilation or low-tidal ventilation with positive end-expiratory pressure (PEEP) during surgery. These patients were undergoing procedures lasting more than 2 hours with a body mass index (BMI) less than 35 and a concern for postoperative pulmonary complications as determined by defined criteria. The concept of low-tidal ventilation has proven to be effective in the intensive care unit (ICU) setting and now is routinely used. The advantages in the ICU probably also exist for intraoperative ventilator support by reducing alveolar overstretching and the resultant lung injury and extrapulmonary dysfunction mediated by inflammatory proteins. In this study, those patients assigned the low-tidal volumes with PEEP had a lower respiratory and overall complication rate (Fig 2). What's more, there was a 3-fold increased need for noninvasive ventilation or intubation for acute respiratory failure among patients receiving traditional high-volume ventilation. These compelling results were found despite no relevant differences between the 2 groups with regard to gas exchange after extubation and on the first postoperative day. Overall, mortality rates were similar between the 2 groups (3% vs 3.5%), but the number of hospital days was nearly 2.5 days shorter in the low tidal volume group. The findings from this study will likely have immediate effects on our patient population. I plan to bring these findings to our anesthesia team and help facilitate a change in intraoperative ventilator management for our patients.

J. Hines, MD

Reference

1. Putensen C, Theuerkauf N, Zinserling J, Wrigge H, Pelosi P. Meta-analysis: ventilation strategies and outcomes of the acute respiratory distress syndrome and acute lung injury. *Ann Intern Med.* 2009;151:566-576.

Current Treatment and Outcome of Esophageal Perforations in Adults: Systematic Review and Meta-Analysis of 75 Studies

Biancari F, D'Andrea V, Paone R, et al (Oulu Univ Hosp, Finland; Univ of Rome "La Sapienza", Italy; et al)

World J Surg 37:1051-1059, 2013

Background.—The current prognosis of esophageal perforation and the efficacy of available treatment methods are not well defined.

Methods.—We performed a systematic review of esophageal perforations published from January 2000 to April 2012 and subjected a proportion of the retrieved data to a meta-analysis. Meta-regression was performed to determine predictors of mortality immediately after esophageal perforation.

Results.—Analysis of 75 studies resulted in a pooled mortality of 11.9 % [95 % confidence interval (CI) 9.7–14.3: 75 studies with 2,971 patients] with a mean hospital stay of 32.9 days (95 % CI 16.9–48.9: 28 studies with 1,233 patients). Cervical perforations had a pooled mortality of 5.9 %, thoracic perforations 10.9 %, and intraabdominal perforations 13.2 %. Mortality after esophageal perforation secondary to foreign bodies was 2.1 %, iatrogenic perforation 13.2 %, and spontaneous perforation 14.8 %. Treatment started within 24 h after the event resulted in a mortality rate of 7.4 % compared with 20.3 % in patients treated later (risk ratio 2.279, 95 % CI 1.632–3.182). Primary repair was associated with a pooled mortality of 9.5 %, esophagectomy 13.8 %, T-tube or any other tube repair 20.0 %, and stent-grafting 7.3 %.

Conclusions.—Results of recent studies indicate that mortality after esophageal perforation is high despite any definitive surgical or conservative strategy. Stent-grafting is associated with somewhat lower mortality rates, but studies may be biased by patient selection and limited experience.

▶ Esophageal perforations are one of the most challenging issues surgeons care for, and the outcomes are potentially fatal. The esophagus is a complex organ because it traverses 3 defined body compartments, each of which have different considerations, surgical approaches, and management options. To more reliably guide us on this condition, the authors have performed a review and meta-analysis of the published series with esophageal perforation. Patients with cervical perforations did better than patients with thoracic and abdominal perforations. Patients managed early (within 24 hours) had a much better outcome than those whose intervention was initiated after this period. Managing these conditions with a drain or T tube is probably not the best choice because 1 in 5 of these patients died. If your local gastroenterologist has the experience and supplies, it appears that esophageal stenting may offer the best outcome, with a mortality of 1 in 14. If this is not available, then primary repair should be the operative choice. The authors did note that these cases are relatively uncommon, with approximately 4 per year among the institutions that reported. It is probably less common at your hospital, which means we simply do not have a lot of experience with esophageal perforation. Early resuscitation, support of the systemic inflammatory response, antibiotics, and closure are the tricks for a reasonable outcome.

J. Hines, MD

Hospital volume, proportion resected and mortality from oesophageal and gastric cancer: a population-based study in England, 2004–2008

Coupland VH, Lagergren J, Lüchtenborg M, et al (King's College London, UK; et al)

Gut 62:961-966, 2013

Objective.—This study assessed the associations between hospital volume, resection rate and survival of oesophageal and gastric cancer patients in England.

Design.—62 811 patients diagnosed with oesophageal or gastric cancer between 2004 and 2008 were identified from a national population-based cancer registration and Hospital Episode Statistics-linked dataset. Cox regression analyses were used to assess all-cause mortality according to hospital volume and resection rate, adjusting for case-mix variables (sex, age, socioeconomic deprivation, comorbidity and type of cancer). HRs and 95% CIs, according to hospital volume, were evaluated for three predefined periods following surgery: <30, 30-365, and >365 days. Analysis of mortality in relation to resection rate was performed among all patients and among the 13 189 (21%) resected patients.

Results.—Increasing hospital volume was associated with lower mortality ($p_{trend} = 0.0001$; HR 0.87, 95% CI 0.79 to 0.95 for hospitals resecting 80+ and compared with <20 patients a year). In relative terms, the association between increasing hospital volume and lower mortality was particularly strong in the first 30 days following surgery ($p_{trend} < 0.0001$; HR 0.52, (0.39 to 0.70)), but a clinically relevant association remained beyond 1 year ($p_{trend} = 0.0011$; HR 0.82, (0.72 to 0.95)). Increasing resection rates were associated with lower mortality among all patients ($p_{trend} < 0.0001$; HR 0.86, (0.84 to 0.89) for the highest, compared with the lowest resection quintile).

Conclusions.—With evidence of lower short-term and longer-term mortality for patients resected in high-volume hospitals, this study supports further centralisation of oesophageal and gastric cancer surgical services in England.

▶ This report reinforces data from the United States that suggests that surgical volume impacts both perioperative and long-term survival for patients undergoing resection for esophageal or gastric cancer. Over a 5-year period ending in 2008, just more than 60 000 patients were diagnosed with these conditions in England. About one-third underwent resection. Centers with higher volumes (> 80 procedures per year) had lower perioperative mortality (4.1 vs 7.3%). The risk of dying over the ensuing 5 years was lower at these high-volume centers (61% vs 69%).

Why have so many studies made this association between volume and outcome? Hospital volume may be an indicator of local resources, but may also reflect referral patterns that influence outcomes. Also, higher volumes could improve the processes of care along defined protocols in a multidisciplinary approach, further the experience in managing postoperative complications, and increase the technical experience of surgeons in performing complex esophageal and gastric cancer surgery. Such factors may contribute to the lower postoperative mortality in high-volume hospitals.

The authors note a curious trend in England of an 8% decrease in resection for curative intent between 1998 and 2005.[1] Whether this is caused by changes in treatment algorithms with new drugs, shrinking resources and physician expertise, or a shift in the disease itself is not delineated.

J. Hines, MD

Reference

1. Palser T, Cromwell D, Van der Meulen J, et al. *National Oesophago-Gastric Cancer Audit: an Audit of the Care Received by People with Oesophago-Gastric Cancer in England and Wales. First Annual Report 2008.* London: The NHS Information Centre; 2008.

A Decade Analysis of Trends and Outcomes of Partial Versus Total Esophagectomy in the United States

Jafari MD, Halabi WJ, Smith BR, et al (Univ of California, Orange)

Ann Surg 258:450-458, 2013

Objective.—To examine the trends and outcomes of partial esophagectomy with an intrathoracic anastomosis compared with total esophagectomy with a cervical anastomosis.

Background.—Controversy exists regarding the optimal surgical approach in the management of esophageal cancer.

Methods.—Using the Nationwide Inpatient Sample database, yearly trends of patients with esophageal cancer who underwent partial and total esophagectomy were analyzed. Multivariate logistic regression analysis was used to analyze serious morbidity and in-hospital mortality between partial and total esophagectomy. In addition, outcomes were analyzed according to hospital volume, with *low-volume centers* defined as those with fewer than 10 cases per year and *high-volume centers* as those with 10 or more cases per year.

Results.—Between 2001 and 2010, 15,190 esophagectomies were performed for cancer. There was an overall increase in the number of esophagectomy procedures performed (1402 to 1975), with a concomitant reduction in the mortality rate (8.3% to 4.2%), particularly for partial esophagectomy. Partial esophagectomy was the predominant operation (76%). Most operations were performed at low-volume centers (62%), with a recent shift of cases to high-volume center. Compared with total esophagectomy, partial esophagectomy was associated with a shorter length of hospital stay (16 ± 6 vs 19 ± 9 days; $P < 0.05$), a lower in-hospital mortality rate (5.8% vs 8.3%; $P < 0.05$), and a lower hospital charge ($119,339 vs $138,496; $P < 0.05$). On multivariate regression analysis, total esophagectomy was associated with higher serious morbidity (odds ratio, 1.39; $P < 0.01$) and in-hospital mortality (odds ratio, 1.67; $P = 0.03$). There were no significant differences in risk-adjusted outcomes between low-volume centers and high-volume center.

Conclusions.—The number of esophagectomies performed for esophageal cancer has increased over the past decade accompanied by an overall reduction in mortality, particularly for the partial esophagectomy approach. The predominant operation in the United States continues to be partial esophagectomy with an intrathoracic anastomosis, which was associated with lower morbidity and in-hospital mortality than total esophagectomy. Hospital volume at a threshold of 10 cases per year was not a predictor of outcome.

▶ No doubt the evaluation, treatment, surgical management, and postoperative care of patients undergoing an esophagectomy require diligence, resources, and expertise. There are several techniques and approaches for this procedure, and the advantages of each is not completely clear. This recent analysis using the National Inpatient Sample database evaluates the safety of partial vs total esophagectomy and includes more than 15 000 patients during a 10-year period ending in 2010. Overall, the study found rates of mortality decreasing over the period and that a partial esophagectomy was safer than a total esophagectomy. These findings are not particularly surprising, but the authors did find that the outcomes there were no different between the low- and high-volume hospitals. This article was presented at the annual American Surgical Association meeting, and a fair amount of discussion focused on the definition of a high-volume center. In this study, a high-volume center was defined as one with 10 or more esophagectomies per year. Many studies that have been published on this subject set the volume cutoff at 30 cases each year. These studies have confirmed an advantage with regard to morbidity and mortality when this more stringent definition is applied. If you are performing esophagectomy in your practice and the outcomes are good, the best advice is to stay with your current techniques rather than change course and risk a higher morbidity and mortality rate for your patients.

J. Hines, MD

Outcomes After Laparoscopic or Open Distal Gastrectomy for Early-Stage Gastric Cancer: A Propensity-Matched Analysis

Yasunaga H, Horiguchi H, Kuwabara K, et al (The Univ of Tokyo, Japan; Kyushu Univ, Fukuoka, Japan; et al)

Ann Surg 257:640-646, 2013

Objective.—In a large nationwide administrative database of hospitalized patients, we investigated postoperative outcomes after laparoscopic or open distal gastrectomy in Japan.

Background.—The benefits of laparoscopic gastrectomy, such as decreased length of stay and morbidity, have typically been evaluated only with limited data on the basis of small samples.

Methods.—Using the Japanese Diagnosis Procedure Combination Database, we identified 9388 patients who were preoperatively diagnosed with stage I and II gastric cancer and underwent laparoscopic (n = 3937) or open (n = 5451) distal gastrectomy between July and December 2010. One-to-one propensity score matching was performed to compare in-hospital mortality, postoperative complication rates, length of stay, total costs, and 30-day readmission rates between the 2 groups.

Results.—Patients with younger age, lower comorbidity index, or stage I cancer were more likely to receive laparoscopic gastrectomy. In the propensity-matched analysis with 2473 pairs, the laparoscopic gastrectomy group in comparison with the open gastrectomy group showed a slight reduction in median postoperative length of stay (13 days vs 15 days, $P < 0.001$) but a slight increase in median total costs (US $21,510 vs $21,024, $P = 0.002$). There were no significant differences in in-hospital mortality (0.36% vs 0.28%, $P = 0.80$), overall postoperative complications (12.9% vs 12.6%, $P = 0.73$), or 30-day readmission rates (3.2% vs 3.2%, $P = 0.94$).

Conclusions.—In this large nationwide cohort of patients with early-stage gastric cancer, laparoscopic gastrectomy was associated with a statistically significant but slight reduction in postoperative length of stay, but no differences between laparoscopic gastrectomy and open gastrectomy were detected in terms of early mortality and morbidity.

► The authors provide a retrospective analysis of a large database evaluating the outcomes from patients undergoing resection for gastric cancer. In general, they observed that laparoscopic operations are offered to patients who are younger, healthier, and burdened with a less aggressive malignancy. Not surprisingly, these patients have statistically fewer postoperative complications, including surgical site infection, sepsis, cardiac events, ileus, and respiratory compromise. When the authors control for these, however, the differences between the open and laparoscopic approach disappear, and they advocate for laparoscopic resection.

We are left with an unanswered question regarding the oncologic outcome for laparoscopic vs open gastrectomy in early-stage gastric cancer. The authors do not address the issues of cancer-free and overall survival between the 2 groups. Until recently, we had no data to support the laparoscopic approach for gastric cancer. Most of the evidence for laparoscopy in gastric cancer has been based on smaller randomized, controlled trials and cohort studies with less clear results. The authors cite a few prospective studies; however, these are limited by size and power.[1] Furthermore, there is virtually no prospective data for laparoscopy in more-advanced-stage gastric cancers detailing our ability to achieve negative margins, adequate nodal harvest, and at least equivalent survival.

Demonstrating perioperative equivalency is not sufficient to categorically change the standard of care for surgical resection of gastric cancer—even early lesions. We have great data for colon and rectal cancer but limited information regarding gastric cancer. Larger randomized trials are certainly needed. Until then, the general surgeon must hold that open gastrectomy remains the gold standard for this disease, and he or she should certainly discuss these issues with their patient if a laparoscopic approach is recommended.

J. Hines, MD

Reference

1. Tanimura S, Higashino M, Fukunaga Y, et al. Laparoscopic with regional lymph node dissection for upper gastric cancer. *Gastric Cancer.* 2003;6:64-68.

Peroral Endoscopic Myotomy Is a Viable Option for Failed Surgical Esophagocardiomyotomy Instead of Redo Surgical Heller Myotomy: A Single Center Prospective Study

Onimaru M, Inoue H, Ikeda H, et al (Showa Univ Northern Yokohama Hosp, Japan)

J Am Coll Surg 217:598-605, 2013

Background.—Surgical Heller myotomy has high rates of successful long-term results, but failed cases still remain. Moreover, the treatment strategy in patients with surgical myotomy failure is controversial. Recently, peroral endscopic myotomy (POEM) was reported to be efficient and safe in primary treatment of achalasia. In this study, we aimed to evaluate the efficacy and safety of POEM for surgical myotomy failure as a rescue second-line treatment, and we discuss the treatment options adapted in achalasia recurrence.

Study Design.—A total of 315 consecutive achalasia patients received POEM from September 2008 to December 2012 in our hospital. Eleven (3.5%) patients who had persistent or recurrent achalasia and had received surgical myotomy as a first-line treatment from other hospitals were included in this study. Patient background, barium swallow studies,

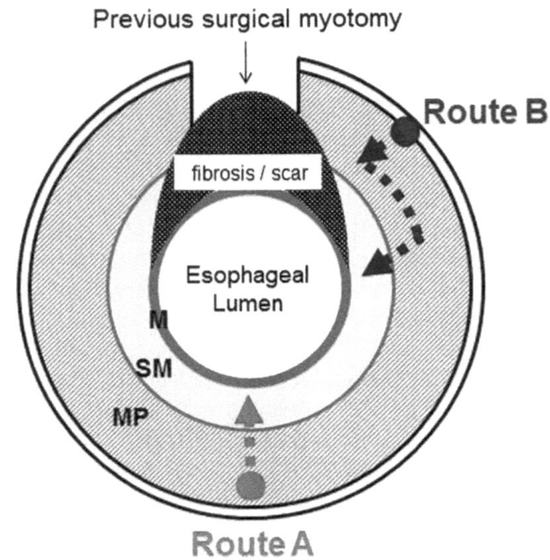

FIGURE 1.—Myotomy routes of the rescue peroral endscopic myotomy. We made the new submucosal tunnel approaching from Route A or Route B. Route A (red arrow), an axis that was different from the previous myotomy from the starting point of the submucosal entry. Route B (blue arrow): beginning at the standard 2 o'clock axis and rotating the axis, avoiding the fibrosis/scar region. M, mucosa; MP, muscularis propia; SM, submucosal. For Interpretation of the references to color in this figure legend, the reader is referred to web version of this article. (Reprinted from the Journal of the American College of Surgeons. Onimaru M, Inoue H, Ikeda H, et al. Peroral endoscopic myotomy is a viable option for failed surgical esophagocardiomyotomy instead of redo surgical Heller myotomy: a single center prospective study. *J Am Coll Surg*. 2013;217:598-605, Copyright 2013, with permission from the American College of Surgeons.)

esophagogastroduodenoscopy (EGD), manometry, and symptom scores were prospectively evaluated. In principle, all patients in whom surgical myotomy failed received pneumatic balloon dilatation (PBD) as the first line "rescue" treatment, and only if PBD failed were patients considered for rescue POEM.

Results.—The PBD alone was effective in 1 patient, and in the remaining 10 patients, rescue POEM was performed successfully without complications. Three months after rescue POEM, significant reduction in lower esophageal sphincter (LES) resting pressures (22.1 ± 6.6 mm Hg vs 10.9 ± 4.5 mm Hg, $p < 0.01$) and Eckardt symptom scores (6.5 ± 1.3 vs 1.1 ± 1.3, $p < 0.001$) were observed.

Conclusions.—Short-term results of POEM for failed surgical myotomy were excellent. Long-term results are awaited (Fig 1).

▶ Achalasia is a rare primary motility disorder of the esophagus for which surgical myotomy (typically laparoscopic Heller myotomy fundoplication) is the most effective and durable treatment for patients who do not respond to pharmacologic therapy. Those who do not respond—either from inadequate myotomy or secondary fibrosis—are highly unlikely to benefit from nonoperative intervention. Secondary surgical intervention consists of redo myotomy or esophagectomy—both of which are associated with considerably increased morbidity and failure rates. Peroral endoscopic myotomy (POEM) is a technique in which an endoscopically created submucosal tunnel is used to perform a longitudinal myotomy extending from above the lower esophageal sphincter (LES) down to the gastric cardia. In this study, the authors investigate POEM as rescue therapy after failed surgical myotomy for achalasia (Fig 1). Eleven patients were studied prospectively after failed surgical myotomy and failed pneumatic balloon dilatation. After esophagogastroduodenoscopy, barium swallow, computed tomography, and manometry, 7 were thought to have had inadequate initial surgical myotomy, the remainder had scarring or fibrosis. POEM was feasible in all patients without any reported complications. At 3 months, all had symptomatic relief; 9 had objective decrease in resting LES pressure. Two conclusions can be drawn from this study. First, the authors have shown that POEM is technically feasible after surgical myotomy. Second, POEM may present an effective and less-invasive alternative to redo myotomy or esophagectomy after an initial surgical myotomy has failed. Unfortunately, the limited sample size and limited follow-up prevent any other firm conclusions from being drawn. Critically, it is unknown whether those with incomplete initial myotomy will have as durable secondary relief with POEM as with redo myotomy. The treatment of achalasia is advancing, and surgeons may want to consider adding POEM to their armamentarium.

J. Hines, MD

Gastric Emptying as a Prognostic Factor for Long-term Results of Total Laparoscopic Fundoplication for Weakly Acidic or Mixed Reflux

Rebecchi F, Allaix ME, Giaccone C, et al (Univ of Turin, Italy)

Ann Surg 258:831-837, 2013

Objectives.—To evaluate the long-term effect of laparoscopic total fundoplication (LTF) on symptoms and reflux control in patients with combined (acidic and weakly acidic) (CR) or weakly acidic reflux (WAR), according to the gastric emptying (GE) rate.

Background.—After LTF, 12% to 15% of patients experience persistent reflux symptoms and 20% and 25% develop gas-related symptoms. Both WAR and inability to belch have been suggestive of these symptoms.

Methods.—Consecutive patients with CR and WAR selected for LTF were included in a prospective clinical study. Gastroesophageal function was assessed by clinical validated questionnaires, upper endoscopy, esophageal manometry, and 24-hour impedance-pH monitoring before and 12 and 60 months after LTF. Gastric scintigraphy was preoperatively performed in all patients to evaluate GE. This trial is registered with ClinicalTrials.gov (no. NCT01741441).

Results.—Between June 2002 and June 2007, a total of 188 patients with CR and WAR underwent LTF; 172 (91.5%) completed the 5-year protocol. Among them, 42 (24.4%) had preoperative mild/moderate delayed GE (DGE). Quality of life at 12 and 60 months improved in patients with normal GE (Gastroesophageal Reflux Disease Health-Related Quality of Life

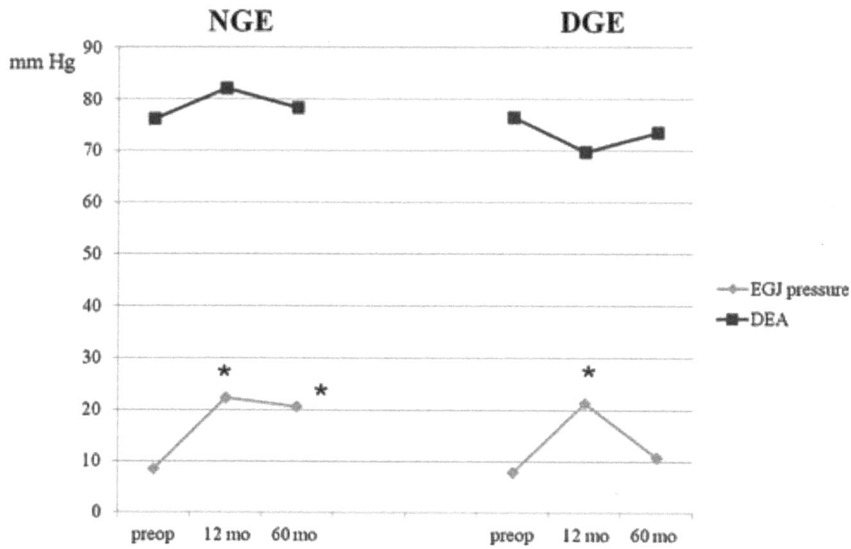

FIGURE 2.—Manometric findings before and after LTF in NGE patients versus DGE patients. preop indicates preoperatively. *$P < 0.001$ compared with preoperative values. (Reprinted from Rebecchi F, Allaix ME, Giaccone C, et al. Gastric emptying as a prognostic factor for long-term results of total laparoscopic fundoplication for weakly acidic or mixed reflux. *Ann Surg*. 2013;258:831-837, Copyright 2013, with permission from Southeastern Surgical Congress.)

score 18.2/2.5, $P < 0.001$; Health-Related Quality of Life score from 52.1 to 68.3, $P < 0.001$) but not in DGE patients. Manometric values of "gastroesophageal junction" significantly increased at 12 and 60 months in all patients with normal GE, whereas the values returned to the baseline at 60 months in 66.7% of DGE patients. Acidic and liquid reflux episodes significantly reduced in both groups, whereas a significant reduction of WAR and mixed (gas + liquid) reflux episodes occurred only in patients with normal GE ($P < 0.001$).

Conclusions.—DGE affects long-term results of LTF in CR and WAR patients (Fig 2).

▶ The causes for failure after fundoplication for gastroesophageal reflux can be difficult to determine and frustrating for the patient. Initial evaluation generally includes radiologic evaluation to be certain that no anatomic change with hernia recurrence or wrap malposition is apparent. Short of that, a new endoscopy or pH study may help to clarify the situation. This article examines the role of preoperative delayed gastric emptying on postoperative success. Generally it is felt that delayed gastric emptying improves after fundoplication for reasons that are unknown. Some routinely evaluate gastric emptying preoperatively with a nuclear medicine test, but others do not if no worrisome symptoms of nausea are present. The follow-up in the study found that, although patients with delayed gastric emptying had increased esophagogastric junction manometric pressures at 12 months, two-thirds of these patients had decreases and normalization of esophagogastric junction pressures at 5 years (Fig 2). In addition to this, these changes had clinical implications with more than 90% of patients back on proton pump inhibitor therapy. Some authors[1] have proposed a pyloroplasty concomitant to fundoplication in patients with severe delayed gastric emptying. However, this procedure is associated with a high incidence of diarrhea, and few data concerning gastroesophageal reflux disease related symptom control over a long follow-up period in patients with mild to moderate delayed gastric emptying are available. These considerations may suggest that most patients being considered for fundoplication should have a preoperative gastric emptying test to properly advise the patient on the expected outcomes.

J. Hines, MD

Reference

1. Khajanchee YS, Dunst CM, Swanstrom LL. Outcomes of Nissen fundoplication in patients with gastroesophageal reflux disease and delayed gastric emptying. *Arch Surg*. 2009;144:823-828.

The Comparative Effectiveness of Sleeve Gastrectomy, Gastric Bypass, and Adjustable Gastric Banding Procedures for the Treatment of Morbid Obesity

Carlin AM, For the Michigan Bariatric Surgery Collaborative (Henry Ford Health System, Detroit, MI; et al)
Ann Surg 257:791-797, 2013

Objective.—To evaluate the comparative effectiveness of sleeve gastrectomy (SG), laparoscopic gastric bypass (RYGB), and laparoscopic adjustable gastric banding (LAGB) procedures.

Background.—Citing limitations of published studies, payers have been reluctant to provide routine coverage for SG for the treatment of morbid obesity.

Methods.—Using data from an externally audited, statewide clinical registry, we matched 2949 SG patients with equal numbers of RYGB and LAGB patients on 23 baseline characteristics. Outcomes assessed included complications occurring within 30 days, and weight loss, quality of life, and comorbidity remission at 1, 2, and 3 years after bariatric surgery.

Results.—Matching resulted in cohorts of SG, RYGB, and LAGB patients that were well balanced on baseline characteristics. Overall complication rates among patients undergoing SG (6.3%) were significantly lower than for RYGB (10.0%, $P < 0.0001$) but higher than for LAGB (2.4%, $P < 0.0001$). Serious complication rates were similar for SG (2.4%) and RYGB (2.5%, $P = 0.736$) but higher than for LAGB (1.0%, $P < 0.0001$). Excess body weight loss at 1 year was 13% lower for SG (60%) than for RYGB (69%, $P < 0.0001$), but was 77% higher for SG

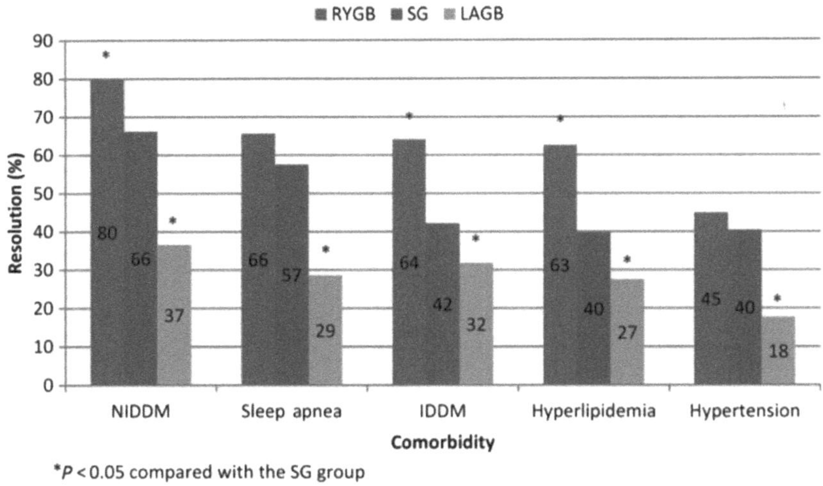

FIGURE 3.—Comorbidity remission at 1-year follow-up by procedure type. *P-value less than 0.05 compared with the SG group. (Reprinted from Carlin AM, For the Michigan Bariatric Surgery Collaborative. The comparative effectiveness of sleeve gastrectomy, gastric bypass, and adjustable gastric banding procedures for the treatment of morbid obesity. *Ann Surg*. 2013;257:791-797, © 2013, Southeastern Surgical Congress.)

than for LAGB (34%, $P < 0.0001$). SG was similarly closer to RYGB than LAGB with regard to remission of obesity-related comorbidities.

Conclusions.—With better weight loss than LAGB and lower complication rates than RYGB, SG is a reasonable choice for the treatment of morbid obesity and should be covered by both public and private payers (Fig 3).

▶ Surgery for morbid obesity has been shown repeatedly to be superior to medical management alone with regard to weight loss, reduction of obesity-associated comorbidities, and patient satisfaction. Compared with the gold standard Roux-en-Y gastric bypass (RYGB), sleeve gastrectomy (SG) is attractive for its relative simplicity, decreased malabsorption risk, and preservation of the pylorus. It also decreases risk of internal hernia and allows future endoscopic access to the foregut. Despite these perceived advantages, both public and private payers have been reluctant to provide routine coverage of SG. This study shows that SG performs admirably when directly compared with RYGB (Fig 3). RYGB shall remain first line for those with the highest degree of obesity and associated comorbidities; however, SG is an effective alternative.

This study was designed to provide additional data to support CMS reimbursement for SG. It makes use of propensity score matching (PSM) to develop matched cohorts for direct comparison. Randomized clinical trials (RCTs) remain the gold standard for evaluating an intervention, as they provide study groups that are theoretically similar in all observed and unobserved manners (ie, any baseline differences between groups are a result of chance and not related to the treatment itself). In contrast, in observational studies, treatment groups usually differ systematically from nontreatment groups, which are therefore ill suited for direct comparison. PSM is a tool that can replicate some of the conditions of an RCT from observational data. Each patient in the treatment (ie, SG) group receives a propensity score based on a logistic regression of predetermined characteristics. Each control patient (ie, RYGB and laparoscopic adjustable gastric banding) patient is then given a propensity score based on the same set of characteristics. The treatment group is matched in a one-to-one fashion with the control group, ensuring similarity between cohorts on the determined baseline characteristics.

There are a few important limitations of PSM, but it is nonetheless a powerful tool. Given the increasing utilization of observation-based, database-driven research, it is important for surgeons to understand the advantages and limitations of this type of study.

J. Hines, MD

Hand-Sewn Versus Mechanical Esophagogastric Anastomosis After Esophagectomy: A Systematic Review and Meta-Analysis

Honda M, Kuriyama A, Noma H, et al (Kyoto Univ, Japan; Kurashiki Central Hosp, Okayama, Japan; The Inst of Statistical Mathematics, Tokyo, Japan; et al)

Ann Surg 257:238-248, 2013

Objective.—To evaluate the risks and benefits of using a circular stapler (CS) compared with the hand-sewn (HS) method for the esophagogastric anastomosis after esophageal resection.

Background Data.—Previous randomized controlled trials (RCTs) indicated that the use of a CS might prevent anastomotic leakage, whereas it was more likely to lead to anastomotic strictures. The relative efficacy of this intervention in comparison with the HS method has not been conclusively determined.

Methods.—A systematic review and meta-analysis of all RCTs that compared HS versus mechanical anastomosis using a CS was conducted regarding the leakage, strictures, operative time, and mortality. The study protocol was established a priori according to the recommendations of the Cochrane Collaboration.

Results.—Twelve RCTs were included with a total of 1407 patients. The use of a CS, compared with the HS method, (1) led to no significant difference in the incidence of anastomotic leakage [risk ratio (RR): 1.02, 95% confidence interval (CI): 0.66–1.59] or postoperative mortality (RR: 1.64, 95% CI: 0.95–2.83), (2) increased the incidence of anastomotic strictures (RR: 1.67, 95% CI: 1.16–2.42), and (3) reduced the length of the operation time (mean: −15.3 minutes, range: −28.1 to −2.39). For these results, a subgroup analysis and a meta-regression analysis yielded no significant differences for the anastomotic site, diameter of the CS, layer, or configuration.

Reference	CS Events	CS Total	HS Events	HS Total	Weight	Risk Ratio [95% Confidence interval]
WSHASG 1991	0	27	1	25	2.0%	0.31 [0.01–7.26]
Craig SR 1996	4	50	3	50	9.2%	1.33 [0.31–5.65]
Valverde A 1996	12	78	12	74	34.3%	0.95 [0.46–1.98]
Law S. 1997	3	61	1	61	3.9%	3.00 [0.32–28.04]
Laterza E. 1999	4	20	1	21	4.4%	4.20 [0.51–34.44]
Walther B 2003	0	42	1	41	1.9%	0.33 [0.01–7.77]
Hsu HH 2004	8	31	7	32	24.0%	1.18 [0.49–2.86]
Okuyama M 2007	1	14	3	18	4.2%	0.43 [0.05–3.69]
Luechakiettisak P 2008	2	58	4	59	7.0%	0.51 [0.10–2.67]
Aquino JL 2009	1	15	5	15	4.7%	0.20 [0.03–1.51]
Zhang YS 2010	6	272	1	244	4.4%	5.38 [0.65–44.39]
Ma RD 2010						
Total	41	**668**	39	**640**	**100.0%**	**1.02 [0.66–1.59]**

Heterogeneity: $\tau^2 = 0.01$; $\chi^2 = 10.14$, $df = 10$ ($P = 0.43$); $I^2 = 1\%$

Test for overall effect: $Z = 0.10$ ($P = 0.92$)

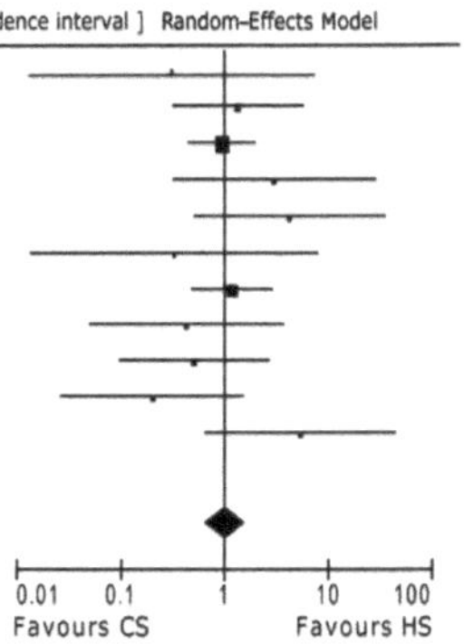

FIGURE 2.—Forest plot for anastomotic leakage. Eleven studies were included. Both clinical and radiological leakages were counted as anastomotic leakages. (Reprinted from Honda M, Kuriyama A, Noma H, et al. Hand-sewn versus mechanical esophagogastric anastomosis after esophagectomy: a systematic review and meta-analysis. *Ann Surg.* 2013;257:238-248, © 2013, Southeastern Surgical Congress.)

Conclusion.—The use of a CS contributed to reducing the length of the operation, but was associated with an increased risk of anastomotic strictures. Both the CS and the HS method are viable alternatives in the reconstruction after esophagectomy (Fig 2).

▶ There is no doubt that the most feared complication after esophagectomy is an anastomotic leak. This event can trigger a series of problems leading to the patient's demise. Many surgeons have advocated particular techniques to prevent leak, and several randomized trials have generally advocated for a stapled anastomosis. This meta-analysis appears to debunk this concept and includes data from 12 randomized, controlled trials and just greater than 1400 patients. The comparison between hand-sewn and circular stapler anastomosis found no advantage in the prevention of leakage with the stapled approach (Fig 2, risk ratio, 1.02). The use of a stapled technique appeared to save an additional 15 minutes of operating time and resulted in 67% higher risk of postoperative stricture formation. This stricture rate did not seem to correlate with that of smaller-diameter staplers and was 32.3% in patients operated on with staplers of diameter ≥ 30 mm. What's more, the mortality within 30 days after surgery was actually higher in the patients who had a stapled anastomosis ($P = .038$). Over the last few years, many have begun to shift to a stapled side-to-side anastomosis that may offer reduced leak and stricture rates. More data will need to be accumulated to know whether this is a clearly superior approach.

J. Hines, MD

The use of laparoscopic ultrasound in difficult cholecystectomy cases significantly decreases morbidity

Gwinn EC, Daly S, Deziel DJ (Rush Univ Med Ctr, Chicago, IL)
Surgery 154:909-917, 2013

Background.—Laparoscopic ultrasound (LUS) is a method of intraoperative bile duct imaging that can be used prior to any potentially hazardous dissection. The purpose of this study was to determine whether LUS could permit safe laparoscopic completion of difficult cholecystectomy (LC) cases and to assess whether its use had any impact on clinical outcome.

Methods.—We identified prospectively 44 patients with severe cholecystitis in whom LUS was considered critical for intraoperative identification of the bile ducts. LC patients were compared, on an intention to treat basis, with 41 contemporaneous patients with severe cholecystitis who had planned open cholecystectomy (OC).

Results.—LUS identified the extrahepatic bile ducts in all cases. Of the cases, 40 (91%) were completed laparoscopically. OC patients had a higher rate of acute cholecystitis and preoperative percutaneous cholecystostomy tubes and a higher mean ASA classification. Intraoperatively, LC patients had significantly less estimated blood loss and fewer drains were placed. Postoperatively, LC patients had significantly fewer total complications, Clavien-Dindo grade 3 complications, biliary complications, biliary reinterventions, intra-abdominal abscesses, and bleeding complications. LC patients had significantly fewer ICU admissions and shorter LOS.

Conclusion.—By allowing identification of the extrahepatic bile ducts during difficult cholecystectomy, LUS results in a high rate of successful laparoscopic completions. Laparoscopic cholecystectomy is associated with better clinical outcomes than OC for patients with severe cholecystitis.

▶ There is no doubt that a laparoscopic cholecystectomy in the case of severe acute cholecystitis and gangrenous cholecystitis is a real challenge. Visualization is difficult, and many times when the operation does not progress, we convert to an open procedure. With all the inherent advantages of a laparoscopic procedure, improvements to help with visualization and lower complications are important and offer the potential to proceed with a laparoscope. This study examined the efficacy of intraoperative ultrasound scan to assist in the identification of the cystic duct and portal anatomy. The authors compared this with a group with similar levels of inflammation but in whom a decision was made preoperatively to perform the operation with an open technique. In all cases, the ultrasound scan was able to identify the cystic duct, common duct, right hepatic artery, and portal vein. More than 90% of the cases were completed laparoscopically, and the complications of abscess, bile duct injury, duodenal injury, and others were avoided and largely confined to the open operation group. The authors noted that the surgeons in this study had extensive experience with intraoperative ultrasound scan with some having performed as many as 600 procedures. Clearly, some experience is required to reliably identify the biliary structures with ultrasound scan. This approach appears to be a real potential adjunct to our ability to perform safe laparoscopic cholecystectomy. This may also decrease hospital charges, as laparoscopic patients are clearly discharged earlier than patients who undergo open operation.

J. Hines, MD

Predictors of Incidental Gallbladder Cancer in Patients Undergoing Cholecystectomy for Benign Gallbladder Disease

Koshenkov VP, Koru-Sengul T, Franceschi D, et al (Univ of Miami Miller School of Medicine, FL)

J Surg Oncol 107:118-123, 2013

Background and Objectives.—Discovery of incidental gallbladder cancer (IGC) has become more frequent due to adoption of laparoscopy. Gallbladder spillage during operation can disseminate cancer and worsen the prognosis.

Methods.—Patients who underwent laparoscopic or open cholecystectomy for benign gallbladder disease January 1996 to August 2011 at two tertiary care facilities were reviewed. Unmatched controls were randomly selected in 2:1 ratio. Preoperative variables were compared between the two groups.

Results.—Sixty-seven patients with IGC were identified and compared to 134 controls. Mean age was 68 for index cases and 49 for controls; 70% of cases and 75% of controls were female. Multivariate analysis showed that higher risk of IGC was significantly associated with age ≥ 65 (OR = 10.61, $P < 0.0001$), dilated bile ducts (OR = 4.76, $P = 0.0028$), and presence of gallbladder wall thickening (OR = 4.39, $P = 0.0003$). This model yielded a very good area under the curve of receiver operating characteristic (AUC = 0.83) for discriminating the patients with IGC from controls.

Conclusions.—IGC is more likely to be found in patients when age is ≥65, with dilated bile ducts and gallbladder wall thickening. Preoperative suspicion of gallbladder cancer should prompt the surgeon to be more careful not to perforate the gallbladder during laparoscopic approach, and to have a lower threshold for conversion if necessary.

► The role of a laparoscopic approach for gallbladder cancer is controversial and largely discouraged. The fear and evidence suggests that violation of the gallbladder wall will lead to spread of the tumor into the abdomen, converting what could be an early and curable stage to a metastatic condition. Certainly, for all but very early tumors, it is unlikely that a proper local excision and node harvest will be performed with a laparoscope. Although the incidence of incidental gallbladder cancer found after 750 000 to 1 000 000 cholecystectomies performed each year in the United States is low, it would be very beneficial if we could predict the likelihood of gallbladder cancer before surgery and potently modifying the technique to properly address the cancer.

This article examines several parameters among patients who were found to have an incidental gallbladder cancer after laparoscopic cholecystectomy and compared theses patients with those who did who did not have cancer. Age ≥ 65, a dilated bile duct (> 8–9 mm), and gallbladder wall thickening increased the likelihood of an incidental gallbladder cancer by 10.6, 4.8, and 4.4 times. Although these data are interesting and helpful, I have many patients with these findings that do not have gallbladder cancer. I am sure you have cared for the older patient with acute cholecystitis, choledocholithiasis, and bile duct obstruction manifesting these 3 parameters. The authors point out that the presence of a large gallstone or porcelain gallbladder does not seem to increase the risk of gallbladder cancer.[1,2] Gallbladder polyps certainly increase the risk of gallbladder cancer, but these are relatively rare and usually alert the surgeon to this possibility.

The take-home message of this report is that we should have a heightened level of concern for patients with the parameters found in this study. If the surgeon is suspicious during the surgery, special care should be taken to not rupture the gallbladder wall, remove the specimen with a bag, and consider the need for conversion to an open operation.

J. Hines, MD

References

1. Shrikhande SV, Barreto SG, Singh S, Udwadia TE, Agarwal AK. Cholelithiasis in gallbladder cancer: coincidence, cofactor, or cause! *Eur J Surg Oncol.* 2010;36: 514-519.
2. Towfigh S, McFadden DW, Cortina GR, et al. Porcelain gallbladder is not associated with gallbladder carcinoma. *Am Surg.* 2001;67:7-10.

Changing Trends and Outcomes in the Use of Percutaneous Cholecystostomy Tubes for Acute Cholecystitis

Smith TJ, Manske JG, Mathiason MA, et al (Gundersen Health System, La Crosse, WI)
Ann Surg 257:1112-1115, 2013

Background.—Percutaneous cholecystostomy tube (PCT) placement serves as a treatment option for acute cholecystitis in elderly and critically ill patients. The objective of this study was to compare PCT and cholecystectomy outcomes over time.

Methods.—PCTs placed from April 1, 1998, to December 31, 2009 (time period 2) were retrospectively reviewed. Patients who underwent cholecystectomies served as matched controls. Institutional data from March 1, 1989, to March 31, 1998 (time period 1) were reviewed to compare trends.

Results.—A total of 143 patients successfully underwent PCT placement in time period 2. When compared with patients undergoing cholecystectomy, PCT patients had a higher rate of cardiovascular disease (66% vs 26%, $P = 0.001$), diabetes (27% vs 13%, $P = 0.001$), and a higher mean Charlson comorbidity index (3.27 vs 1.07, $P = 0.001$). Compared with the first time period, patients undergoing PCT in the second time period had lower American Society of Anesthesiologist's classifications (American

Society of Anesthesiologist's class I, II: 0% vs 18%, $P = 0.001$). Thirty-day mortality decreased from 36% to 12% in patients undergoing PCT ($P = 0.001$).

Conclusions.—Among patients with acute cholecystitis, percutaneous cholecystostomy tubes were placed in older patients with increased comorbidities compared to cholecystectomy. Mortality rates after PCT decreased over time.

▶ No randomized data exist that directly compare percutaneous cholecystostomy (PCT) with cholecystectomy in the treatment of acute cholecystitis, nor is it likely that any such study will be conducted. As a technique for urgent biliary decompression, this study documents the expanding demographics as well as the increasing frequency and success with which PCT is being used.

Accordingly, general surgeons are increasingly being called on to manage PCTs—both acutely and in the clinic. This study is useful insofar as it details the outcomes and complications to be expected after PCT placement. Ninety-one percent of patients acutely improved with PCT; those that did not, have a guarded prognosis regardless (85% mortality reported). Approximately 15% experience a complication, most commonly dislodgement, bile leak, occlusion, pain, and infection. These may be treated either with replacement, observation, or interval cholecystectomy depending on surgeon preference. Finally, the surgeon must be aware that previous PCT placement is not a contraindication to a laparoscopic approach, as evidenced by the 78% success rate reported here.

The authors worry about the increasing frequency of PCT use in (relatively) healthier patients; however, the 8% PCT rate and 88% cholecystectomy rate seem laudable. The point is, nevertheless, well taken, and it must be stressed that the best outcomes (decreased morbidity and mortality) for acute cholecystitis are achieved with early laparoscopic cholecystectomy. PCT—despite its increasing popularity—remains an effective therapy as a bridge to definitive therapy only in those patients ill suited for surgery.

J. Hines, MD

Improved Outcomes of Bile Duct Injuries in the 21st Century

Pitt HA, Sherman S, Johnson MS, et al (Indiana Univ School of Medicine, Indianapolis; et al)

Ann Surg 258:490-499, 2013

Objective.—The objectives of this analysis were to compare the outcomes of bile duct injuries by specialist over time and the role of management timing and biliary stents.

Background.—Postoperative bile duct injuries require multidisciplinary management. In recent years, advancements have occurred in patient evaluation and in timing and type of therapy.

Methods.—A multidisciplinary team managed 528 patients over 18 years. Mean age was 52 years; 69% were women and 95% had a

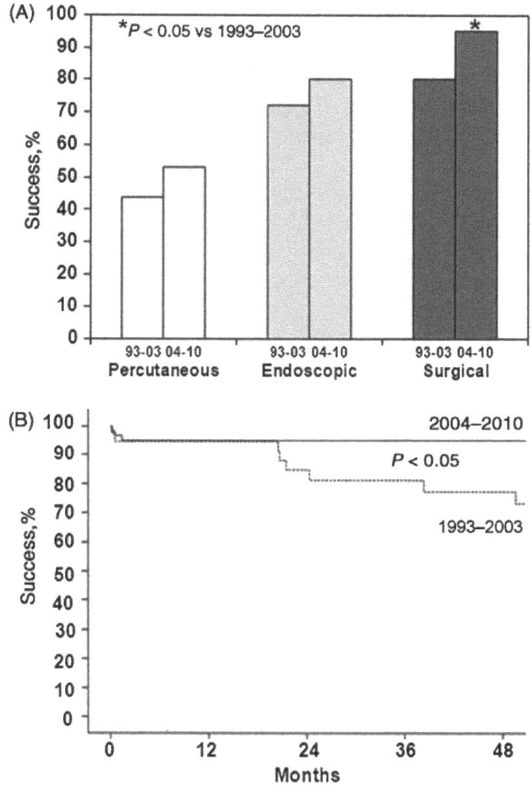

FIGURE 3.—(A) Outcomes by time period (Strasberg B→E). (B) Outcomes by time period over time for surgery (Strasberg B→E). (Reprinted from Pitt HA, Sherman S, Johnson MS, et al. Improved outcomes of bile duct injuries in the 21st century. *Ann Surg*. 2013;258:490-499, Copyright 2013, with permission from Southeastern Surgical Congress.)

cholecystectomy and/or bile duct exploration. Patients were classified by the Strasberg system as having bile leaks (type A, n = 239, 45%) or bile duct injuries (types B-E, n = 289, 55%). Injury outcomes from 1993 to 2003 (n = 132) were compared with those from 2004 to 2010 (n = 157). A successful outcome was defined as no need for further intervention after the initial 12 months of therapy. Standard statistical methods were employed.

Results.—Patients with bile leaks were managed almost exclusively by endoscopists (96%) with a 96% success rate. Patients with bile duct injuries were managed most often by endoscopists (N = 115, 40%) followed by surgeons (N = 104, 36%) and interventional radiologists (N = 70, 24%). Overall success rates were best for surgery (88%, $P < 0.05$) followed by endoscopy (76%) and interventional radiology (50%) and improved over time (78% vs 69%). Outcomes were best for surgery in recent years (95% vs 80%, $P < 0.05$) and for patients stented for more than 6 months ($P < 0.01$) (Fig 3).

Conclusions.—Almost all bile leaks and many bile duct injuries can be managed successfully by endoscopists. Selected proximal injuries can be treated by interventional radiologists with modest success. Outcomes of bile duct injuries are best with surgical management and in patients who are stented for more than 6 months.

▶ Those of us who perform laparoscopic cholecystectomy still fear the possibility of a bile duct injury. When that happens, the patient care is extended sometimes for months, and the need for multiple interventions is not uncommon. This group examined their experience with bile duct injuries in more than 500 patients. Interestingly, only a third of bile duct injuries was recognized intraoperatively. Those patients who simply had a bile duct leak without partial or complete transaction were effectively managed by endoscopic stent placement alone. Of the patients with more than just a bile leak, interventions included both transhepatic radiologic management and surgical reconstruction. Seven of these patients died within 3 months. Outcomes were worse in endoscopically managed patients who presented relatively late (2–6 months) and patients who underwent surgery 2 to 4 weeks after the injury when inflammation is peaking rather than waiting some additional time before operation. It appears that the successful management is improving with time, however, as we have developed multidisciplinary teams with expertise in this area (Fig 3). This modern experiential review is helpful and typifies the current management of bile duct injury.

J. Hines, MD

Comparison of laparoscopic common bile duct exploration and endoscopic retrograde cholangiopancreatography plus laparoscopic cholecystectomy for choledocholithiasis: a prospective randomized study

Koc B, Karahan S, Adas G, et al (Okmeydani Training and Res Hosp, Turkey)
Am J Surg 206:457-463, 2013

Background.—Endoscopic retrograde cholangiopancreatography and laparoscopic common bile duct exploration are safe and efficient methods that have recently been used for the treatment of bile duct stones. The aim of this study was to compare the efficacy, safety, and surgical outcomes of the laparoscopic common bile duct exploration plus laparoscopic cholecystectomy (LCBDE+LC) and endoscopic retrograde cholangiopancreatography plus laparoscopic cholecystectomy (ERCP+LC).

Methods.—One hundred twenty patients were prospectively randomized into 2 groups: LCBDE with LC in a single intervention and LC after ERCP.

Results.—The success rate of the LCBDE+LC group (96.5%) was found to be higher than for the ERCP+LC group (94.4%). Complication rates of the LCBDE+LC and ERCP+LC group were 7% and 11.1%,

TABLE 4.—Complications of Interventions

Complications	No. of Patients (%)
LCBDE	
Bile leak	2 (3.5)
Bile leak + retained stones	2 (3.5)
ERCP/S+LC	
Duodenal perforation	1 (1.8)
Retained stones	3 (5.5)
Pancreatitis	2 (3.7)

ERCP/S+LC = endoscopic retrograde cholangiopancreatography sphincterotomy plus laparoscopic cholecystectomy; LCBDE+LC = laparoscopic common bile duct exploration plus laparoscopic cholecystectomy.

respectively. Complications requiring ERCP in the postoperative period after LCBDE+LC have been noted in 3.5% of cases.

Conclusions.—Laparoscopic CBD exploration provides an alternative therapeutic approach that has less morbidity, is cost-effective, and allows earlier recovery with a reduced period of short-term disability (Table 4).

▶ In the United States, we have largely pushed the management of common bile duct stones to the gastroenterologist. The efficacy as measured by successful extraction is high and reliable in most sites. A handful of surgeons have instead managed common duct stones with laparoscopic bile exploration and stone extraction. This technique requires additional skill above that of a laparoscopic cholecystectomy. This surgical group randomly assigned their patients with preoperative suspicion of common bile duct stones to either preoperative endoscopic retrograde cholangiopancreatography and stone extraction followed by laparoscopic cholecystectomy or to laparoscopic cholecystectomy and common bile duct exploration. All procedures were performed by the surgical group, and by all signs it appears this group is quite facile with all of these techniques. In their hands, the completely laparoscopic group fared as well as the endoscopic group and had fewer complications (Table 4). Patients who leaked after common bile duct exploration most commonly leaked because of retained bile duct stones. Clearance of the duct was 96% and 95%, respectively—equally effective. In addition, hospital stay was shorter in the laparoscopic group. Developing the skill set to perform laparoscopic common bile duct exploration will require some dedication and equipment (best to use a flexible scope than a traditional rigid scope). But this could be an option for our patients if we dedicated some time to learning about these techniques. Until then, most of us will rely on the expertise of our local gastroenterologist to comanage patients with gallstones.

J. Hines, MD

Laparoscopic cholecystectomy for biliary dyskinesia: Which patients have long term benefit?

Wybourn CA, Kitsis RM, Baker TA, et al (Loyola Univ Med Ctr, Maywood, IL)
Surgery 154:761-768, 2013

Purpose.—Biliary dyskinesia (BD) is described as biliary colic in the absence of gallstones. The diagnosis relies on imaging studies and decreased excretion of bile in response to cholecystokinin during quantitative cholescintigraphy. The purpose of this study was to evaluate the success of laparoscopic cholecystectomy (LC) for relieving symptoms in patients diagnosed with BD and correlate gallbladder ejection fraction (EF) with symptom relief.

Methods.—A retrospective review was performed at a single institution of all patients who underwent LC for BD from January 2005 through January 2012. The diagnosis of BD was determined by a normal gallbladder as viewed with ultrasonography and cholescintigraphy with a gallbladder EF less than or equal to 45%. Data collection included demographics, results of imaging studies, pathologic diagnosis, and early postoperative pain relief. Patients were contacted by phone after being discharged from the surgeon's care for evaluation of symptom relief. Data were analyzed with nonparametric statistical methods, including Mann–Whitney U test, receiver operator characteristic, Fisher exact test, and χ^2 test. All data are expressed as median and 25th and 75th percentile range.

Results.—There were 126 patients who had a LC for BD during the study period. The median biliary EF was 20% (10–29%). The most common pathologic finding was chronic cholecystitis ($n = 95$; 75%). Median length of follow-up in the perioperative period was 11 days (8–17), during which time 98 patients (78%) had relief of symptoms. Phone interviews ($n = 53$; 42%) confirmed 66% ($n = 35$) of patients remained free of pain. There was no difference in the mean EF among those with resolution of pain 20% (10–29%) compared with patients with persistent pain 23% (11–29%), $P = .62$. Obese patients were more likely to have persistent symptoms in the perioperative period with a shift to lower body mass index at the time of the phone survey. Receiver operator characteristic characteristic for the association between scintigraphic EF and resolution of postoperative pain demonstrated no association, with the area under the curve equal to 0.47.

Conclusion.—The majority of patients in this series with BD had resolution of symptoms with LC. However, cholescintigraphy EF did not correlate with outcome. Further studies are needed to better identify patients diagnosed with BD who will benefit from LC (Fig).

▶ Whether biliary dyskinesia is a real entity may be a moot point, as the concept exists on the Internet, and patients find this information. The real issue for us as surgeons is to know how to evaluate and counsel these patients. We have all had patients who present with classic symptoms of biliary colic, but the evaluation reveals no evidence of gallstones. We might have a gastroenterologist evaluate

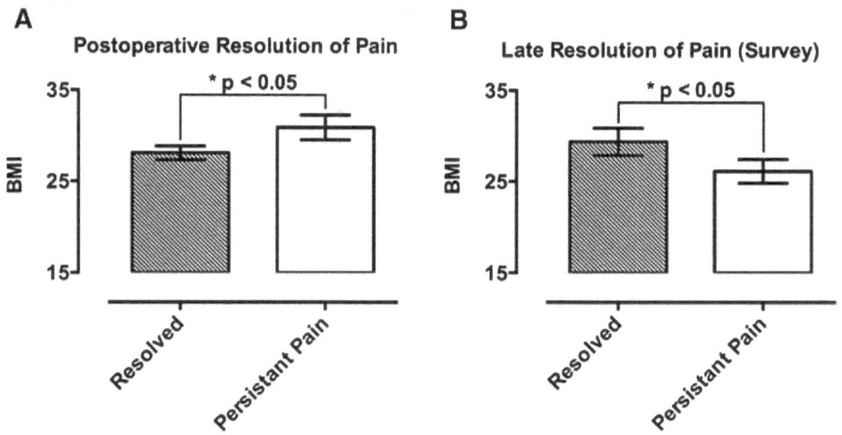

FIGURE.—Correlation of BMI with relief of pain. The median BMI was significantly greater for the group with persistent pain at the initial postoperative visit (*A*). In contrast, the median BMI for the group who had relief of pain at the time of the phone survey was significantly greater for the group who had no recurrence of preoperative pain compared to the group with persistent pain (*B*). (Reprinted from Surgery. Wybourn CA, Kitsis RM, Baker TA, et al. Laparoscopic cholecystectomy for biliary dyskinesia: Which patients have long term benefit? *Surgery*. 2013;154:761-768, Copyright 2013, with permission from Elsevier.)

the patient and have an endoscopy performed to rule out peptic disease. Many have advocated the use of scintography to determine gallbladder function and predict outcomes from cholecystectomy. But the truth is this is a difficult group of patients. This study looked at a case series of patients who underwent cholecystectomy for biliary dyskinesia. Scintography had no ability to predict relief of pain after cholecystectomy for these patients. About two-thirds were relieved of their pain, but this was less consistent in patients with a higher body mass index (Fig). This remains a difficult group of patients, so the patient must fully understand the limited benefit compared to patients with documented gallstones.

J. Hines, MD

Partial Anterior vs Partial Posterior Fundoplication Following Transabdominal Esophagocardiomyotomy for Achalasia of the Esophagus: Meta-regression of Objective Postoperative Gastroesophageal Reflux and Dysphagia

Kurian AA, Bhayani N, Sharata A, et al (Providence Portland Cancer Ctr, Portland, OR; Oregon Clinic Gastrointestinal and Minimally Invasive Surgery Division, Portland)
JAMA Surg 148:85-90, 2013

Objectives.—To review transabdominal esophagocardiomyotomy (surgical treatment of achalasia) of the esophagus and to compare outcomes of partial anterior vs partial posterior fundoplication.

TABLE 4.—Estimated Postoperative Event Rates

Group	Dysphagia		GERD	
	Odds (95% CI)	Rate (95% CI), %	Odds (95% CI)	Rate (95% CI), %
Myotomy only	0.06 (0.03-0.12)	6.38 (3.69-10.81)	0.37 (0.12-1.08)	27.12 (11.39-51.87)
Myotomy with anterior fundoplication	0.11 (0.09-0.14)	10.12 (8.27-12.33)	0.16 (0.11-0.24)	14.3 (10.43-19.37)
Myotomy with posterior fundoplication	0.06 (0.04-0.08)	5.85 (4.12-8.22)	0.18 (0.13-0.25)	15.82 (12.27-20.15)

Abbreviation: GERD, gastroesophageal reflux disease.

Data Sources.—An electronic search was conducted among studies published between January 1976 and September 2011 using the keywords *achalasia, myotomy, antireflux surgery,* and *fundoplication.*

Study Selection.—Prospective studies of transabdominal esophagocardiomyotomy were selected.

Data Extraction.—Outcomes selected were recurrent or persistent postoperative dysphagia and an abnormal 24-hour pH test result. Studies were divided into the following 3 groups: myotomy only, myotomy with anterior fundoplication, and myotomy with posterior fundoplication. Studies were weighted by the number of patients and by the follow-up duration. Event rates were calculated using meta-regression of the log-odds with the inverse variance method.

Data Synthesis.—Thirty-nine studies with a total of 2998 patients were identified. The odds of postoperative dysphagia were 0.06 (95% CI, 0.03-0.12) for myotomy only, 0.11 (95% CI, 0.09-0.14) for myotomy with anterior fundoplication, and 0.06 (95% CI, 0.04-0.08) for myotomy with posterior fundoplication. The odds of a postoperative abnormal 24-hour pH test result were 0.37 (95% CI, 0.12-1.08) for myotomy only, 0.16 (95% CI, 0.11-0.24) for myotomy with anterior fundoplication, and 0.18 (95% CI, 0.13-0.25) for myotomy with posterior fundoplication. The increased odds of postoperative dysphagia in the group undergoing myotomy with anterior fundoplication compared with the group undergoing myotomy with posterior fundoplication were statistically significant ($P < .001$). However, the incidence of a postoperative abnormal 24-hour pH test result was statistically similar.

Conclusion.—Partial posterior fundoplication when combined with an esophagocardiomyotomy may be associated with significantly lower reintervention rates for postoperative dysphagia, while providing similar reflux control compared with partial anterior fundoplication (Table 4)

▶ The minimally invasive group at the Oregon Clinic has analyzed the available reports of esophagomyotomy for achalasia with the intent of determining the best method for fundoplication combined with this procedure. To prevent postoperative gastroesophageal reflux, options for a fundoplication after this procedure include an anterior, posterior, or 360° wrap. Most would agree that a complete wrap is not appropriate given the significant dysmotility these patients have and the high rate of dysphagia associated with this approach. The advantages of an anterior wrap include the ease of this technique, the coverage of the mucosa with gastric serosa, and preservation of the phrenoesophageal ligament. The posterior wrap results in fewer angulations of the gastroesophageal junction and may help to keep the edges of the myotomy separated. This study includes a meta-analysis of 39 studies and nearly 3000 patients. The rate of gastroesophageal reflux as documented by pH study was 27.1% in the myotomy-alone group. The rate of postoperative dysphagia was similar between patients who underwent a myotomy alone and those that also had a posterior fundoplication (Table 4). An anterior fundoplication significantly increased the rate of dysphagia over the other 2 approaches. The anterior and posterior approaches were equally effective in decreasing the incidence of postoperative gastroesophageal reflux disease. Even though it takes more operating time and more time to create a posterior fundoplication, this is probably the correct wrap to perform after an esophagomyotomy.

J. Hines, MD

Laparoscopic Resection of Gastric and Small Bowel Gastrointestinal Stromal Tumors: 10-Year Experience at a Single Center

Tabrizian P, Sweeney RE, Uhr JH, et al (Icahn School of Medicine at Mount Sinai, NY)

J Am Coll Surg 218:367-373, 2014

Background.—Complete curative resection remains the treatment of choice for nonmetastatic gastrointestinal stromal tumors (GISTs). The safety and feasibility of laparoscopy in the treatment of this disease has been shown, however, the long-term oncologic outcomes of this technique remain unclear.

Study Design.—An ongoing prospectively maintained database including all laparoscopically resected gastric and small bowel GISTs (n = 116) at Mount Sinai Medical Center from July 1999 to December 2011 was retrospectively analyzed. Recurrence and survival outcomes were calculated using the Kaplan-Meier method and compared with log-rank test.

Results.—Tumors were of gastric (77.6%) and small bowel (22.4%) origins. Overall mean tumor size was 4.0 cm (± 2.7 cm) and R0 resection was achieved in 113 (97.4%) cases. Overall perioperative complication rate was 14.7%, with a reoperative rate of 4.3% at 90 days. When comparing gastric with small bowel GISTs, a more acute presentation requiring emergent resections was noted in patients with small bowel GISTs ($p = 008$). However tumor size, operative data, and perioperative outcomes were comparable in both groups ($p = \text{NS}$). At a median follow-up of 56.4 months (range 0.1 to 162.4 months), recurrence rate was 7.8% and comparable in both gastric and small bowel GISTs ($p = \text{NS}$). Risk factors for recurrence on univariate analysis were presence of ulceration/necrosis ($p < 0.001$) and tumor size >5 cm ($p = 0.05$). Overall 10-year survival rate

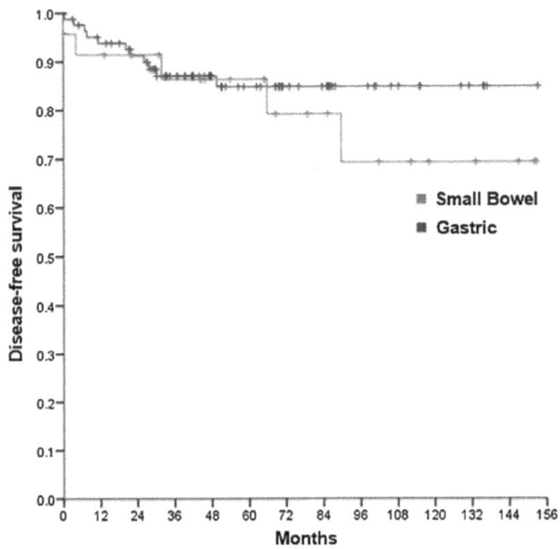

FIGURE 3.—Disease-free survival of gastric (n = 89) versus small bowel (n = 26) Gastrointestinal Stromal Tumors (p = NS). (Reprinted from the Journal of the American College of Surgeons. Tabrizian P, Sweeney RE, Uhr JH, et al. Laparoscopic resection of gastric and small bowel gastrointestinal stromal tumors: 10-year experience at a single center. *J Am Coll Surg*. 2014;218:367-373, Copyright 2014, with permission from the American College of Surgeons.)

was 90.8%. Gastric and small bowel overall survival rates were similar (90.7% vs 91.3%, respectively). Overall 10-year disease-free survival was 80.0% (84.3% gastric vs 71.6% small bowel; p = NS).

Conclusions.—Our series demonstrates the safety and feasibility of laparoscopy in patients undergoing resection of small bowel and gastric GISTs. Comparable long-term oncologic outcomes with a 10-year survival of 90.8% were achieved (Fig 3).

▶ Although laparoscopic approaches are used for many abdominal procedures and allow for faster recovery of bowel function, better immunologic response, and overall accelerated recovery for the patient, the use of laparoscopy for cancer surgery is still a matter of some discussion. For patients with cancer, questions remain about the immunologic implications of laparoscopic surgery, the adequacy and standardization of laparoscopic techniques, the risk for disease recurrence, and the impact on survival. The safety and efficacy of laparoscopic surgery for colorectal cancer has certainly been established, but the same rigorous approach to other cancers has yet to be reported. Gastrointestinal stromal tumors (GISTs) are stromal tumors characterized by mutations in the tyrosine-kinase gene, and they stain positive for CD117. They are often located in the stomach but can occur in any portion of the alimentary tract. The goals of operation include a segmental resection with an intact pseudo-capsule and a thorough exploration of the abdomen for metastasis. Lymphadenectomy is unnecessary because nodal metastases are rare. This article reports on a large case series of gastric and small intestinal GISTs resected laparoscopically. The results are solid and suggest these can be resected safely laparoscopically with 10-year survivals of more than 90% of patients (Fig 3). Size greater than 5 cm and tumor ulceration were associated with recurrence. Mitotic index and a positive margin did not have an impact on survival. Several new oral drugs (imatinib) are available for the treatment of these tumors, and many advocate preoperative treatment for larger GISTs and postoperative treatment for tumors with unfavorable characteristics.[1] In this study, it does not appear that many patients received treatment; despite this, the recurrence rate was relatively low. We have found that preoperative treatment can provide significant tumor shrinkage, allowing for a technically simpler operation with a potential therapeutic outcome. A modern approach to large GISTs includes the use of advanced therapeutics and timed laparoscopic resection when maximal response has been reached.

J. Hines, MD

Reference

1. Bednarski BK, Araujo DM, Yi M, et al. Analysis of prognostic factors impacting oncologic outcomes after neoadjuvant tyrosine kinase inhibitor therapy for gastrointestinal stromal tumors. *Ann Surg Oncol.* 2014 Mar 18 [Epub ahead of print].

Definitive Surgical Treatment Of Enterocutaneous Fistula: Outcomes of a 23-Year Experience

Owen RM, Love TP, Perez SD, et al (Emory Univ School of Medicine, Atlanta, GA)

JAMA Surg 148:118-126, 2013

Objective.—To analyze postoperative outcomes, morbidity, and mortality following enterocutaneous fistula (ECF) takedown.

Design, Setting, and Patients.—Retrospective review of the complete medical records of patients who presented to a single tertiary care referral center from December 24, 1987, to June 18, 2010, and subsequently underwent definitive surgical treatment for ECF originating from the stomach, small bowel, colon, or rectum.

Main Outcome Measures.—Postoperative fistula recurrence and mortality.

Results.—A total of 153 patients received operative intervention for ECF. Most ECFs were referred to us from outside institutions (75.2%), high output (52.3%), originating from the small bowel (88.2%), and iatrogenic in cause (66.7%). Successful ECF closure was ultimately achieved in 128 patients (83.7%). Six patients (3.9%) died within 30 days of surgery, and overall 1-year mortality was 15.0%. Postoperative complications occurred in 134 patients, for an overall morbidity rate of 87.6%. Significant risk factors for fistula recurrence were numerous, but postoperative ventilation for longer than 48 hours, organ space surgical site infection, and blood transfusion within 72 hours of surgery carried the most considerable impact (relative risks, 4.87, 4.07, and 3.91, respectively; $P < .05$). Risk of 1-year mortality was also associated with multiple risk factors, the most substantial of which were postoperative pulmonary and infectious complications. Closure of abdominal fascia was protective against both recurrent ECF and mortality (relative risks, 0.47 and 0.38, respectively; $P < .05$).

Conclusions.—Understanding risk factors both associated with and protective against ECF recurrence and postoperative morbidity and mortality is imperative for appropriate ECF management. Closure of abdominal fascia is of utmost importance, and preventing postoperative complications must be prioritized to optimize patient outcomes.

▶ Enterocutaneous fistula (ECF) is one of the most feared complications after gastrointestinal surgery. The initial push for these patients should not be a return to the operating room, but rather aggressive local and systemic sepsis control, nutritional optimization (yes, they can eat), and expert wound care. The goal is to wait 9 to 12 months before reoperation, although we agree with the authors that there is likely no benefit in waiting longer.

This thorough retrospective review out of Emory University Hospital documents the outcomes of all patients undergoing definitive surgical treatment of ECF by the hands of a single, experienced surgeon from 1987 to 2010. An initial closure rate of 76.5% after one attempt, and overall closure rate of 83.7% after 3 attempts, is consistent with the literature.

Notably missing in the secondary analyses is any documentation of albumin and prealbumin levels at the time of surgery, markers commonly used by surgeons to assess nutritional status. Finally, the single-surgeon, single-center experience limits the generalizability of the conclusions. However, this excellently compiled data should influence surgeons in 3 important ways: (1) patient selection optimization is paramount, (2) resection of involved segment should be performed unless not technically feasible, and (3) by all means close the fascia!

J. Hines, MD

A Prospective, Randomized, Noninferiority Trial of Steroid Dosing After Major Colorectal Surgery

Zaghiyan K, Melmed GY, Berel D, et al (Cedars Sinai Med Ctr, Los Angeles, CA)
Ann Surg 259:32-37, 2014

Objective.—To evaluate the safety of perioperative low-dose steroids (LDS) versus high-dose steroids (HDS) in steroid-treated patients with inflammatory bowel disease (IBD) undergoing major colorectal surgery.

Background.—Corticosteroid-treated patients undergoing major colorectal surgery are commonly prescribed HDS to prevent perioperative adrenal insufficiency and cardiovascular collapse. There is little evidence to support this practice.

Methods.—We performed a single-blinded noninferiority trial to compare perioperative hemodynamic instability in 92 steroid-treated IBD patients undergoing major colorectal surgery. Patients were randomly assigned to receive perioperative high-dose corticosteroids (HDS; hydrocortisone, 100 mg, intravenously 3 times daily, followed by taper) or low-dose corticosteroids (LDS; intravenous hydrocortisone equivalent to presurgical oral dosing, followed by taper). The primary outcome was the absence of postural hypotension on postoperative day 1, defined as a decrease in systolic blood pressure by 20 mm Hg after sitting from a supine position.

Results.—The primary outcome, absence of postural hypotension on postoperative day 1, occurred in 95% of those randomized to receive high doses of corticosteroids compared with 96% of those who received low doses (noninferiority 95% confidence interval = −0.08 to 0.09; $P = 0.007$).

Conclusions.—In IBD patients undergoing abdominal surgery, the incidence of postural hypotension or adrenal insufficiency is similar among those receiving high doses or low doses of corticosteroids in the perioperative period. To reduce complications associated with unnecessarily high doses of steroids, steroid-treated IBD patients undergoing major colorectal surgery should be treated with low doses of steroids in the perioperative period. (Clinicaltrials.gov ID# NCT01559675)

► Who knows if bolusing steroids at the time of surgery is the right thing to do. We have been taught that patients on steroids or who have taken steroids within the past year should receive a big dose at the time of surgery and a taper postoperatively to prevent adrenal insufficiency in the perioperative period—this is standard. The practice began after 2 case reports in the 1950s describing the death of surgical patients whose steroids were abruptly discontinued.[1,2] We do know that steroids increase perioperative complications such as infections, impaired wound healing, hyperglycemia, hypertension, and mental hyperactivity. This study evaluated inflammatory bowel disease surgery patients who were on steroids or recently tapered off steroids and randomized them to traditional high doses or a lower-dose protocol. Although the patients were not specifically studied with an ACTH stimulation test to be certain adrenal function was intact, the clinical surrogates of adrenal insufficiency, including hemodynamic instability, were evaluated. The low-dose group showed no increase in the number of episodes of hypotension and tachycardia. What's more, there was a trend toward lower infectious complications in the low-dose group (4 vs 16%, $P = 0.11$). So maybe it is time to stop bombarding our patients with steroids with the hope that we will see lower complication rates and less need for interventions to manage the side effects of high-dose steroids.

J. Hines, MD

References

1. Fraser CG, Preuss FS, Bigford WD. Adrenal atrophy and irreversible shock associated with cortisone therapy. *JAMA*. 1952;149:1542-1543.
2. Lewis L, Robinson RF, Yee J, Hacker LA, Eisen G. Fatal adrenal cortical insufficiency precipitated by surgery during prolonged continuous cortisone treatment. *Ann Intern Med*. 1953;39:116-126.

Risk adjusted benchmarking of abdominoperineal excision for rectal adenocarcinoma in the context of the Belgian PROCARE improvement project

Penninckx F, on behalf of PROCARE (UZ Gasthuisberg, Leuven, Belgium; et al)

Gut 62:1005-1011, 2013

Objective.—The abdominoperineal excision (APE) rate, a quality of care indicator in rectal cancer surgery, has been criticised if not adjusted for confounding factors. This study evaluates variability in APE rate between centres participating in PROCARE, a Belgian improvement initiative, before and after risk adjustment. It also explores the effect of merging the Hartmann resections (HR) rate with that of APE on benchmarking.

Design.—Data of 3197 patients who underwent elective radical resection for invasive rectal adenocarcinoma up to 15 cm were registered between January 2006 and March 2011 by 59 centres, each with at least 10 patients in the registry. Variability of APE or merged APE/HR rates between centres was analysed before and after adjustment for gender, age, ASA score (3 or more), tumour level (rectal third), depth of tumour invasion (cT4) and preoperative incontinence.

Results.—The overall APE rate was 21.1% (95% CI 19.7 to 22.5%). Significant variation of the APE rate was observed before and after risk adjustment ($p < 0.0001$). For cancers in the lower rectal third, the overall APE rate increased to 45.8% (95% CI 43.1 to 48.5%). Also, variation between centres increased. Risk adjustment influenced the identification of outliers. HR was performed in only 2.6% of patients. However, merging of risk adjusted APE and HR rates identified other centres with outlying definitive colostomy rates than APE rate alone.

Conclusion.—Significant variation of the APE rate was observed. Adjustment for confounding factors as well as merging HR with APE rates were found to be important for the assessment of performances.

▶ We are experiencing a rapid coalescence of quality assessment and improvement across the country. With time, all surgeons will be evaluated by outcomes and benchmarked against their peers. This should allow individual surgeons to move toward improved care after understanding the status of their practice. The indicators of quality for specific procedures are still in evolution and will continue to be refined as ever-higher levels of efficiency and quality are achieved.

This study examines the rate of abdominoperineal excision (resection) for rectal cancer across dozens of centers in Belgium. This rate has been proposed as a quality indicator for rectal cancer surgery, as this approach probably offers the most complete oncologic resection for this disease. The decision for an abdominoperineal resection rather than a low anterior resection requires the consideration of many factors, including the location of the tumor, relationship of the tumor to the anal sphincters, response to neoadjuvant treatment, and patient-specific conditions. The overall rate of abdominoperineal resection was just one-fifth of all patients with rectal cancer but was nearly one-half for lower-third rectal cancers. After risk adjustment, the authors noted significant variability in the rate of abdominoperineal resection among centers, suggesting that the decision making among surgeons was highly variable.

The authors point out that one method to fix the rate of abdominoperineal resection would be to centralize these procedures to a single or regional center. However, it is clear that this is not a reasonable option in a country the size of the United States or with a disease as common as rectal cancer. Instead, the authors suggest that procedures such as this be limited to those surgeons with documented "oncological surgical proficiency" at each site. Once data like these become available to all of us, every center and surgeon should be rushing to improve and achieve a high standard of quality for their patients.

J. Hines, MD

Predictors of mortality after emergent surgery for acute colonic diverticulitis: Analysis of National Surgical Quality Improvement Project data

Ballian N, Rajamanickam V, Harms BA, et al (Univ of Wisconsin School of Medicine and Public Health, Madison)

J Trauma Acute Care Surg 74:611-616, 2013

Background.—The surgical treatment of acute colonic diverticulitis is associated with significant morbidity and mortality. However, patient and operative characteristics associated with mortality in this patient population are unclear. We hypothesize that demographic and perioperative variables can be used to predict postoperative mortality. The purpose of this study was to identify perioperative variables predictive of postoperative mortality after emergent surgery for acute diverticulitis.

Methods.—Patients with diverticulitis undergoing colostomy and/or partial colectomy with or without primary anastomosis were retrieved from the American College of Surgeons National Surgical Quality Improvement Program database for years 2005 to 2008 inclusive. Only patients undergoing emergent surgery for acute diverticulitis were included. Univariate analyses were performed to compare demographic characteristics, preoperative laboratory values, comorbidities, and intraoperative variables. Variables with a significant ($p < 0.10$) difference between survivors and nonsurvivors were included in a stepwise logistic regression model to determine predictors of 30-day mortality. Concordance indices (*c* indices) for postoperative mortality were calculated using 2005 to 2008 data to determine predictive accuracy and validated on 2009 data.

Results.—A total of 2,214 patients met inclusion criteria. Mean age was 61 years, and 50% of patients were male. Thirty-day mortality was 5.1%. Nine preoperative variableswere significantly associated with postoperative mortality on multivariable analysis. The c index of this nine-variable model was 0.901. Renal dysfunction, hypoalbuminemia, American Society of Anesthesiologists class, and age were chosen to create a simpler model, with a c index of 0.886 for 2005 to 2008 data and 0.893 for 2009 data.

Conclusion.—Four readily available perioperative variables can be used to predict 30-day mortality after emergent surgery for acute diverticulitis.

▶ The general surgeon faces 2 critical questions when treating a patient with acute diverticulitis, namely: (1) do I need to operate now (alternatively, should I not operate) and (2) if I operate, should I perform a primary anastomosis? Most agree that in the absence of free perforation or fecal peritonitis, hemodynamic instability, obstruction, or an abscess not amenable to percutaneous drainage, nonoperative management is preferred.

This thorough review of the American College of Surgeons National Surgical Quality Improvement Program (NSQIP) data identifies 9 independent risk factors for 30-day mortality after emergency surgery (specifically colonic resection) for acute diverticulitis. It ultimately establishes a 4-variable model—age, American Society of Anesthesiologists class, serum creatinine, and serum albumin—that the authors demonstrate to be highly accurate. When uniformly absent, this model predicts a 0.2% mortality rate; when all 4 are present, this increases to 54%. This information provides a quick reference tool for the surgeon and can guide patient and surgeon expectation as well as patient counseling. Surgeon-dependent factors, such as choice and length of operation, did not independently predict mortality.

As an NSQIP database study limited to patients who have undergone the operation, this database is fundamentally unable to address the questions stated above. In each case, the reason the surgeon chose to operate was not available to the authors. To that end, it would be useful to understand the risk factors for mortality after nonoperative management. Finally, using the same methodology to predict outcomes in patients after Hartmann's or primary anastomosis might guide the surgeon in appropriate choice of operation.

J. Hines, MD

Current management of acute malignant large bowel obstruction: a systematic review

Frago R, Ramirez E, Millan M, et al (Univ of Barcelona, Spain; et al)

Am J Surg 207:127-138, 2014

Background.—The management of colonic obstruction has changed in recent years. In distal obstruction, optimal treatment remains controversial, particularly after the appearance and use of colonic endoluminal stents. The purpose of this study was to review the current treatment of acute malignant large bowel obstruction according to the level of evidence of the available literature.

Methods.—A systematic search was conducted in PubMed, MEDLINE, Embase, and Google Scholar for articles published through January 2013 to identify studies of large bowel obstruction and colorectal cancer. Included studies were randomized and nonrandomized controlled trials, reviews, systematic reviews, and meta-analysis.

TABLE 3.—Keys Points

Diagnostic tools	Computed tomography with endovenous and rectal contrast
Right colectomy + loop ileostomy	Proximal colonic obstruction in the presence of risk factors
Left colectomy + primary anastomosis	Distal colonic obstruction in selected patients
Subtotal colectomy	Distal colonic obstruction in selected patients with proximal colonic lesions
Hartmann's procedures	Distal colonic obstruction in the presence of high-risk factors, other options of treatment not available, lack of surgeon's experience in colorectal emergency surgery
Left colectomy + primary anastomosis + loop ileostomy	Distal colonic obstruction in the presence of high-risk factors
Stent as a bridge to surgery	Distal colonic obstruction in presence of high-risk factors or lack of surgeon's experience in colorectal emergency surgery
Definitive stents	Patients with limited overall survival

Results.—After a literature search of 1,768 titles and abstracts, 218 were selected for full-text assessment; 59 studies were ultimately included. Twenty-five studies of the diagnosis and treatment of obstruction and 34 studies of the use of stents were assessed.

Conclusions.—In view of the various alternatives and the lack of high-grade evidence, the treatment of distal colonic obstruction should be individually tailored to each patient (Table 3).

▶ Colonic stents for large bowel obstruction have come onto the scene and gastroenterologists are working through the establishment of appropriate use of these quite expensive devices. The concept is simple—place a stent to avoid surgery. Many reports have been published discussing feasibility of stent deployment and efficacy. Unfortunately, the definition of efficacy varies and all too often is simply judged to be that the stent was placed. The details of specific indications and the long-term utility are relatively uncertain. This group has attempted to comb the literature looking for these answers. Can colonic stents decrease the need for surgery and stoma and bridge the time to operation when the patient's condition has been maximized? After examining more than 1700 publications on the subject, the answer is, we do not know. The authors conclude "in view of the various alternatives and the lack of high-grade evidence, the treatment of distal colonic obstruction should be individually tailored to each patient"; otherwise known as, we do not know. The authors have made some reasonable recommendations, although based on current surgical approaches and common sense (Table 3). Generally, colonic stents should not be used long term, as ultimately these become obstructed, and the patient is back with a large bowel obstruction. Stents can be used for patients with a short life expectancy or as a bridge to definitive operation. Once deployed, it is virtually impossible to remove these endoscopically, and with time the stent will erode through the bowel wall. So for now we should follow the authors' recommendation and tailor the treatment plan to each patient.

J. Hines, MD

Comparison between oral antibiotics and probiotics as bowel preparation for elective colon cancer surgery to prevent infection: Prospective randomized trial

Sadahiro S, Suzuki T, Tanaka A, et al (Tokai Univ, Isehara, Japan; et al)
Surgery 155:493-503, 2014

Background.—We have already reported that, for patients undergoing elective colon cancer operations, perioperative infection can be prevented by a single intravenous dose of an antibiotic given immediately beforehand if mechanical bowel preparation and the administration of oral antibiotics are implemented. Synbiotics has been reported to reduce the rate of infection in patients after pancreatic cancer operations. The effectiveness of oral antibiotics and probiotics in preventing postoperative infection in elective colon cancer procedures was examined in a randomized controlled trial.

Methods.—Three hundred ten patients with colon cancer randomly were assigned to one of three groups. All patients underwent mechanical bowel preparation and received a single intravenous dose of flomoxef immediately before operation. Probiotics were administered in Group A; oral antibiotics were administered in Group B; and neither probiotics nor oral antibiotics were administered in Group C. Stool samples were collected 9 and 2 days before and 7 and 14 days after the procedure. Clostridium difficile toxin and the number of bacteria in the intestine were determined.

Results.—The rates of incisional surgical-site infection were 18.0%, 6.1%, and 17.9% in Groups A, B, and C, and the rates of leakage were 12.0%, 1.0%, and 7.4% in Groups A, B, and C, respectively, indicating that both rates were lesser in Group B than in Groups A and C ($P = .014$ and $P = .004$, respectively). The detection rates of C. difficile toxin were not changed among the three groups.

Conclusion.—We recommend oral antibiotics, rather than probiotics, as bowel preparation for elective colon cancer procedures to prevent surgical-site infections (Table 3).

▶ Everyone seems focused on surgical site infections these days, rapidly collecting data and making plans to lower the rate of this complication. With lower rates comes less expense and need for readmission. Colon surgery is particularly impacted by surgical site infections, and some report that as many as a third of patients experience this. Since a report in the 1970s,[1] many surgeons have routinely utilized both preoperative mechanical and oral antibiotic bowel preparation. But recently, some data have been published, suggesting that this is not necessary and may actually increase the rates of infections by altering the normal gut flora. In addition, there is evidence from studies conducted on patients undergoing pancreatic surgery that probiotics may decrease infectious complications. This group randomly divided more than 300 patients undergoing colon surgery to receive a bowel preparation, probiotics, or nothing. All groups received a single preoperative dose of intravenous antibiotics, and the bowel preparation group took 2 liters of polyethylene glycol solution along with 0.5 g

TABLE 3.—Postoperative Infectious Diseases and Other Complications

	Group A ($n = 100$)	Group B ($n = 99$)	Group C ($n = 95$)	P value
Incisional SSI	18 (18.0%)	6 (6.1%)	17 (17.9%)	.014
	Adj-P = 1.00	Adj-P = .028	–	
Organ/space SSI	4 (4.0%)	4 (4.0%)	5 (5.3%)	.88
	Adj-P = .93	Adj-P = .93	–	
Remote infection	2 (2.0%)	1 (1.0%)	2 (2.1%)	.88
	Adj-P = 1.00	Adj-P = .85	–	
Total	24 (24.0%)	11 (11.1%)	24 (25.3%)	
Leakage	12 (12.0%)	1 (1.0%)	7 (7.4%)	.004
	Adj-P = .56	Adj-P = .06	–	
Leakage (abscess free)	11 (11.0%)	1 (1.0%)	5 (5.0%)	.008

Adj-P, Adjusted *P* value by Dunn-Sidak method of Fisher's exact test compared to Group C; *P*, Fisher exact test; *SSI*, surgical-site infection.

of kanamycin and metronidazole at 1 PM, 2 PM, and 11 PM the night before surgery. Taking probiotics offered no advantage over taking nothing. But the bowel preparation group had a third of the surgical site infections compared with the no-intervention and probiotic group (Table 3). In addition to this important finding, the anastomotic leak rate was significantly lower in the bowel preparation group. A recent report indicated that only a third of surgeons are administering preoperative bowel preparations for their colon patients.[2] Given the striking data from this randomized trial, it may be time to reconsider the use of preoperative bowel preparation in patients scheduled for colon resection.

J. Hines, MD

References

1. Clarke JS, Condon RE, Bartlett JG, Gorbach SL, Nichols RL, Ochi S. Preoperative oral antibiotics reduce septic complications of colon operations: results of prospective, randomized, double-blind clinical study. *Ann Surg*. 1977;186:251-259.
2. Hendren S, Fritze D, Banerjee M, et al. Antibiotic choice is independently associated with risk of surgical site infection after colectomy: a population-based cohort study. *Ann Surg*. 2013;257:469-475.

A Novel Nomogram Accurately Quantifies the Risk of Mortality in Elderly Patients Undergoing Colorectal Surgery

Kiran RP, Attaluri V, Hammel J, et al (Cleveland Clinic, OH)
Ann Surg 257:905-908, 2013

Objective.—The ability to accurately predict postoperative mortality is expected to improve preoperative decisions for elderly patients considered for colorectal surgery.

Methods.—Patients undergoing colorectal surgery were identified from the National Surgical Quality Improvement Program database (2005–2007) and stratified as elderly (>70 years) and nonelderly (<70 years).

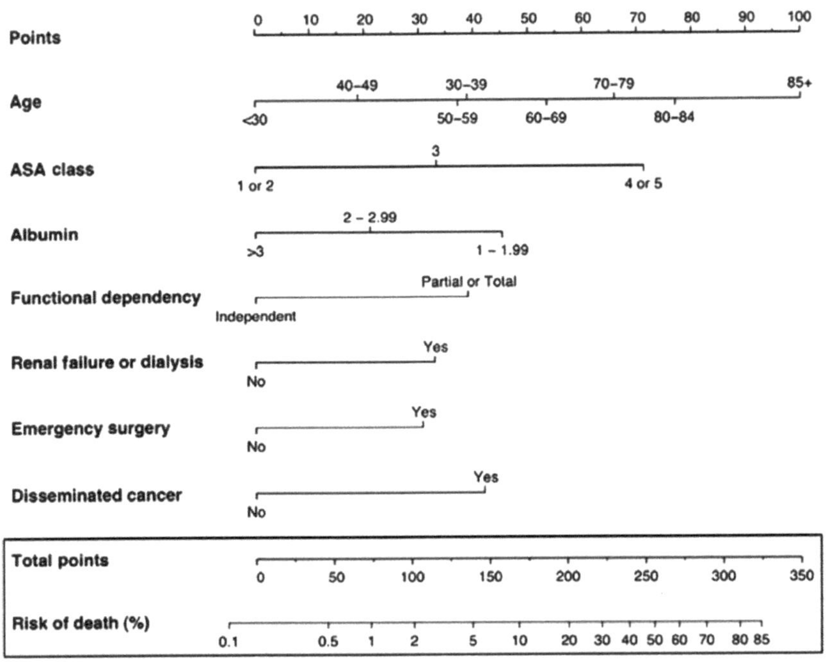

FIGURE 2.—Nomogram predicting 30-day mortality following colorectal surgery. (Reprinted from Kiran RP, Attaluri V, Hammel J, et al. A novel nomogram accurately quantifies the risk of mortality in elderly patients undergoing colorectal surgery. *Ann Surg*. 2013;257:905-908, © 2013, Southeastern Surgical Congress.)

Univariate analysis of preoperative risk factors and 30-day mortality and morbidity were analyzed on 70% of the population. A nomogram for mortality was created and tested on the remaining 30%.

Results.—Of 30,900 colorectal cases, 10,750 were elderly (>70 years). Mortality increased steadily with age (0.5% every 5 years) and at a faster rate (1.2% every 5 years) after 70 years, which defined "elderly" in this study. Elderly (mean age: 78.4 years) and nonelderly patients (52.8 years) had mortality of 7.6% versus 2.0% and a morbidity of 32.8% versus 25.7%, respectively. Elderly patients had greater preoperative comorbidities including chronic obstructive pulmonary disease (10.5% vs 3.8%), diabetes (18.7% vs 11.1%), and renal insufficiency (1.7% vs 1.3%). A multivariate model for 30-day mortality and nomogram were created. Increasing age was associated with mortality [age >70 years: odds ratio (OR) = 2.0 (95% confidence interval (CI): 1.7–2.4); >85 years: OR = 4.3 (95% CI: 3.3–5.5)]. The nomogram accurately predicted mortality, including very high-risk (>50% mortality) with a concordant index for this model of 0.89.

Conclusions.—Colorectal surgery in elderly patients is associated with significantly higher mortality. This novel nomogram that predicts postoperative mortality may facilitate preoperative treatment decisions (Fig 2).

▶ With the advent of large national databases, highly reliable models predicting the outcome of patients from particular operations can be created. The value of these models is to use the information when counseling patients on the risks and benefits of an operation so that the patient can be fully informed. These types of data can be very helpful in cases in which palliative care or end-of-life decisions are being considered.

This article has pulled data from the American College of Surgeons National Surgical Quality Improvement Program (NSQIP). Just more than 30 000 patients undergoing colorectal surgery were evaluated to predict preoperative mortality. Overall mortality rate increased from 2.4% to 7.6% for patients older than the age of 70. These parameters along with others were used to create a monogram (Fig 2).

This nomogram can be used now in your practice to counsel patients. As an example, let's consider a planned right hemicolectomy for local cancer in a 76-year-old woman with an American Society of Anesthesiologists (ASA) class of 2, with an albumen level of 2.8, who is independent with regard to activities of daily life, and with normal renal function. These parameters would give a score of 88 and a risk of mortality of 1.8%. With this information, you could discuss with the patient and her family that it is very likely that she will have an excellent outcome from the operation. This would be a very different discussion for the 85-year-old dependent patient with and ASA class of 4, with an albumen level of 1.8, on dialysis, needing an emergency operation for a perforated colon cancer. The chance of death for this patient is greater than 85%. Whether patients or their families will accept or use this type of information in the urgent/emergent situation is unknown.

J. Hines, MD

Equal Efficacy of Endoscopic and Surgical Cystogastrostomy for Pancreatic Pseudocyst Drainage in a Randomized Trial

Varadarajulu S, Bang JY, Sutton BS, et al (Univ of Alabama at Birmingham; James A. Haley Veterans Affairs Med Ctr, Tampa, FL)

Gastroenterology 145:583-590.e1, 2013

Background & Aims.—Although surgery is the standard technique for drainage of pancreatic pseudocysts, use of endoscopic methods is increasing. We performed a single-center, open-label, randomized trial to compare endoscopic and surgical cystogastrostomy for pancreatic pseudocyst drainage.

Methods.—Patients with pancreatic pseudocysts underwent endoscopic (n = 20) or surgical cystogastrostomy (n = 20). The primary end point was pseudocyst recurrence after a 24-month follow-up period. Secondary end points were treatment success or failure, complications, re-interventions, length of hospital stay, physical and mental health scores, and total costs.

Results.—At the end of the follow-up period, none of the patients who received endoscopic therapy had a pseudocyst recurrence, compared with 1 patient treated surgically. There were no differences in treatment successes, complications, or re-interventions between the groups. However, the length of hospital stay was shorter for patients who underwent endoscopic cystogastrostomy (median, 2 days, vs 6 days in the surgery group; $P < .001$). Although there were no differences in physical component scores and mental health component scores (MCS) between groups at baseline on the Medical Outcomes Study 36-Item Short-Form General Survey questionnaire, longitudinal analysis showed significantly better physical component scores ($P = .019$) and mental health component scores ($P = .025$) for the endoscopy treatment group. The total mean cost was lower for patients managed by endoscopy than surgery ($7011 vs $15,052; $P = .003$).

Conclusions.—In a randomized trial comparing endoscopic and surgical cystogastrostomy for pancreatic pseudocyst drainage, none of the patients in the endoscopy group had pseudocyst recurrence during the follow-up period, therefore there is no evidence that surgical cystogastrostomy is superior. However, endoscopic treatment was associated with shorter hospital stays, better physical and mental health of patients, and lower cost. Trial Registration: ClinicalTrials.gov: NCT00826501 (Fig. 1).

▶ Operation for bowel obstruction is a common occurence, and over the past century, the decision tree for patients undergoing this procedure has evolved. Before the availability of high-quality imaging, the concept of early operation made sense because we had a limited ability to gage intestinal ischemia. Clear clinical signs of a systemic inflammatory response and abdominal examination findings can certainly push us toward early operation. Now high-resolution computed tomography (CT) scanning can give us some assurance that the bowel is not ischemic. But frequently patients do not present this way, and a large percentage of bowel obstructions will resolve with hydration, bowel rest, and nasogastric tube decompression. Now it is common to have a trial of conservative management for 3 to 5 days before a decision is made to operate. This study examined the National Surgical Quality Improvement Program database and found that delaying operation past 24 hours significantly increased mortality, surgical site infections, pneumonia, and sepsis (Fig. 1). With each additional day of observation, these rates increased. In addition, early-operation patients had 5 fewer hospital days. What we do not know from this study is what happened to the patients who did not require an operation. So the trick is finding a way to predict early on which patients will require operation. Two meta-analyses suggest that the presence of water-soluble contrast in the colon within 24 hours of admission predicts the resolution of bowel obstruction with 97% sensitivity and as high as 98% specificity.[1,2] We should consider changing our algorithm for patients with nonischemic bowel obstruction to start with a water-soluble oral-contrast CT scan of the abdomen and pelvis at the time of presentation, close observation with serial examinations in the first 24 hours, and a

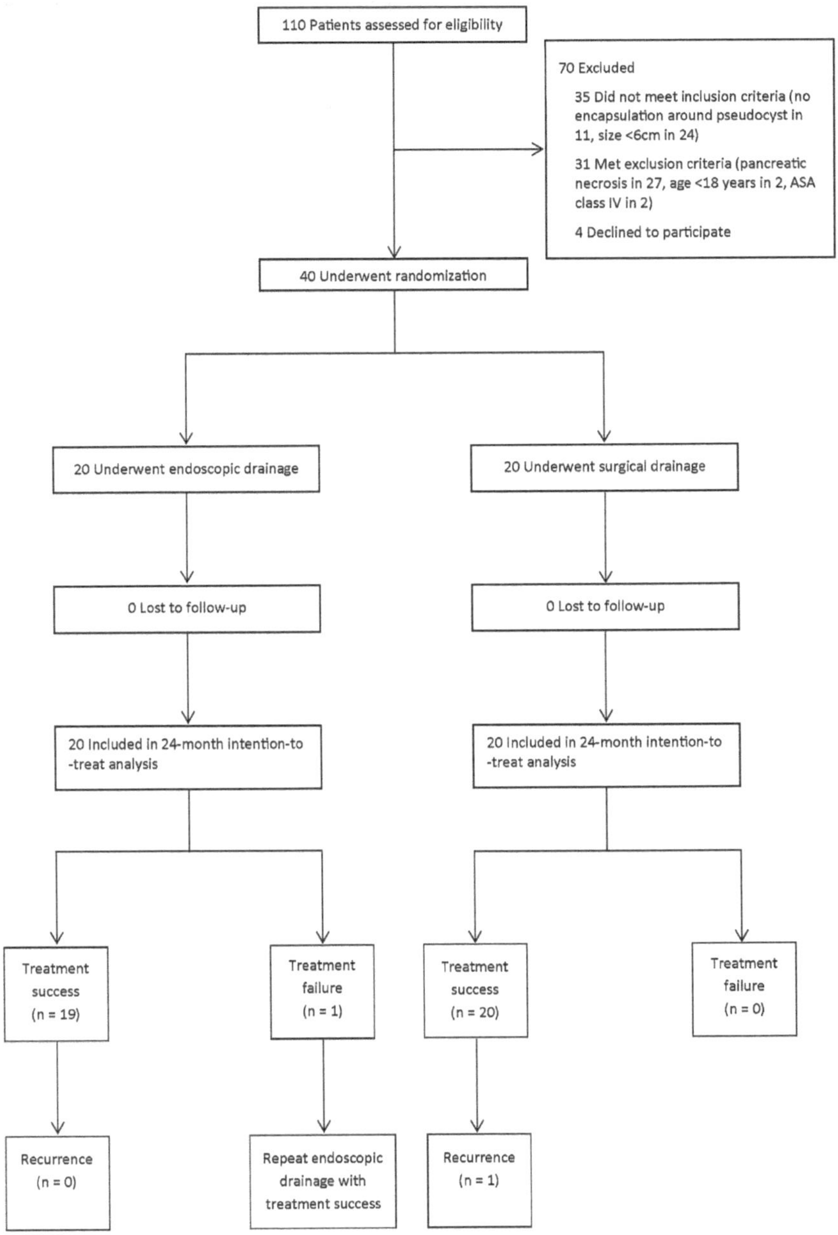

FIGURE 1.—Diagrammatic illustration of participant screening, enrollment, randomization, and follow-up evaluation. ASA, American Society of Anesthesiologists. (Reprinted from Varadarajulu S, Bang JY, Sutton BS, et al. Equal efficacy of endoscopic and surgical cystogastrostomy for pancreatic pseudocyst drainage in a randomized trial. *Gastroenterology.* 2013;145:583-590.e1, Copyright 2013, with permission from AGA Institute.)

new x-ray at the end of this period. Based on these studies, if there is no evidence of contrast in the colon at this point, then we should proceed with surgical exploration.

J. Hines, MD

References

1. Branco BC, Barmparas G, Schnüriger B, et al. Systematic review and meta-analysis of the diagnostic and therapeutic role of water-soluble contrast agent in adhesive small bowel obstruction. *Br J Surg.* 2010;97:470-478.
2. Abbas S, Bissett IP, Parry BR. Oral water soluble contrast for the management of adhesive small bowel obstruction. *Cochrane Database Syst Rev.* 2005;(25): CD004651.

Postoperative Outcomes After Laparoscopic Splenectomy Compared With Open Splenectomy

Musallam KM, Khalife M, Sfeir PM, et al (American Univ of Beirut Med Ctr, Lebanon; et al)
Ann Surg 257:1116-1123, 2013

Objective.—To evaluate 30-day postoperative outcomes in laparoscopic (LS) versus open splenectomy (OS).

Summary Background Data.—LS has generally been associated with lower rates of postoperative complications than OS. However, evidence mainly comes from small studies that failed to adjust for the confounding effects of the underlying indication or clinical condition that may have favored the use of one technique over the other.

Methods.—A retrospective cohort study of patients undergoing splenectomy in 2008 and 2009 using data from the American College of Surgeons National Surgical Quality Improvement Program database (n = 1781). Retrieved data included 30-day mortality and morbidity (cardiac, respiratory, central nervous system, renal, wound, sepsis, venous thromboembolism, and major bleeding outcomes), demographics, indication, and preoperative risk factors. We used multivariate logistic regression to assess the adjusted effect of the splenectomy technique on outcomes.

Results.—A total of 874 (49.1%) cases had LS and 907 (50.9%) had OS. After adjusting for all potential confounders including the indication and preoperative risk factors, LS was associated with decreased 30-day mortality [OR (odds ratio): 0.39, 95% CI: 0.18–0.84] and postoperative respiratory occurrences (OR: 0.46, 95% CI: 0.27–0.76), wound occurrences (OR: 0.37, 95% CI: 0.11–0.79), and sepsis (OR: 0.52, 95% CI: 0.26–0.89) when compared with OS. Patients who underwent LS also had a significantly shorter total length of hospital stay and were less likely to receive intraoperative transfusions compared with patients who underwent OS.

Conclusions.—LS is associated with more favorable postoperative outcomes than OS, irrespective of the indication for splenectomy or the patient's clinical status.

▶ The utility of laparoscopic splenectomy has been known for some time and is documented with many published case series. This publication includes several cases from the American College of Surgeons National Surgical Quality Improvement Program database. Nearly 1800 patients who underwent either a laparoscopic or open splenectomy were analyzed. Laparoscopic splenectomy resulted in fewer blood transfusions, lower risk of pulmonary and wound complications, less sepsis, half the number of days in the hospital, and lower mortality.

The 2 groups, however, were not comparable with regard to indication. Patients undergoing laparoscopic splenectomy were more likely to be having this performed for hematologic conditions. This makes sense because one common indication for a planned splenectomy is idiopathic thrombocytopenia—a condition characterized by a small spleen. Although it has been shown that very large spleens can be removed laparoscopically, these are clearly a challenge. I have found that preoperative splenic artery embolization on the day of surgery decreases blood loss and leads to a lower chance of conversion to an open operation. Embolization the day before or earlier often results in significant pain and may initiate a systemic inflammatory response requiring intensive monitoring.

J. Hines, MD

Randomized Clinical Trial of Intestinal Ostomy Takedown Comparing Pursestring Wound Closure vs Conventional Closure to Eliminate the Risk of Wound Infection

Camacho-Mauries D, Rodriguez-Díaz JL, Salgado-Nesme N, et al (Instituto Nacional de Ciencias Médicas y Nutrición Salvador Zubirán, Mexico)

Dis Colon Rectum 56:205-211, 2013

Background.—The use of temporary stomas has been demonstrated to reduce septic complications, especially in high-risk anastomosis; therefore, it is necessary to reduce the number of complications secondary to ostomy takedowns, namely wound infection, anastomotic leaks, and intestinal obstruction.

Objective.—To compare the rates of superficial wound infection and patient satisfaction after pursestring closure of ostomy wound vs conventional linear closure.

Design.—Patients undergoing colostomy or ileostomy closure between January 2010 and February 2011 were randomly assigned to linear closure ($n = 30$) or pursestring closure ($n = 31$) of their ostomy wound. Wound infection within 30 days of surgery was defined as the presence of purulent discharge, pain, erythema, warmth, or positive culture for bacteria. Patient satisfaction, healing time, difficulty managing the wound, and limitation of activities were analyzed with the Likert questionnaire.

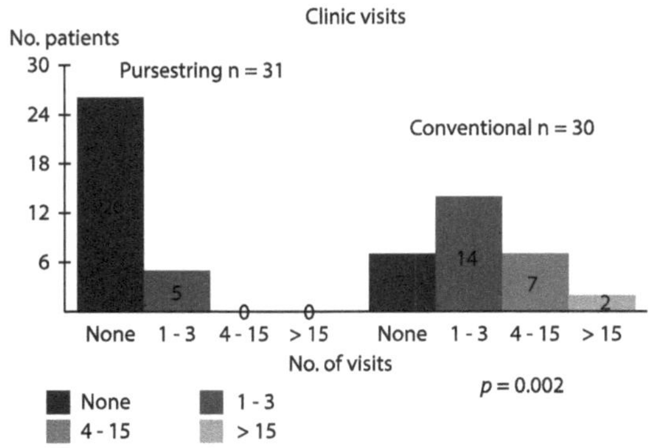

FIGURE 5.—Number of outpatient additional clinic visits to address wound issues. (Reprinted from Camacho-Mauries D, Rodriguez-Díaz JL, Salgado-Nesme N, et al. Randomized clinical trial of intestinal ostomy takedown comparing pursestring wound closure vs conventional closure to eliminate the risk of wound infection. *Dis Colon Rectum.* 2013;56:205-211, with permission from The ASCRS 2013.)

TABLE 3.—Results

Variables	Pursestring (n = 31)	Conventional (n = 30)	*P*
Healing time, wk	3.8	5.9	0.0001
Wound infection	0/31	11/30	0.0001
Morbidity			
Anastomotic leaks	0/31	1/30	0.3
Midline infection	2/13	3/15	0.75
Postincisional hernia	0/31	2/30	0.14
Intestinal obstruction	3/31	2/30	0.66

Results.—The infection rate for the control group was 36.6% (n = 11) vs 0% in the pursestring closure group (p < 0.0001). Healing time was 5.9 weeks in the linear closure group and 3.8 weeks in the pursestring group (p = 0.0002). Seventy percent of the Patients with pursestring closure were very satisfied in comparison with 20% in the other group (p = 0.0001).

Limitations.—This study was limited by the heterogeneity in the type of stoma in both groups.

Conclusion.—The pursestring method resulted in the absence of infection after ostomy wound closure (shorter healing time and improved patient satisfaction) (Fig 5, Table 3).

▶ Surgical site infection (SSI) is a particularly challenging problem in colorectal surgery, including the management of the ostomy site after reversal. National reporting guidelines for hospitals are now focused on SSI in this patient population. Lowering SSI in colorectal surgery patients provides a real opportunity for improved outcome and lower cost. This study details a randomized, prospective trial that may, in part, address these issues for the practicing surgeon.

The purse string technique, as described, involves dissecting circularly around the stoma, then closing the wound with a single, running subcuticular

0-0 polypropylene suture. This effectively decreases the size of the defect (a 3- to 4-mm orifice will remain), while allowing for drainage. This technique was compared with a traditional linear closure comprised of interrupted 2-0 polypropylene sutures.

The authors report an astonishing 0% SSI rate in the purse string group in contrast to a somewhat higher-than-expected 33% SSI rate in the linear group (Table 3). They also note a significantly decreased healing time in the purse string group, although this may reflect the lag time required to diagnose and open the wounds closed in the linear group. Most impressively, the authors note that the number of unplanned postoperative clinic visits was significantly lower in the purse string group (Fig 5). This is perhaps related to the ease with which patients with a purse string closure can manage the wound at home, and it could have a huge impact for the individual surgeon's clinic flow and resource utilization.

Regardless of technique, the mainstay of treatment for grossly contaminated wounds remains frequent examination, early detection and drainage, culture-driven antibiotic treatment when necessary, and patient education. The purse string closure could be an excellent choice.

J. Hines, MD

Randomized Prospective Study to Compare Laparoscopic Appendectomy Versus Umbilical Single-Incision Appendectomy

Frutos MD, Abrisqueta J, Lujan J, et al (Hospital Universitario "Virgen de la Arrixaca," Murcia, Spain)

Ann Surg 257:413-418, 2013

Introduction.—The use of single-incision laparoscopic surgery may represent an improvement over conventional laparoscopic surgery. In recent years, more and more articles have been published demonstrating the feasibility of this approach. Hence, for this reason, we present this randomized prospective study to compare the 2 techniques.

Methods.—Between September 2009 and December 2010, a total of 184 patients with a diagnosis of acute appendicitis and indicated for surgery were included in the study, of whom, 91 received an appendectomy via a single umbilical incision and 93 via conventional laparoscopy. The study protocol was approved by the ethical committee of the Virgen de la Arrixaca University Hospital (Murcia). The study was registered on ClinicalTrials.gov with inscription number NCT0151529. All the operations were performed by the same team of surgeons.

Results.—As far as the demographical results of the study population are concerned, there were no significant differences between the 2 groups for age, weight, sex, body mass index, and removed appendix type. Operating time was longer with the single-port approach: 38.13 ± 13.49 versus 32.12 ± 12.44 minutes ($P = 0.02$). Significant differences were observed for postoperative pain, which was measured on the visual analog scale, with less pain reported in the single-incision group: 2.76 ± 1.64 versus

TABLE 2.—Operative and Postoperative Results

	Single-Incision Laparoscopic Surgery (n = 91)	Conventional (n = 93)	*P*
Operating time, mean ± standard deviation, min	38.13 ± 13.49	32.12 ± 12.44	0.02
Scale of pain (range, 1–10), mean ± standard deviation	2.76 ± 1.64	3.78 ± 1.76	<0.001
Reoperation, %	0/91	1/93	0.08
Early complications, %	4/91	4/93	0.52
Late complications, %	1/91	0/93	0.31
Length of hospital stay, mean ± standard deviation, h	18.86 ± 9.77	21.32 ± 11.72	0.12

3.78 ± 1.76 ($P < 0.001$). There were no significant differences between the 2 groups for early and late complications and lengths of hospital stay measured in postoperative hours.

Conclusions.—The transumbilical single-port approach is seen as a feasible technique for performing appendectomy. It does not increase the rate of complications and represents a possible alternative to conventional laparoscopic appendectomy (Table 2).

► Despite its relative simplicity, the management of acute appendicitis continues to receive considerable attention. Nationally, there are groups interested in the nonoperative approach of acute pancreatitis with antibiotics alone. Several randomized studies are in the process of examining this concept. Until then, we continue to refine our operative techniques, and this randomized trial from Spain investigated the utility of single-port (Covidien) vs conventional laparoscopic appendectomy. Overall, the results were comparable with a slightly longer operating time and the need for an additional port in only one patient who underwent the single-port approach. One patient in this group also had an incisional hernia. The single-port group did experience less postoperative pain, and one patient in the conventional group required a reoperation for injury and bleeding from the inferior epigastric artery (Table 2). Whether the single-port approach actually reduces postoperative pain is not clear. Other prospective studies report equivalent pain scores or even increased pain scores with the use of a large umbilical port.[1] And to create a suitable working angle between instruments, it is best to use special instruments that rotate between 0° and 80° at their distal end like the Endodissect Roticulator. The use of a single port for appendectomy will probably be based on surgeon preference unless a significant cost differential develops between the 2 techniques.

J. Hines, MD

Reference

1. St Peter SD, Adibe OO, Juang D, et al. Single incision versus standard 3-port laparoscopic appendectomy: a prospective randomized trial. *Ann Surg*. 2011;254: 586-590.

Short and Long-Term Mortality After Appendectomy in Sweden 1987 to 2006. Influence of Appendectomy Diagnosis, Sex, Age, Co-morbidity, Surgical Method, Hospital Volume, and Time Period. A National Population-Based Cohort Study

Andersson RE (Ryhov County Hosp, Jönköping, Sweden)

World J Surg 37:974-981, 2013

Background.—Avoiding mortality is the ultimate goal when managing patients with suspected appendicitis. Previous studies have shown high mortality after negative appendectomy. This national cohort study analyzes short- and long-term mortality after appendectomy in relation to appendectomy diagnosis, age, co-morbidity, surgical method, hospital volume, and time period.

Method.—A total of 223,543 appendectomy patients treated from 1987 to 2006 were identified from the Swedish National Patient Register and followed up via the Swedish Cause of Death Register. Analysis of mortality was conducted as Standardized Mortality Ratio (SMR) and by Cox multivariate regression.

Results.—Negative appendectomy was followed by a higher mortality in the short term (30-day Standardized Mortality Ratio (SMR_{30d}) 8.95, confidence interval (CI) 6.68–12.61) than after perforated appendicitis (SMR_{30d} 6.39, CI 5.44–7.48), and remained increased for up to 5 years (SMR_{5yr} 1.31, CI 1.16–1.47). Non-perforated appendicitis had a lower than expected long-term mortality (SMR_{5yr} 0.72, CI 0.68–0.76). These differences remained after adjustment for covariates. Laparoscopic appendectomy had similar short-term mortality as open appendectomy but lower than expected long-term morality (SMR_{5yr} 0.70, CI 0.62–0.78). Mortality was decreasing during the study period. Hospital volume had no influence on mortality.

Conclusions.—Negative appendectomy is associated with excess short- and long-term mortality that remains after adjustment for known confounders, suggesting an association with underlying undetected morbidity. This motivates an improved preoperative diagnosis to avoid the additional trauma from unnecessary surgical interventions, but further studies are needed to investigate the cause of the increased long-term mortality and if this can be prevented by an improved follow-up of patients with negative appendectomy. Laparoscopic and open appendectomy have similar short-term mortality. The lower long-term mortality after non-perforated appendicitis and laparoscopic appendectomy suggest selection of healthier patients for these interventions. This possibility should be taken into account when comparing mortality after open and laparoscopic appendectomy.

▶ Appendectomy is a standard procedure for general surgery, and the management and outcome are relatively predictable. The controversies surrounding the use of imaging and rates of negative appendectomy have been discussed at length. The long-term implications for our patients, however, are rarely considered. What is the outcome for patients who have a negative appendectomy, and is a source for the pain ever identified? This article reviews the outcome of more than 200 000 appendectomy patients in Sweden and examines the long-term outcomes, particularly for patients who had a negative appendectomy. Short-term mortality in patients with a normal appendiceal pathology was higher by 8-fold, and this effect was seen up to 5 years after the appendectomy. This is a curious finding and suggests that these patients may have serious undiscovered diagnoses responsible for their presentation and ultimate outcome, or that these patients simply have a higher incidence of comorbid conditions that have yet to have been identified. The authors suggest that patients with a negative appendectomy may need closer follow-up and additional investigation to correct this discrepancy in mortality. As surgeons, we usually are a bit worried when we remove an appendix that is normal thinking that we subjected the patient to a potentially unnecessary operation. Most of these patients recover without difficulty and leave our care relatively quickly. However, we may want to reconsider the implications of a negative appendectomy with the results of this study and work with our medicine colleagues more closely to close the loop and improve the outlook for this group of patients.

J. Hines, MD

Among 1,706 cases of abdominal wall reconstruction, what factors influence the occurrence of major operative complications?

Fischer JP, Wink JD, Nelson JA, et al (Hosp of the Univ of Pennsylvania, Philadelphia)

Surgery 155:311-319, 2014

Background.—Abdominal wall reconstruction (AWR) poses a substantial operative challenge, often in the setting of multiple failed attempts at repair in high-risk patients. Our aim was to assess risk factors for major operative morbidity after AWR using the American College of Surgeons-National Surgical Quality Improvement Program (ACS-NSQIP) patient database.

Methods.—A review of the ACS-NSQIP database of outcomes from 2005 to 2010 was performed to identify patients undergoing AWR utilizing Current Procedural Terminology codes for ventral hernia repair and a concomitant component separation. Independent variables included patient demographics, medical comorbidities, and operative considerations. Major operative complication (deep wound infection, graft or prosthetic loss, or unplanned return to the operating room within 30 days) was used as our dependent variable. Stepwise, multivariate logistic regression was performed to evaluate patient risk factors influencing the occurrence of major operative complications.

Results.—We identified 1,706 patients with an average age of 55.9 ± 12.8 years with 30.1% undergoing concurrent intra-abdominal procedures and 57.1% undergoing mesh repair. Notable medical comorbidities included obesity (63.4%), smoking (24.9%), hypertension (53.1%), diabetes (19.9%), and anemia (22.6%). Average operative time was

211.7 ± 105.0 minutes. Regression analysis determined that prolonged operative time (odds ratio [OR], 2.7; $P < .001$) and American Society of Anesthesiologists >2 (OR, 1.8; $P = .009$) were positively associated, whereas advanced age (OR, 0.5; $P = .005$) was negatively associated with the occurrence of major operative complications.

Conclusions.—Greater operative times and overall patient health are important prognostic factors for individuals undergoing AWR. The increased physiologic stress of a greater operative duration on patients who often have multiple comorbidities seems to play a significant role in predicting negative outcomes after AWR.

▶ Abdominal wall reconstruction for incisional and ventral hernias and traumatic defects can be quite complex, and the results are variable. We now have multiple options with regard to method and materials for reconstruction with no clear standardized approach assuring the best outcomes. This series, which may be the largest examining abdominal wall reconstruction, examines the National Surgical Quality Improvement Program database and includes more than 1700 patients. Interestingly, more than 70% of the patients underwent a concomitant procedure, including 25 patients who had a colon procedure. This is concerning, given the fear of increased infection. One hundred fifty-one patients experienced a superficial wound infection, and 135 patients had a deep or organ space infection. Not much information is available regarding the type of prosthetic material used, but 18% of the patients did have acellular dermal matrix implanted. The risk of complications correlated with the length of operation and American Society of Anesthesiologists class. The authors suggest that a long operation is a surrogate for a difficult procedure and that these patients receive additional fluid impacting bowel edema, intra abdominal pressure, and infection risk. This report is included this year because it provides a modern state-of-the-art assessment of this common procedure in our country and can be used as a comparison with your results.

J. Hines, MD

Glue Versus Suture Fixation of Mesh During Open Repair of Inguinal Hernias: A Systematic Review and Meta-Analysis

Colvin HS, Rao A, Cavali M, et al (Western General Hosp, Edinburgh UK; Ninewells Hosp, Dundee, UK; Univ of Insubria, Milano, Italy; et al)

World J Surg 37:2282-2292, 2013

Background.—Glue fixation of mesh has been explored for some time as a strategy for reducing postoperative chronic groin pain. Previous studies have come to different conclusions about the superiority of one method over another. We conducted a meta-analysis of randomized control trials comparing the performance of glue versus suture fixation of mesh in open inguinal hernioplasty.

Methods.—Studies published up to November 2012 were searched using PubMed, EMBASE, MEDLINE, Cochrane Library, and the international

Study or Subgroup	Glue Fixation Events	Glue Fixation Total	Suture Fixation Events	Suture Fixation Total	Weight	Odds Ratio M-H, Fixed, 95% CI
Campanellin 2012	4	149	9	155	20.7%	0.45 [0.13, 1.49]
Dabrowiecki 2012	0	20	0	21		Not estimable
Kim-Fuchs 2012	3	111	10	118	22.8%	0.30 [0.08, 1.12]
Mikhail 2012	3	101	10	97	23.9%	0.27 [0.07, 1.00]
Paajane 2011	17	144	11	141	0.0%	1.58 [0.71, 3.51]
Shen 2012	0	51	2	51	6.0%	0.19 [0.01, 4.11]
Sozen 2012	0	62	5	54	14.1%	0.07 [0.00, 1.33]
Testini 2010	0	108	2	59	7.7%	0.11 [0.01, 2.25]
Wong 2011	2	29	2	25	4.8%	0.85 [0.11, 6.53]
Total (95% CI)		**631**		**580**	**100.0%**	**0.30 [0.16, 0.55]**
Total events	12		40			

Heterogeneity: $Chi^2 = 2.93$, df = 6 (P = 0.82); $I^2 = 0\%$
Test for overall effect: Z = 3.82 (P = 0.0001)

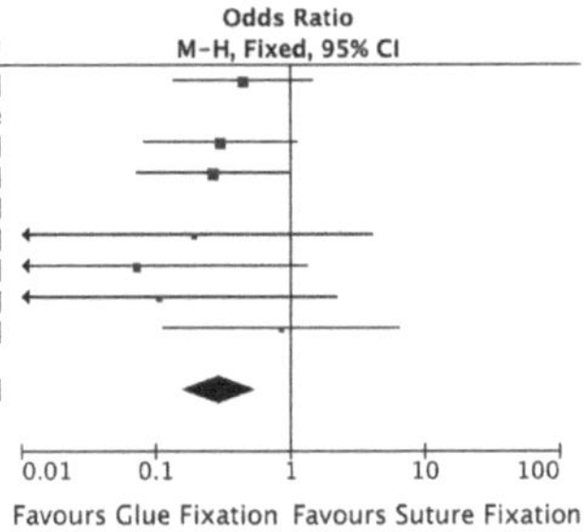

FIGURE 2.—Forrest plot comparing chronic groin pain following glue fixation versus suture fixation of mesh during open inguinal hernia repair. A Mantel–Haenszel random effect model was used for the meta-analysis. Odds ratios are charted with 95 % confidence intervals. (With kind permission from Springer Science+Business Media. Colvin HS, Rao A, Cavali M, et al. Glue versus suture fixation of mesh during open repair of inguinal hernias: a systematic review and meta-analysis. *World J Surg.* 2013;37:2282-2292, with permission from Société Internationale de Chirurgie.)

standard randomised controlled trials number (ISRCTN) register. Mean differences (MDs) were derived from secondary continuous outcomes and pooled risk ratios (RRs) for categoric outcomes. Meta-analysis was conducted utilizing the random-effects and fixed-effects models as appropriate.

Results.—Ten randomized controlled studies were selected, with a total of 1,623 patients. Glue fixation for open inguinal hernioplasty reduced chronic groin pain (RR 0.46, 95 % confidence interval (CI) 0.22–0.97), hematoma (RR 0.56, 95 % CI 0.34–0.90), acute postoperative pain (MD −7.92, 95 % CI, −13.17 to −2.66), and time taken to return to normal activities (MD −1.39, 95 % CI, −2.58 to −0.21). There was no evidence of an increase in adverse outcomes including recurrence with glue fixation (RR 0.83, 95 % CI 0.30–2.35).

Conclusions.—Glue fixation of mesh for open inguinal hernioplasty is superior in many outcomes including the reduction of chronic groin pain. Glue fixation was not associated with an increased risk of hernia recurrence (Fig 2).

▶ Issues regarding recurrence and return to work have been largely addressed by modern surgical approaches to inguinal hernia repair. A percentage of patients do, however, experience chronic pain after surgery. Solutions to this are inconsistent and range from anti-inflammatory medications to complex neurectomy procedures. Many of the patients will never recover from chronic pain, and efforts to minimize this are important. Some have advocated the use of glue rather than suture or tacking to minimize the possibility of this complication. Two products are available: Tisseel (Baxter, Deerfield, IL, USA) and N-butyl cyanoacrylate (Dermabond, Ethicon, Cincinnati, OH, USA). This group performed a meta-analysis of current randomized trials evaluating glue versus suture fixation of mesh during open hernia repair. Consistently, the group identified a pattern of advantage for glue with regard to both acute and chronic pain (Fig 2), hematoma occurrence, and return to normal activities. The occurrence of hematoma may have been less simply because there was no suturing in the glue group. This analysis includes a fairly large group of patients (1623) and randomized data, so the conclusions are probably reliable. For some surgeons, it may be difficult to convert to glue because it is somewhat of a leap of faith to imagine that glue will keep the mesh in place until it is fully incorporated. However, the incidence of recurrence was no different between the 2 groups. Glue is certainly more expensive than suture, and so the risk-benefit analysis for any health system will need to account for this compared with the expense incurred from patients who go on to have chronic pain after suture fixation.

J. Hines, MD

A systematic review and meta-analysis evaluating the effectiveness of lightweight mesh against heavyweight mesh in influencing the incidence of chronic groin pain following laparoscopic inguinal hernia repair

Sajid MS, Kalra L, Parampalli U, et al (Worthing Hosp, UK)
Am J Surg 205:726-736, 2013

Background.—A systematic analysis was conducted of randomized controlled trials (RCTs) comparing lightweight mesh (LWM) with heavyweight mesh in laparoscopic inguinal hernia repair.

Methods.—Data extracted from the included RCTs were analyzed according to the principles of meta-analysis.

Results.—Eleven RCTs encompassing 2,189 patients were analyzed. In a fixed-effects model, operating time, postoperative pain, and recurrence rate were statistically similar between LWM and heavyweight mesh. LWM was associated with fewer perioperative complications and a reduced risk for developing chronic groin pain. There was also a reduced risk for developing other groin symptoms, such as foreign body sensations, but it was not statistically significant.

Conclusions.—The use of LWM for laparoscopic inguinal hernia repair is not associated with an increased risk for hernia recurrence. LWM reduces the incidence of chronic groin pain, groin stiffness, and foreign body

	LWM			HWM				Mean Difference
Study or Subgroup	Mean	SD	Total	Mean	SD	Total	Weight	IV, Fixed, 95% CI
Bringman [35]	9	7.25	69	11	15.25	70	2.8%	-2.00 [-5.96, 1.96]
Chowbey [37]	7.2	4.5	191	7.52	4.75	211	54.5%	-0.32 [-1.22, 0.58]
Heikkinen [39]	15	18	68	13	7.25	69	2.1%	2.00 [-2.61, 6.61]
Langenbach [40]	33.5	4.1	30	35.3	4.1	60	13.8%	-1.80 [-3.60, -0.00]
Langenbach [41]	33.5	4.1	58	35.3	4.1	117	26.8%	-1.80 [-3.09, -0.51]
Total (95% CI)			**416**			**527**	**100.0%**	**-0.92 [-1.59, -0.25]**

Heterogeneity: Chi² = 6.23, df = 4 (P = 0.18); I² = 36%
Test for overall effect: Z = 2.70 (P = 0.007)

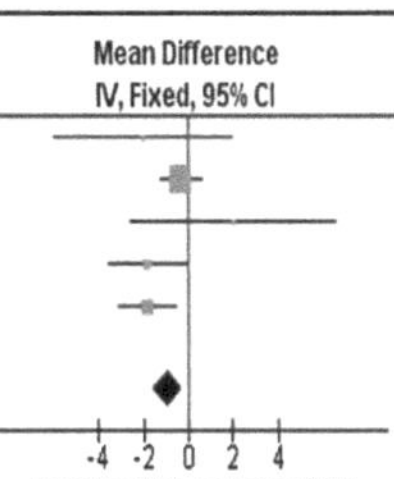

FIGURE 6.—Time to return to work. IV = Inverse Variance. (Reprinted from The American Journal of Surgery. Sajid MS, Kalra L, Parampalli U, et al. A systematic review and meta-analysis evaluating the effectiveness of lightweight mesh against heavyweight mesh in influencing the incidence of chronic groin pain following laparoscopic inguinal hernia repair. *Am J Surg*. 2013;205:726-736, Copyright 2013, with permission from Elsevier.)

Study or Subgroup	LWM Events	LWM Total	HWM Events	HWM Total	Weight	Risk Ratio M-H, Fixed, 95% CI
Bittner [33]	9	150	13	150	23.3%	0.69 [0.31, 1.57]
Bittner [34]	14	450	12	150	32.2%	0.39 [0.18, 0.82]
Bringman [35]	0	69	1	70	2.7%	0.34 [0.01, 8.16]
Champault [36]	3	51	11	66	17.2%	0.35 [0.10, 1.20]
Chowbey [37]	3	191	10	211	17.0%	0.33 [0.09, 1.19]
Langenbach [41]	0	58	2	117	3.0%	0.40 [0.02, 8.20]
Peeters [42]	5	39	2	20	4.7%	1.28 [0.27, 6.03]
Total (95% CI)		**1008**		**784**	**100.0%**	**0.48 [0.31, 0.75]**
Total events	34		51			

Heterogeneity: Chi² = 3.24, df = 6 (P = 0.78); I² = 0%
Test for overall effect: Z = 3.27 (P = 0.001)

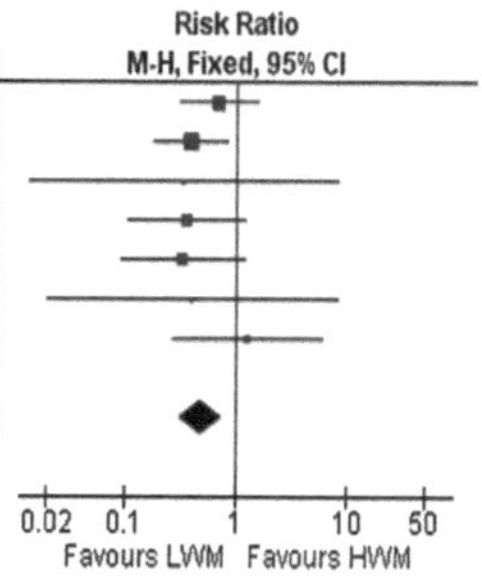

FIGURE 8.—Chronic groin pain. M-H = Mantel-Haenszel. (Reprinted from The American Journal of Surgery. Sajid MS, Kalra L, Parampalli U, et al. A systematic review and meta-analysis evaluating the effectiveness of lightweight mesh against heavyweight mesh in influencing the incidence of chronic groin pain following laparoscopic inguinal hernia repair. *Am J Surg*. 2013;205:726-736, Copyright 2013, with permission from Elsevier.)

sensations. Therefore, LWM may routinely be used in laparoscopic inguinal hernia repair. However, high-quality RCTs with longer follow-up periods are required to validate these findings (Figs 6 and 8).

▶ When inguinal hernias are fixed, there are several choices for the type of mesh and the approach of repair. Much progress has been made with regard to lowering recurrence rates and improving recovering, but we remain faced with the problem of chronic pain in our patients. You may have your favorite mesh and know that your technique is superior to all others. A few years ago, lightweight mesh products became available and were developed with the concept that less foreign material and larger pore sizes might reduce postoperative pain. It appears this is the case when it comes to laparoscopic inguinal hernia repair. This meta-analysis included 11 randomized trials and almost 2200 patients. The use of lightweight mesh resulted in fewer perioperative complications, a feeling of groin stiffness, and lower incidence of chronic pain (Fig 8). In addition, patients who received lightweight mesh had a quicker return to work (Fig 6). Some surgeons have feared a high chance of recurrence, but this was not the case—the recurrence rate was equal. So maybe it is time to switch to lightweight mesh for your patients.

J. Hines, MD

Laparoscopic component separation reduces postoperative wound complications but does not alter recurrence rates in complex hernia repairs

Fox M, Cannon RM, Egger M, et al (Univ of Louisville, KY)

Am J Surg 206:869-875, 2013

Background.—The purpose of this study was to evaluate and compare the incidence of wound complications after laparoscopic component separation (LCS) vs open component separation (OCS) in patients with complex abdominal wall hernias.

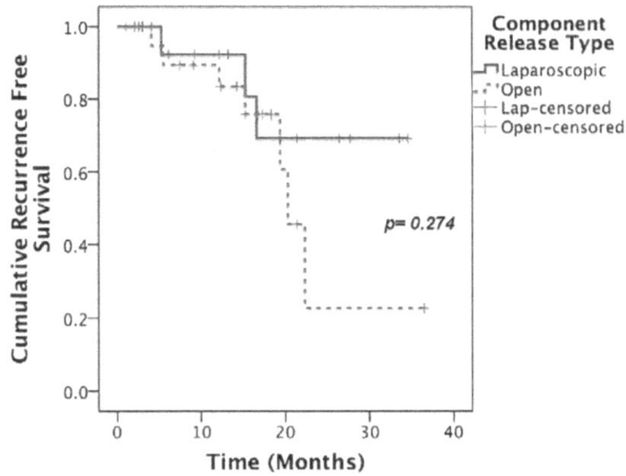

FIGURE 3.—Kaplan-Meier curve demonstrating cumulative recurrence free survival in OCS and LCS. (Reprinted from The American Journal of Surgery. Fox M, Cannon RM, Egger M, et al. Laparoscopic component separation reduces postoperative wound complications but does not alter recurrence rates in complex hernia repairs. *Am J Surg*. 2013;206:869-875, Copyright 2013, with permission from Elsevier.)

Methods.—A retrospective review was performed of all patients who underwent LCS or OCS for repair of a complex abdominal wall hernia at a single institution between 2009 and 2011. Charts were reviewed to identify postoperative wound complications. A computed tomographic scan or physical examination was used for the determination of hernia recurrence. Categoric variables were compared using the Fisher exact test. Univariate and multivariate analyses were performed using linear and Cox regression. Recurrence rates were compared using log-rank tests (Kaplan-Meier method).

Results.—A total of 44 patients underwent LCS (n = 18) or OCS (n = 26). There was no statistically significant difference between categoric variables. Multivariate analysis using wound complications as the dependent variable showed a statistically significantly lower rate of wound complications in the LCS group.

Conclusions.—LCS is associated with a lower rate of wound complications when compared with OCS but yields comparable recurrence rates (Fig 3).

▶ The repair of complex incisional hernias is one of the most challenging operations because the outcomes are generally variable and the complications significant. Over the last several years, the concept of component separation has been popularized and offers several advantages. Namely, the procedure utilizes native tissue to repair the defect and may result in lower recurrence rates. Initial approaches utilized an open technique, but more recently many advocate a laparoscopic operation. The laparoscopic technique maintains better blood supply to the fascial/muscular compartment because the small perforating vessels are not compromised. This case series examined the experience of this approach versus an open approach to component separation. The group found a lower wound complication rate, which is common to laparoscopic operations but may also be due to vascular preservation. Despite the component approach, more than a quarter of the open procedure patients and 17% of the laparoscopic patients experienced a hernia recurrence (Fig 3). Because there is no standard and reliable operative choice for the repair of incisional hernias, surgeons should have a large array of capabilities to tackle these. Learning how to properly perform a component separation repair is not particularly challenging but can offer your patients one additional and probably more reliable option. Your patients may also benefit from a laparoscopic procedure with all the inherent advantages described by this report.

J. Hines, MD

A meta-analysis examining the use of tacker mesh fixation versus glue mesh fixation in laparoscopic inguinal hernia repair

Sajid MS, Ladwa N, Kalra L, et al (Worthing Hosp, West Sussex, UK)
Am J Surg 206:103-111, 2013

Background.—The aim of this study was to systematically analyze the randomized trials comparing tacker mesh fixation with glue mesh fixation (GMF) in laparoscopic inguinal hernia repair (LIHR).

Methods.—Standard electronic database were searched to retrieve relevant randomized trials comparing tacker mesh fixation with GMF in LIHR, which were analyzed systematically using RevMan.

Results.—Five randomized controlled trials encompassing 1,001 patients were retrieved from the electronic databases. In a random-effects model, operating time, postoperative pain, postoperative complications, length of hospital stay and risk for hernia recurrence were statistically comparable between the 2 techniques of mesh fixation in LIHR. However, GMF was associated with a reduced risk for developing chronic groin pain.

Conclusions.—GMF in LIHR does not increase the risk for hernia recurrence and reduces the risk for developing chronic groin pain. It is comparable with tacker mesh fixation in terms of operation time, postoperative

	TMF		GMF			Risk Ratio
Study or Subgroup	**Events**	**Total**	**Events**	**Total**	**Weight**	**M-H, Fixed, 95% CI**
Boldo	0	11	0	11		Not estimable
Lau	8	47	5	46	80.2%	1.57 [0.55, 4.43]
Lovisetto et al	6	98	0	99	7.9%	13.13 [0.75, 229.98]
Olmi et al	29	450	0	150	11.9%	19.75 [1.21, 321.33]
Total (95% CI)		**606**		**306**	**100.0%**	**4.64 [1.85, 11.66]**
Total events	43		5			

Heterogeneity: Chi² = 5.73, df = 2 (P = 0.06); I² = 65%
Test for overall effect: Z = 3.27 (P = 0.001)

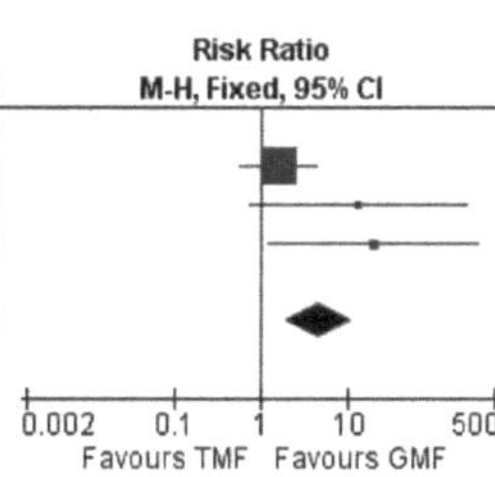

FIGURE 6.—Forest plot for chronic groin pain after the use of TMF and GMF in LIHR. RRs are shown with 95% CIs. M-H = Mantel-Haenszel. (Reprinted from The American Journal of Surgery. Sajid MS, Ladwa N, Kalra L, et al. A meta-analysis examining the use of tacker mesh fixation versus glue mesh fixation in laparoscopic inguinal hernia repair. *Am J Surg*. 2013;206:103-111, Copyright 2013, with permission from Elsevier.)

Study or Subgroup	TMG Events	TMG Total	GMF Events	GMF Total	Weight	Risk Ratio M-H, Fixed, 95% CI
Boldo	2	11	3	11	48.0%	0.67 [0.14, 3.24]
Fortelny et al	1	45	1	44	16.2%	0.98 [0.06, 15.15]
Lau	0	47	0	46		Not estimable
Lovisetto et al	0	98	1	99	23.9%	0.34 [0.01, 8.17]
Olmi et al	3	450	0	150	12.0%	2.34 [0.12, 45.11]
Total (95% CI)		**651**		**350**	**100.0%**	**0.84 [0.27, 2.59]**
Total events	6		5			

Heterogeneity: $Chi^2 = 0.87$, $df = 3$ ($P = 0.83$); $I^2 = 0\%$
Test for overall effect: $Z = 0.31$ ($P = 0.76$)

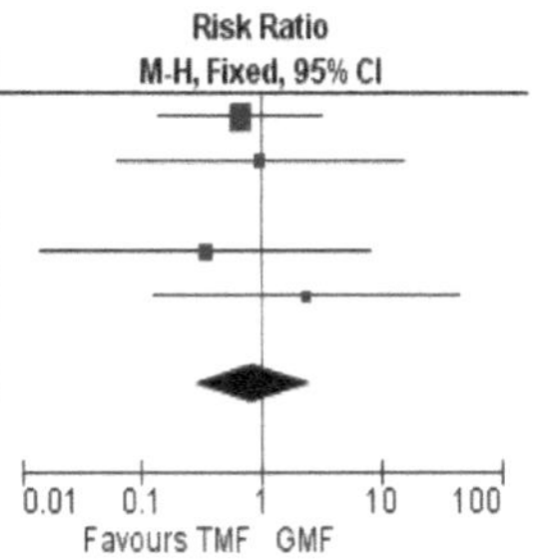

FIGURE 7.—Forest plot for recurrence after the use of TMF and GMF in LIHR. RRs are shown with 95% CIs. M-H = Mantel-Haenszel. (Reprinted from The American Journal of Surgery. Sajid MS, Ladwa N, Kalra L, et al. A meta-analysis examining the use of tacker mesh fixation versus glue mesh fixation in laparoscopic inguinal hernia repair. *Am J Surg*. 2013;206:103-111, Copyright 2013, with permission from Elsevier.)

pain, postoperative complications, length of hospital stay, and risk for hernia recurrence (Figs 6 and 7).

▶ For many surgeons, laparoscopic inguinal hernia repair has become a standard approach, especially for recurrent and bilateral inguinal hernias. Some have advocated glue for mesh fixation to prevent chronic pain postoperatively. We have worried about the risk of recurrence without using a tacking device to secure the mesh in position. This meta-analysis examines the randomized data of 5 studies examining glue vs tack fixation of mesh during laparoscopic inguinal hernia repair. Four of the studies were performed transabdominally and one extraperitoneally. Although the trials were somewhat heterogeneous, the data regarding recurrence (Fig 7) and chronic pain (Fig 6) are fairly clear. From this analysis, glue fixation appears to have an equal recurrence rate to tack fixation with a lower incidence of chronic pain (relative risk, 4.64; $P < .001$). Despite this analysis, several outstanding issues remain. Currently, glue (Tisseel) is not approved for this indication. Additionally, larger hernias may not be appropriate for glue alone, and the confounding factors of the number and positioning of tacks need standardization. Further follow-up to assess for recurrence is still needed.

J. Hines, MD

11 Oncology

Breast

Long-term effects of continuing adjuvant tamoxifen to 10 years versus stopping at 5 years after diagnosis of oestrogen receptor-positive breast cancer: ATLAS, a randomised trial

Davies C, for the Adjuvant Tamoxifen: Longer Against Shorter (ATLAS) Collaborative Group (Univ of Oxford, UK; et al)

Lancet 381:805-816, 2013

Background.—For women with oestrogen receptor (ER)-positive early breast cancer, treatment with tamoxifen for 5 years substantially reduces the breast cancer mortality rate throughout the first 15 years after diagnosis. We aimed to assess the further effects of continuing tamoxifen to 10 years instead of stopping at 5 years.

Methods.—In the worldwide Adjuvant Tamoxifen: Longer Against Shorter (ATLAS) trial, 12,894 women with early breast cancer who had completed 5 years of treatment with tamoxifen were randomly allocated to continue tamoxifen to 10 years or stop at 5 years (open control). Allocation (1:1) was by central computer, using minimisation. After entry (between 1996 and 2005), yearly follow-up forms recorded any recurrence, second cancer, hospital admission, or death. We report effects on breast cancer outcomes among the 6846 women with ER-positive disease, and side-effects among all women (with positive, negative, or unknown ER status). Long-term follow-up still continues. This study is registered, number ISRCTN19652633.

Findings.—Among women with ER-positive disease, allocation to continue tamoxifen reduced the risk of breast cancer recurrence (617 recurrences in 3428 women allocated to continue vs 711 in 3418 controls, $p = 0{\cdot}002$), reduced breast cancer mortality (331 deaths vs 397 deaths, $p = 0{\cdot}01$), and reduced overall mortality (639 deaths vs 722 deaths, $p = 0{\cdot}01$). The reductions in adverse breast cancer outcomes appeared to be less extreme before than after year 10 (recurrence rate ratio [RR] 0·90 [95% CI 0·79–1·02] during years 5–9 and 0·75 [0·62–0·90] in later years; breast cancer mortality RR 0·97 [0·79–1·18] during years 5–9 and 0·71 [0·58–0·88] in later years). The cumulative risk of recurrence during years 5–14 was 21·4% for women allocated to continue versus 25·1% for controls; breast cancer mortality during years 5–14 was

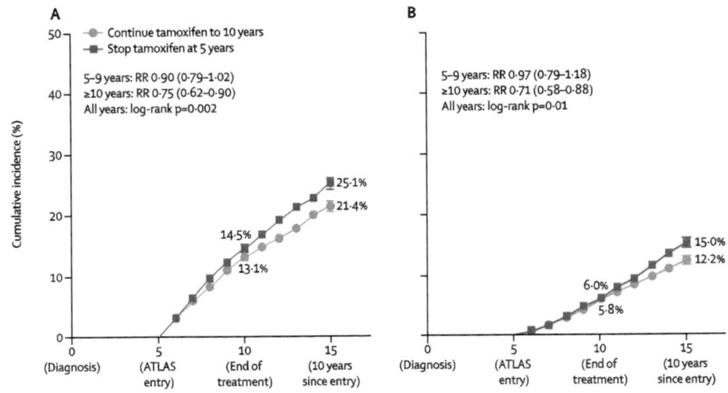

	A: 5–9 years	A: 10–14 years	A: ≥15 years	B: 5–9 years	B: 10–14 years	B: ≥15 years
Continue tamoxifen to 10 years	2·83% (428/15 115)	1·96% (165/8439)	2·54% (24/945)	1·17% (SE 0·09)	1·38% (SE 0·12)	1·64% (SE 0·39)
Stop tamoxifen at 5 years	3·16% (471/14 889)	2·66% (214/8038)	3·03% (26/859)	1·21% (SE 0·09)	2·01% (SE 0·15)	2·29% (SE 0·47)
Rate ratio, from (O–E)/V	0·90 (SE 0·06)	0·74 (SE 0·09)	0·85 (SE 0·26)	0·97 (SE 0·10)	0·70 (SE 0·10)	0·79 (SE 0·27)
Log-rank O–E and variance V	−24·8/224·7	−29·1/94·7	−2·1/12·5	−3·2/94·0	−27·2/77·5	−2·5/10·6

FIGURE 3.—Recurrence (A) and breast cancer mortality (B) by treatment allocation for 6846 women with ER-positive disease Bars show SE. Recurrence rates are percentage per year (events/patient-years of follow-up). Death rates (overall rate-rate in women without recurrence) are percentage per year (SE). ATLAS = Adjuvant Tamoxifen: Longer Against Shorter. (Reprinted from The Lancet. Davies C, for the Adjuvant Tamoxifen: Longer Against Shorter (ATLAS) Collaborative Group. Long-term effects of continuing adjuvant tamoxifen to 10 years versus stopping at 5 years after diagnosis of oestrogen receptor-positive breast cancer: ATLAS, a randomised trial. *Lancet.* 2013;381:805-816 Copyright 2013, with permission from Elsevier.)

12·2% for women allocated to continue versus 15·0% for controls (absolute mortality reduction 2·8%). Treatment allocation seemed to have no effect on breast cancer outcome among 1248 women with ER-negative disease, and an intermediate effect among 4800 women with unknown ER status. Among all 12,894 women, mortality without recurrence from causes other than breast cancer was little affected (691 deaths without recurrence in 6454 women allocated to continue versus 679 deaths in 6440 controls; RR 0·99 [0·89–1·10]; $p = 0·84$). For the incidence (hospitalisation or death) rates of specific diseases, RRs were as follows: pulmonary embolus 1·87 (95% CI 1·13–3·07, $p = 0·01$ [including 0·2% mortality in both treatment groups]), stroke 1·06 (0·83–1·36), ischaemic heart disease 0·76 (0·60–0·95, $p = 0·02$), and endometrial cancer 1·74 (1·30–2·34, $p = 0·0002$). The cumulative risk of endometrial cancer during years 5–14 was 3·1% (mortality 0·4%) for women allocated to continue versus 1·6% (mortality 0·2%) for controls (absolute mortality increase 0·2%).

Interpretation.—For women with ER-positive disease, continuing tamoxifen to 10 years rather than stopping at 5 years produces a further reduction in recurrence and mortality, particularly after year 10. These results, taken together with results from previous trials of 5 years of tamoxifen treatment versus none, suggest that 10 years of tamoxifen treatment can approximately halve breast cancer mortality during the second decade after diagnosis (Fig 3).

► It has been found that women with estrogen receptor (ER)-positive breast cancer who take tamoxifen for 5 years after diagnosis will have reduced risk of breast cancer recurrence and mortality. Interestingly, these benefits seem to extend for 15 years, and what is not clear is whether patients might benefit from taking 10 years of tamoxifen versus 5 years. This trial, called the ATLAS (Adjuvant Tamoxifen Longer Against Shorter) Trial, was designed to address this issue. Women with early breast cancers who had been receiving tamoxifen for several years and who were clinically free of disease were eligible for the trial, which assembled patients between 1996 and 2005 from 36 countries. After 5 years of tamoxifen, women were randomly assigned to receive another 5 years of tamoxifen or no treatment; no placebo was given to the control group. This trial enrolled women who were ER positive, ER negative, and ER unknown. The ER-positive patients were the ones in whom the most meaningful results were obtained; however, the entire group was useful for seeing complications from the therapy. In the ER-positive women, there were 617 recurrences in the treatment group versus 711 in the control group, for a relative risk of 0.84 with the treatment, which was highly significant. There was a reduced risk of breast cancer mortality and overall mortality in the treatment group as well, both of which were highly significant. This translated into a risk of recurrent disease of 21.4% in the treatment group between years 5 and 14 versus 25.1% in the control group (Fig 3). There were twice as many recurrences in the first 5 years than the second 5 years after randomization. Furthermore, there was no significant risk of death from other causes in the entire group from the treatment. However, there was an increased risk of pulmonary embolism (relative risk of 1.87) and endometrial cancer (relative risk of 1.74) with treatment; however, treatment reduced the risk from ischemic heart disease to 0.76. This trial shows that continuing tamoxifen for 10 years instead of the previously recommended 5 years continues to protect against recurrent breast cancer and breast cancer death. This effect lasted into the second decade after the treatment had ended. The risk of endometrial cancer and pulmonary embolism was far outweighed by the decrease in breast cancer mortality; therefore, it appears that 10 years of tamoxifen is more protective than 5 years in women with ER-positive breast cancer.

J. Howe, MD

The UK Standardisation of Breast Radiotherapy (START) trials of radiotherapy hypofractionation for treatment of early breast cancer: 10-year follow-up results of two randomised controlled trials

Haviland JS, on behalf of the START Trialists' Group (The Inst of Cancer Res, Sutton, UK; et al)

Lancet Oncol 14:1086-1094, 2013

Background.—5-year results of the UK Standardisation of Breast Radiotherapy (START) trials suggested that lower total doses of radiotherapy delivered in fewer, larger doses (fractions) are at least as safe and effective as the historical standard regimen (50 Gy in 25 fractions) for women after primary surgery for early breast cancer. In this prespecified analysis, we report the 10-year follow-up of the START trials testing 13 fraction and 15 fraction regimens.

Methods.—From 1999 to 2002, women with completely excised invasive breast cancer (pT1–3a, pN0–1, M0) were enrolled from 35 UK radiotherapy centres. Patients were randomly assigned to a treatment regimen after primary surgery followed by chemotherapy and endocrine treatment (where prescribed). Randomisation was computer-generated and stratified by centre, type of primary surgery (breast-conservation surgery or mastectomy), and tumour bed boost radiotherapy. In START-A, a regimen of 50 Gy in 25 fractions over 5 weeks was compared with 41·6 Gy or 39 Gy in 13 fractions over 5 weeks. In START-B, a regimen of 50 Gy in 25 fractions over 5 weeks was compared with 40 Gy in 15 fractions over 3 weeks. Eligibility criteria included age older than 18 years and no immediate surgical reconstruction. Primary endpoints were local-regional tumour relapse and late normal tissue effects. Analysis was by intention to treat. Follow-up data are still being collected. This study is registered as an International Standard Randomised Controlled Trial, number ISRCTN59368779.

Findings.—START-A enrolled 2236 women. Median follow-up was 9·3 years (IQR 8·0–10·0), after which 139 local-regional relapses had occurred. 10-year rates of local-regional relapse did not differ significantly between the 41·6 Gy and 50 Gy regimen groups (6·3%, 95% CI 4·7–8·5 *vs* 7·4%, 5·5–10·0; hazard ratio [HR] 0·91, 95% CI 0·59–1·38; $p = 0{\cdot}65$) or the 39 Gy (8·8%, 95% CI 6·7–11·4) and 50 Gy regimen groups (HR 1·18, 95% CI 0·79–1·76; $p = 0{\cdot}41$). In START-A, moderate or marked breast induration, telangiectasia, and breast oedema were significantly less common normal tissue effects in the 39 Gy group than in the 50 Gy group. Normal tissue effects did not differ significantly between 41·6 Gy and 50 Gy groups. START-B enrolled 2215 women. Median follow-up was 9·9 years (IQR 7·5–10·1), after which 95 local-regional relapses had occurred. The proportion of patients with local-regional relapse at 10 years did not differ significantly between the 40 Gy group (4·3%, 95% CI 3·2–5·9) and the 50 Gy group (5·5%, 95% CI 4·2–7·2; HR 0·77, 95% CI 0·51–1·16; $p = 0{\cdot}21$). In START-B, breast shrinkage, telangiectasia, and breast oedema were significantly less common normal tissue effects in the 40 Gy group than in the 50 Gy group.

Interpretation.—Long-term follow-up confirms that appropriately dosed hypofractionated radiotherapy is safe and effective for patients with early breast cancer. The results support the continued use of 40 Gy in 15 fractions, which has already been adopted by most UK centres as

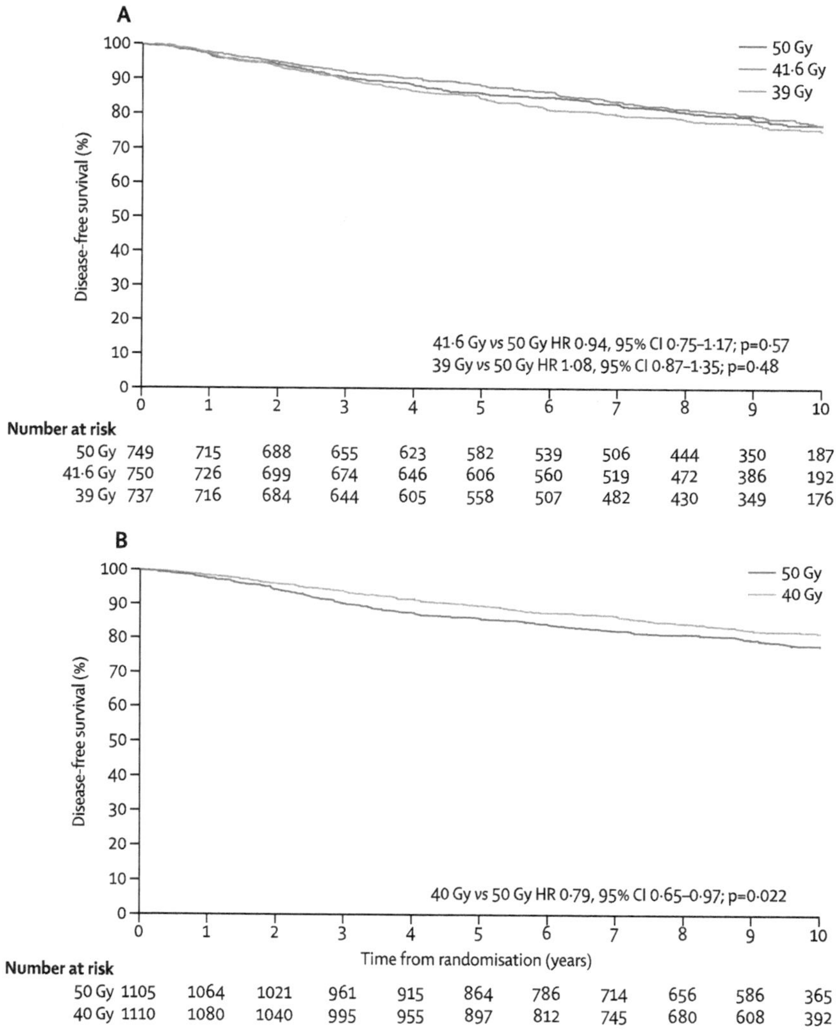

FIGURE 2.—Kaplan-Meier analysis of disease-free survival. In START-A (A) and START-B (B). (Reprinted from Haviland JS, on behalf of the START Trialists' Group. The UK Standardisation of Breast Radiotherapy (START) trials of radiotherapy hypofractionation for treatment of early breast cancer: 10-year follow-up results of two randomised controlled trials. *Lancet Oncol.* 2013;14:1086-1094.)

the standard of care for women requiring adjuvant radiotherapy for invasive early breast cancer (Fig 2).

▶ In the United Kingdom, the standard dose of radiation to the breast after surgery for breast cancer was 50 Gy delivered in 25 fractions of 2 Gy each over 5 weeks. It is unclear whether higher individual doses of radiation given over the same or shorter period would result in increases in local recurrence and changes to normal adjacent tissues. Retrospective studies from Canada and the United Kingdom in the early 1990s suggested that a lower total dose with less fractions given, but higher doses per fraction, was a reasonable alternative to the standard method. In 1998 in the United Kingdom, 2 trials were begun to evaluate this, one called START-A and the other START-B. These were begun at the same time but in different centers. They randomly assigned women who had T1 to T3A, pN0 to N1, M0 breast cancers to have radiation with 50 Gy over 25 fractions over 5 weeks as the control arm in both trials; in START-A, they compared giving 39 Gy in 13 fractions or 41.6 Gy in 13 fractions over 5 weeks with the control, and for START-B, giving 40 Gy in 15 fractions over 3 weeks. The patients were randomly assigned to stratification for a number of variables, and patients were eligible to get boost radiation to the tumor bed before randomization, so that the number of patients was equal in both groups. Five-year results showed that there was no significant difference in local recurrence, and this report now represents 10 years of follow-up. For the START-A trial, there were no differences in local recurrence or overall survival between the 50-Gy and the 39- and 41.6-Gy treatment arms. There was an improvement in the breast tissue effects in the 39-Gy arm, but there was a slightly higher incidence of local relapse, which was not significant. In the START-B trial, there was no difference in local recurrence between the 50-Gy and the 40-Gy fractions; however, there was a significantly higher disease-free and overall survival advantage in the 40-Gy group (Fig 2), as well as reduced incidence of breast shrinkage, telangiectasia, and breast edema. These trials, which together included more than 4400 women, found that giving lower doses of radiation in fewer fractions resulted in no difference in local recurrence, and potentially there may be a benefit for the 40-Gy fractionation over 3 weeks in terms of overall survival and breast cosmesis. Therefore, this is a safe alternative and may even show an improvement over previous regimens of radiation therapy. Whether the effects seen in the United Kingdom are translatable to the United States remains to be seen, but the American Society for Radiation Oncology has suggested that hypofractionated therapy is a reasonable option for patients with pT1 to T2pN0 breast cancer who have not received chemotherapy.

J. Howe, MD

Effect of MRI on the Management of Ductal Carcinoma In Situ of the Breast

Pilewskie M, Kennedy C, Shappell C, et al (Northwestern Univ, Chicago IL)

Ann Surg Oncol 20:1522-1529, 2013

Introduction.—The accuracy of breast magnetic resonance imaging (MRI) for detection of ductal carcinoma in situ (DCIS) has prompted recommendations for its routine preoperative use, but its clinical benefit is debated. We reviewed our experience with MRI in DCIS patients to assess the utility of MRI for surgical planning.

Methods.—DCIS patients (2008–2010) were identified through a prospectively maintained database and grouped into MRI and no-MRI groups. The rates of additional biopsies, altered surgical management, and reoperation were compared. Additionally, DCIS size ascertained by mammography, MRI, and final pathology was compared.

Results.—Of 352 DCIS patients, 217 received MRI and 135 did not. The type of initial operation and number of reoperations were similar between the two groups, but successful breast conservation was more frequent in the no-MRI group ($p = 0.06$). The additional biopsy rate was 38 % in the MRI group versus 7 % in the no-MRI group; ≥2 additional biopsies were performed in 18 % of the MRI group and 2 % of the no-MRI group ($p < 0.0001$). These yielded a cancer diagnosis in 26 % of MRI and 33 % of no-MRI patients ($p = 0.73$). MRI was not superior to mammogram in detecting size of DCIS lesions preoperatively; 52 % of mammograms were accurate (within 1 cm) compared with 41 % of MRIs.

Conclusions.—DCIS patients who undergo preoperative breast MRI are far more likely to undergo additional biopsies. Unless these can be demonstrated to lead to improved long-term outcomes, the utility of routine preoperative MRI in DCIS patients remains questionable.

▶ Ductal carcinoma in situ (DCIS) has been diagnosed by mammography, but magnetic resonance imaging (MRI) has been increasingly performed over the last decade. On mammography, the characteristic findings would be microcalcification; however, DCIS may extend beyond the area of microcalcification; therefore, MRI may have some diagnostic advantages. This study set out to examine whether patients who had DCIS diagnosed and had MRI performed had differences in the number of biopsies performed, local recurrence, and contralateral lesions identified. This single institutional study reviewed patients between 2008 and 2010 who had a core needle biopsy showing DCIS. Of these 352 women, 217 had MRI and mammography, and the entire group had mammography performed. Groups without MRI and those with MRI were not equally matched, and there was a higher propensity to get an MRI in patients who were younger or pre- or perimenopausal; there was a higher incidence of prior breast cancer in patients without MRI. No abnormality was seen in the mammogram-only group in 2.3% of cases, but in 9.3% of cases no imaging abnormality was seen on MRI. The average size of the lesions seen on MRI was approximately a centimeter larger than those by mammography. Women who had MRI had a significantly higher incidence of second biopsies performed (38.3%), which was 6.7% in the no-MRI group. Eighteen percent of women had a third biopsy performed in the MRI group versus only 2.2% in the no-MRI group. In the MRI group, 3.2% of patients had a contralateral breast finding that resulted in the diagnosis of malignant disease. In addition, the success of breast conservation therapy was decreased in the MRI group by 9%. The authors concluded that MRI results in more unnecessary biopsies, nonbeneficial changes in surgical management, and prior studies have not shown any differences in local recurrence. One advantage of the MRI is the discovery of contralateral breast lesions; however, longer-term follow-up will be necessary to determine whether there is improved survival as a result.

J. Howe, MD

Preoperative Axillary Ultrasound in Breast Cancer: Safely Avoiding Frozen Section of Sentinel Lymph Nodes in Breast Conserving Surgery

Ibrahim-Zada I, Grant CS, Glazebrook KN, et al (Univ of Arizona, Tucson; Mayo Clinic, Rochester, MN)

J Am Coll Surg 217:7-16, 2013

Background.—The American College of Surgeons Oncology Group Z0011 trial results provided convincing evidence that completion axillary lymph node dissection (CALND) was unnecessary in selected patients with 1 to 2 positive sentinel lymph nodes (SLNs). We hypothesized that preoperative axillary ultrasound (AUS) with fine-needle aspiration is sufficiently sensitive to detect worrisome macrometastasis to preclude the need for frozen-section pathology of SLNs.

Study Design.—We conducted a retrospective single-institution study at a tertiary academic referral center. A total of 1,140 T1 to 2 breast cancer patients who underwent SLN biopsy with or without CALND from January 1, 2007 to December 31, 2010 were reviewed. All patients had negative preoperative AUS with or without fine-needle aspiration.

Results.—One hundred forty-four (13%) patients were node positive at surgery. Mean age, tumor size, histology, and estrogen receptor and progesterone receptor status were similar comparing 996 SLN-negative with 144 (13%) SLN-positive patients. Of the SLN-positive patients, 25% were premenopausal, 9% were estrogen receptor–negative, and 19% had additional lymph nodes at CALND. Only 19 (2%) patients had SLN metastasis ≥6 mm, 10 (1%) had metastasis >7 mm, and only 1 patient had ≥3 positive SLNs.

Conclusions.—The addition of preoperative AUS with or without fine-needle aspiration to management of patients who meet American College of Surgeons Oncology Group Z0011 trial eligibility criteria reduced the risk of macrometastasis measuring ≥6 mm to only 2%; very few of these patients would be premenopausal, have estrogen receptor–negative tumors, or ≥3 positive SLNs. With the addition of AUS with or without fine-needle aspiration, we endorse the conclusions of the American College of Surgeons Oncology Group Z0011 trial to avoid CALND, and see marginal gain in frozen-section analysis of SLNs.

▶ This study reviews a single institution's use of preoperative axillary ultrasonography to help in the management of axillary disease in breast cancer patients. They selected patients with T1 or T2 cancers without palpable lymphadenopathy to undergo preoperative axillary ultrasound scan. If suspicious lymph nodes were seen, then a fine-needle aspiration was performed. In this study, they looked at 1140 patients who had a negative preoperative axillary ultrasound scan to determine whether there was sentinel lymph node involvement so that perhaps frozen sections could be eliminated. Of 1140 patients with negative axillary ultrasound scans, 12.6% were found to have positive sentinel lymph nodes. Of these 144 patients, 100 underwent completion axillary lymph node dissection, and, of these, 27% had additional nonsentinel lymph nodes that had metastases. Only

19 patients had macrometastases greater than 6 mm. The significant findings from this study were that the addition of preoperative axillary ultrasound scan reduced the number of patients who had macrometastases, and these women were more frequently found to be premenopausal or estrogen receptor negative. Therefore, the population of patients who might be at a higher risk for axillary recurrence was reduced. Criticisms of the study are that the ACOSOG Z0011 study has shown that axillary node dissection can be avoided in patients with T1 and T2 tumors even when 1 to 2 lymph nodes were positive, as long as they receive breast irradiation or adjuvant therapy. Therefore, the utility of this study is in question besides the potential benefit of reducing the population of higher-risk patients by doing ultrasound scan on all patients. However, a trial in Europe may abandon sentinel lymph node biopsy altogether if axillary ultrasound scan is negative, and perhaps it will find a role back into the management of breast cancer in the future.

J. Howe, MD

When is a Lymph Node Dissection a Lymph Node Dissection? The Number of Lymph Nodes Resected in Sentinel and Axillary Lymph Node Dissections

Olaya W, Wong J, Wong J, et al (Loma Linda Univ School of Medicine, CA; East Carolina Univ, Greenville, NC; et al)
Ann Surg Oncol 20:627-632, 2013

Purpose.—We sought to compare the number of lymph nodes (LN) resected in axillary lymph node dissections (ALND) and sentinel lymph node dissections (SLND), and to assess the validity of registry reporting for axillary staging in breast cancer.

Methods.—Women in the California Cancer Registry who underwent surgical axillary staging for T1/T2, M0 breast cancer between 2004 and 2008 were evaluated. The number of LN resected in patients reported as having SLND+ALND and ALND were assessed for compliance with 6 and 10 LN threshold definitions for ALND. The proportion of patients with $\leq$3 LN removed was assessed for patients receiving SLND only.

Results.—Of 71,907 patients, 45.5 % had SLND, 24.0 %, SLND+ALND, and 30.5 %, ALND. The median number of LN resected with SLND cases was 2 (range 1–41); SLND+ALND, 9 (range 1–63); and ALND, 11 (range 1–81) ($p < 0.0001$). Of patients undergoing ALND, 56.7 % had $\geq$10 LN removed; 46.2 % of patients with SLND+ALND had $\geq$10 LN removed ($p < 0.0001$). Overall, 75.5 % of patients with ALND had $\geq$6 LN removed and 67.8 % of patients with SLND+ALND had $\geq$6 LN removed ($p < 0.0001$). Of those receiving only SLND, 83.4 % had $\leq$3 LN removed.

Conclusions.—A significant proportion of patients did not meet the minimum LN count thresholds for full ALND or had excess LN removed in a SLND. Further investigation is required to determine whether absolute LN

number or reported operative procedure and implied surgical technique better defines axillary staging in a registry database.

▶ Quality indicators for sentinel lymph node biopsy (SLNB) with axillary lymph node dissection (ALND) and ALND alone for breast cancer have had several standards proposed. The National Surgical Adjuvant Breast and Bowel Project (NSABP) B32 trial established that the mean number of lymph nodes resected during SNLB was 3, and the Danish Breast Cancer Cooperative Group suggested that a minimum of 10 lymph nodes should be removed for a complete axillary lymph node dissection; this latter number was also endorsed in the American College of Surgeons Oncology Group (ACOSOG) Z11 study. The previous NSABP B32 protocol defined an ALND as >6 nodes having been removed. The current study reviewed patients in the California Cancer Registry with T1–T2/N0 breast cancers who were treated between 2004 and 2008. The authors reviewed the database for patients receiving SLNB and looked at the number of nodes, as well as SNLB and ALND together and ALND alone. What they found was the median number of lymph nodes removed in SLNB was 2; in SLNB plus ALND, 9; and in ALND alone, 11. Of patients undergoing ALND, the standard of having 10 or more lymph nodes removed was achieved in 57% of cases, whereas in those with both SLND and ALND, this was only achieved in 46% of cases. If one reduces the threshold to 6 lymph nodes, then 76% of ALND patients, and 68% of those having SLND and ALND, met this criterion. The authors point out that there was a lot of variability in the number of nodes removed, and indeed even in the SNLB category, the lowest number removed was 1 and the greatest 41. This raises the question of whether some of the procedures entered into the database were correct. In other words, perhaps some of the patients listed as having SNLB had a larger dissection performed, whereas some who had SNLB alone may have been misclassified as having ALND or SNLB and ALND. Because of this, the Commission on Cancer recommended in 2012 that cancer registrars should rely on the operative report, rather than the pathology report alone, for coding the type of surgical procedure. Also interesting from this study was that fewer nodes were generally removed in Commission on Cancer–approved programs, but one explanation for this could be the use of other modalities, such as axillary irradiation instead of larger node dissections and possibly early adoption of the recommendation of the ACOSOG Z11 study, which showed that no additional axillary surgery may be necessary after SNLB. Certainly this study raises questions about the adequacy of lymph node dissection performed in a variety of hospitals, but it is still difficult to understand what fraction of this is due to surgical technique as opposed to misclassification by cancer registrars or the efforts of pathologists.

J. Howe, MD

An Extended Phase II Trial of Iodine-125 Methylene Blue for Sentinel Lymph Node Identification in Women with Breast Cancer

Harkrider WW, Diebold AE, Maloney T, et al (Univ Med Ctr, Lafayette, LA; Louisiana State Univ Health Sciences Ctr, New Orleans, Iso-Tex Diagnostics Inc, Friendswood, TX)

J Am Coll Surg 216:599-605, 2013

Background.—The aim of this study was to determine if an intraoperative injection of iodine-125—labeled methylene blue (^{125}I-MB) is a sensitive and effective method for detecting SLNs in women with breast cancer.

Study Design.—Sixty-two women were enrolled in an extended phase II trial using ^{125}I-MB to guide SLNB. All patients were anesthetized and then injected subcutaneously with 1 mCi ^{125}I-MB in the outer quadrant of the areola.

Results.—Radioactivity was detected in the axilla within 3 to 5 minutes. Fifty-eight of 62 (94%) patients had SLNs detected during their procedure. Mean (± SD) number of SLNs per patient was 1.8 ± 1.3 (range 0 to 6). A total of 112 nodes were dissected from 58 women; 110 of these nodes were considered sentinel. One hundred and eight (98%) nodes were hot, 98 (89%) nodes were blue, and 96 (87%) nodes were both hot and blue. Two women had complications; 1 had superficial skin staining and 1 had a superficial skin slough. Both healed uneventfully. No allergic reactions were observed. No radioactive uptake in the thyroid was seen.

Conclusions.—Iodine-125—labeled methylene blue can be mixed and administered in the operating room, improving hospital efficiency. Patient satisfaction is higher with ^{125}I-MB than with the technetium 99m sulfur colloid procedure because ^{125}I-MB does not produce localized burning and other adverse reactions associated with the traditional method, and 125I-MB is administered with the patient under anesthesia. Iodine-125 emits a lower-energy gamma ray than technetium 99m, lowering the surgeon's radiation exposure. Iodine-125—labeled methylene blue SLN identification is safe, cost effective, and produces equivalent outcomes compared with the traditional technique, making it an attractive alternative.

▶ Sentinel lymph node mapping is a very useful staging procedure for both melanoma and breast cancer. The current method of sentinel lymph node mapping usually involves injection of technetium-99—labeled sulfur colloid when the patient is awake, lymphoscintigraphy, followed by injection of blue dye in the operating room. In this study, the group attempted to consolidate the injection of radionuclide with methylene blue in the operating room when the patient was asleep. For this they used iodine-125—labeled methylene blue, which has a much longer shelf life than Technetium-99 of 120 days. They sought to determine the results using this compound in sentinel lymph node biopsy for breast cancer. They recruited 62 women and, using this procedure, injected 1 mCi of iodine-125 diluted in methylene blue into a subareolar upper outer quadrant. They found that they could identify the sentinel lymph node in 94% of patients. They found that of the sentinel nodes, 98% had high specific activity, which they defined as greater than 10 counts per second; 89% had a blue color; and 87% were both hot and blue. The overall rate of positivity in their sentinel lymph nodes was 19%. Two patients had complications from this procedure, one with staining at the site in the skin and one with superficial skin ulceration. They concluded that this combined procedure had several advantages over the typical sentinel lymph node mapping that most centers do today. These were a combined injection of dye and isotope, not requiring a visit to nuclear medicine (and therefore ease of scheduling), similar accuracy in finding the sentinel lymph nodes, and a longer shelf life of the radionuclide. They did additional studies to determine the radiation exposure and found that it was significantly less with iodine-125 than technetium because of attenuation through human fat. They concluded that this was a useful procedure with several advantages over the classical technique. One drawback is that because iodine is used, it could have an effect on the thyroid, and therefore they had to give the patients Lugol's solution 2 days before and 2 days after the procedure. Critics would say that using the standard procedure that sentinel lymph node identification rates approach nearly 100% in experienced centers, and questions could be raised about the specific activity of nodes and whether this made them more difficult to find. Nevertheless, this technique does appear to be a useful alternative for sentinel lymph node biopsy in breast cancer.

J. Howe, MD

Randomized Controlled Trial to Reduce Bacterial Colonization of Surgical Drains After Breast and Axillary Operations

Degnim AC, Scow JS, Hoskin TL, et al (Mayo Clinic, Rochester, MN)
Ann Surg 258:240-247, 2013

Objective.—To determine whether bacterial colonization of drains can be reduced by local antiseptic interventions.

Background.—Drains are a potential source of bacterial entry into surgical wounds and may contribute to surgical site infection after breast surgery.

Methods.—After institutional review board approval, patients undergoing total mastectomy and/or axillary lymph node dissection were randomized to standard drain care (control) or drain antisepsis (treated). Standard drain care comprised twice daily cleansing with alcohol swabs. Antisepsis drain care included (1) a chlorhexidine disc at the drain exit site and (2) irrigation of the drain bulb twice daily with dilute sodium hypochlorite (Dakin's) solution. Culture results of drain fluid and tubing were compared between control and antisepsis groups.

Results.—Overall, 100 patients with 125 drains completed the study with 48 patients (58 drains) in the control group and 52 patients (67 drains) in the antisepsis group. Cultures of drain bulb fluid at 1 week were positive (1+ or greater growth) in 66% (38/58) of control drains compared with 21% (14/67) of antisepsis drains ($P = 0.0001$). Drain tubing cultures demonstrated more than 50 colony-forming units in 19% (8/43) of control drains versus 0% (0/53) of treated drains ($P = 0.004$). Surgical site infection was diagnosed in 6 patients (6%)—5 patients in the control group and 1 patient in the antisepsis group ($P = 0.06$).

Conclusions.—Simple and inexpensive local antiseptic interventions with a chlorhexidine disc and hypochlorite solution reduce bacterial colonization of drains. Based on these data, further study of drain antisepsis and its potential impact on surgical site infection rate is warranted (ClinicalTrials.gov Identifier: NCT01286168).

► Surgical drains are commonly used after procedures, such as mastectomy and axillary dissection. The benefit of drains is to decrease seroma formation; however they can also be a conduit for bacterial colonization. This study randomized patients undergoing total mastectomy with or without axillary node dissection into 2 groups, 1 with surgical drains, would be stripped twice daily and the skin exit site cleansed with 70% isopropyl alcohol swabs. The treatment group was assigned for cleansing the drain exit sites with alcohol followed by placing a chlorhexidine gluconate disc dressing, which were changed every 3 days, as well as twice daily 10-mL irrigation of 0.0125% sodium hypochlorite solution. Cultures were taken of the drain fluid and the drain tubing at day 7 and/or the day of drain removal. The patients were monitored for surgical site infections. One hundred patients were randomized to the trial, and the median duration of drains was 7 days, with a median output of approximately 23 mL the 24 hours before removal. The 2 groups showed significant differences in colonization of the drain bulb fluid, with 65% of patients in the control arm having 1+ or greater growth of bacteria from the drain fluid, vs 25% in those with the antisepsis regimen. With respect to drain tubing cultures, none of the treatment group had positive cultures greater than 50 colony forming units, whereas 19% of the control group did. Surgical site infections developed in 5 patients in the control group and 1 patient in the antisepsis group, but this difference was not statistically significant ($P = .06$). The other differences in colonization of the fluid in the drain tubing were significant. This study showed that the antisepsis regimen of flushing the drain and local skin care with chlorhexidine reduced the incidence of colonization in the drain fluid and the drain tubing in a well-controlled trial. Although statistical significance was not reached for reduction of surgical site infections, it should be noted that the 1 patient in the treatment group who developed an infection did so at 31 days postoperatively, after the first week of chemotherapy. These findings could be carried over to other situations in which drains may need to be placed in potentially high-risk situations, such as groin dissections, ventral hernia repairs with mesh, and reconstructive breast surgery.

J. Howe, MD

Colon

Current Use and Surgical Efficacy of Laparoscopic Colectomy in Colon Cancer

Sticca RP, Alberts SR, Mahoney MR, et al (Univ of North Dakota School of Medicine and Health Sciences, Grand Forks; Mayo Clinic, Rochester, MN; et al)
J Am Coll Surg 217:56-63, 2013

Background.—The Clinical Outcomes in Surgical Therapy trial demonstrated that laparoscopic colectomy (LC) was equivalent to open colectomy (OC) for 30-day mortality, time to recurrence, and overall survival in colon cancer (CC) patients. Current use of LC for CC is not well known.

Study Design.—Surgical data were reviewed for all patients randomized into a national phase III clinical trial for adjuvant therapy in stage III CC (North Central Cancer Treatment Group trial N0147). Colon resections were grouped as open (traditional laparotomy) or laparoscopic, including laparoscopic; laparoscopic assisted; hand assisted; and laparoscopic converted to OC. Statistical methods included nonparametric methods, categorical analysis, and logistic regression modeling.

Results.—A total of 3,393 evaluable patients were accrued between 2004 and 2009; 53% were male, median age was 58 years, 86% were white, and 70% had a body mass index >25 kg/m^2. Two thousand one hundred thirteen (62%) underwent OC. One thousand two hundred eighty (38%) were initiated as laparoscopic procedures, 25% (n = 322) were laparoscopic, 32% (n = 410) were laparoscopic assisted, 26% (n = 339) were hand assisted, and 16% (n = 209) were LC converted to OC. Significant predictors of LC (vs OC) in multivariate models were T stage (T1 or T2 vs T3 or T4; $p = 0.0286$), and absence of perforation, bowel obstruction, or adherence to surrounding organs ($p < 0.01$ each). Increasing rates of LC were observed over time, with LC eclipsing OC in 2009 ($p < 0.0001$). Surgical efficacy, measured by lymph node retrieval, was similar, with the mean number of lymph nodes retrieved higher in the LC group (20.6 vs 19.5 nodes; $p = 0.0006$).

Conclusions.—This study demonstrated a steadily increasing use of LC for the surgical treatment of CC between 2004 and 2009, with LC preferred by study completion. Surgical efficacy was similar in stage III CC patients.

► Publication of the results of the Clinical Outcomes in Surgery Trial (COST) in 2004 showed that laparoscopic and open colectomy were equivalent in terms of complication and recurrence rates. Since then, more and more surgeons are adopting a laparoscopic approach for resection of colon cancer. This study by Sticca et al tried to look for differences between patients having laparoscopic vs open procedure for colon cancer. They took advantage of the NCCTG N0147 trial, in which patients with stage 3 colon cancer were randomly assigned to various chemotherapy regimens. The randomization was performed after their surgical procedure; therefore, this was an ideal patient population in which to study the use of open vs laparoscopic colectomy. Many interesting things emerged from this trial, which was performed between 2004 and 2009. One was that over this period, 1280 patients underwent a laparoscopic colectomy vs 2113 having an open colectomy for cancer, and by the year 2009 laparoscopic colectomy had become more common than open colectomy. Other factors more commonly associated with having laparoscopic vs open colectomy on multivariate analyses included a higher incidence of open procedures done in patients with bowel obstruction, bowel perforation, T3 or T4 tumors, or adherence to surrounding organs. Patients with cecal tumors had a higher percentage of laparoscopic procedures, whereas those patients with transverse colon lesions and descending colon lesions were more likely to have open colectomy. Interestingly, the number of lymph nodes removed were very similar for each group, with a mean of 20.6 in the laparoscopic vs 19.5 in the open group. Because this is a measure of quality of resection, the conclusion was that not only was laparoscopic colectomy being performed at a higher rate with each increasing year, but that the quality of these resections appeared equivalent to those in open colectomy. This study did not look at complication rates or length of stay but clearly showed that laparoscopic colectomy became the most popular approach for resection of colon cancer over this study period, without any sacrifice in nodal clearance.

J. Howe, MD

Nodal Status, Number of Lymph Nodes Examined, and Lymph Node Ratio: What Defines Prognosis after Resection of Colon Adenocarcinoma?

Gleisner AL, Mogal H, Dodson R, et al (St Louis Univ School of Medicine, MO; The Johns Hopkins Univ School of Medicine, Baltimore, MD)

J Am Coll Surg 217:1090-1100, 2013

Background.—Lymph node ratio (LNR) has been proposed as an optimal staging variable for colorectal cancer. However, the interactive effect of total number of lymph nodes examined (TNLE) and the number of metastatic lymph nodes (NMLN) on survival has not been well characterized.

Study Design.—Patients operated on for colon cancer between 1998 and 2007 were identified from the Surveillance, Epidemiology, and End Results database (n = 154,208) and randomly divided into development (75%) and validation (25%) datasets. The association of the TNLE and NMLN on survival was assessed using the Cox proportional hazards model with terms for interaction and nonlinearity with restricted cubic spline functions. Findings were confirmed in the validation dataset.

Results.—Both TNLE and NMLN were nonlinearly associated with survival. Patients with no lymph node metastasis had a decrease in the risk of death for each lymph node examined up to approximately 25 lymph nodes, while the effect of TNLE was negligible after approximately 10 negative lymph nodes (NNLN) in those with lymph node metastasis. The hazard ratio varied considerably according to the TNLE for a given LNR when LNR ≥ 0.5, ranging from 2.88 to 7.16 in those with an

LNR = 1. The independent effects of NMLN and NNLN on survival were summarized in a model-based score, the N score. When patients in the validation set were categorized according to the N stage, the LNR, and the N score, only the N score was unaffected by differences in the TNLE.

Conclusions.—The effect of the TNLE on survival does not have a unique, strong threshold (ie, 12 lymph nodes). The combined effect of NMLN and TNLE is complex and is not appropriately represented by the LNR. The N score may be an alternative to the N stage for prognostication of patients with colon cancer because it accounts for differences in nodal samples.

► A quality measure that has been in use for some time has been the recommendation that 12 lymph nodes be removed at the time of surgery for colon cancer. This has worked its way into becoming a measure upon which institutions and surgeons are judged for the quality of their colon cancer care. This article seeks to address whether this is a reasonable cutoff or whether other factors, such as the number of metastatic lymph nodes found, or even the more recently popular lymph node ratio of metastatic vs total nodes would be a more appropriate factor to examine. This study looked at a development and validation set from the Surveillance, Epidemiology, and End Results database, which included a total of 154 000 patients. Complex statistical analyses were carried out to judge the performance of various metrics concerning lymph nodes and their relationship to patient survival. The important findings were that there was no discrete cutoff for the total number of lymph nodes examined above or below which there was significant difference in survival, and rather, that the risk of death decreased for each negative lymph node up to a threshold of 20 to 25 lymph nodes that were examined. The risk of death increased with the number of metastatic lymph nodes found, which was a factor independent of the total number examined. Separately, if 10 to 12 nodes were found to be negative, then the addition of more negative nodes did not change the risk of death. The notion that the lymph node ratio is more accurate than other measures because it incorporates both the total number of lymph nodes examined and the number of metastatic lymph nodes was not borne out in this study. They found that survival differed by as much as 3-fold in patients with the same lymph node ratio, depending on the total number of lymph nodes that were examined, with worse survival as more nodes were examined. The authors did come up with a good predictor, which they called the end score, but the score is difficult to calculate and may not turn out to be a very useful measure for most clinicians. The value of this study is that it explored in detail the importance of total number of lymph nodes examined vs number of metastatic lymph nodes examined vs the ratio and showed the importance of each. They could not conclude that 12 is indeed the magic number, but it still appears that this is a reasonable benchmark to separate adequate from potentially inadequate nodal examination. Furthermore, this study showed that lymph node ratio may not be as promising as some have suggested it might be.

J. Howe, MD

Bevacizumab in Stage II-III Colon Cancer: 5-Year Update of the National Surgical Adjuvant Breast and Bowel Project C-08 Trial

Allegra CJ, Yothers G, O'Connell MJ, et al (Natl Surgical Adjuvant Breast and Bowel Project, Pittsburgh, PA)

J Clin Oncol 31:359-364, 2013

Purpose.—The National Surgical Adjuvant Breast and Bowel Project trial C-08 was designed to investigate the safety and efficacy of adding bevacizumab to fluorouracil, leucovorin, and oxaliplatin (FOLFOX6) for the adjuvant treatment of patients with stage 2-3 colon cancer. Our report summarizes the primary and secondary end points of disease-free and overall survival, respectively, with 5 years median follow-up time.

Patients and Methods.—Patients received modified FOLFOX6 once every 2 weeks for a 6-month period (control group) or modified FOLFOX6 for 6 months plus bevacizumab (5 mg/kg) once every 2 weeks for a 12-month period (experimental group). The primary end point of the study was disease-free survival (DFS) and overall survival (OS) was a secondary end point.

Results.—Of 2,673 analyzed patients, demographic factors were well-balanced by treatment. With a median follow-up of 5 years, the addition of bevacizumab to mFOLFOX6 did not result in an overall significant increase in DFS (hazard ratio [HR], 0.93; 95% CI, 0.81 to 1.08; $P = .35$). Exploratory analyses found that the effect of bevacizumab on DFS was different before and after a 1.25-year landmark (time-by-treatment interaction P value $<.0001$). The secondary end point of OS was no different between the two study arms for all patients (HR, 0.95; 95% CI, 0.79 to 1.13; $P = .56$) and for those with stage 3 disease (HR, 1.0; 95% CI, 0.83 to 1.21; $P = .99$).

Conclusion.—Bevacizumab for 1 year with modified FOLFOX6 does not significantly prolong DFS or OS in stage 2-3 colon cancer. We observed no evidence of a detrimental effect of exposure to bevacizumab. A transient effect on disease-free survival was observed during bevacizumab exposure in the study's experimental arm.

▶ Chemotherapy regimens for colorectal cancer are generally tried in the adjuvant setting after they have shown benefit in patients with metastatic disease. The most active chemotherapy for colorectal cancer, FOLFOX (5 fluorouracil, leucovorin, and oxaliplatin) was combined with bevacizumab (humanized antibody to vascular endothelial growth factor) and found to be beneficial in patients with metastatic colorectal cancer, with improved overall survival from 10.8 to 12.9 months in the ECOG E3200 trial. Another trial by Saltz et al found no significant difference in response rates or overall survival of FOLFOX6 versus FOLFOX6 plus bevacizumab in metastatic colorectal cancer, but there was a significant improvement in disease-free survival (DFS). In this study, the NSABP C08 trial, the objective was to look at survival and toxicity of FOLFOX6 versus FOLFOX6 and bevacizumab in the treatment of stage 2 and stage 3 colon cancer in the adjuvant setting. The FOLFOX6 was given for 6 months, whereas bevacizumab was given for a full 12 months. More than 2700 patients were randomly assigned to the 2 arms (with 25% of patients being stage 2 and 75% stage 3), and there was a median follow-up of 4.9 years. Bevacizumab did not increase mortality, and there is no significant difference in toxicity. Examination of the endpoint of DFS found that there was no significant improvement with the addition of bevacizumab to FOLFOX6. There was a significant improvement of DFS with bevacizumab at 15 months (hazard ratio, 0.61), but this did not hold up at 5 years. There was no significant difference in overall survival between the 2 groups (Fig 3 in the original article). Patients who relapsed after treatment appeared to have more rapid death if they had been treated with bevacizumab versus just chemotherapy. The study concluded that there was no benefit to adding bevacizumab to the regimen of FOLFOX 6 in the adjuvant setting. Survival was not improved, and this is a very expensive treatment regimen ($35–50 000). Reasons for potentially improved DFS when noted at 15 months could have been the effect of bevacizumab on vascularity (perhaps making computed tomography scans less sensitive), and an explanation for hastened mortality after relapse could be that treatment with the vascular endothelial growth factor inhibitor leads to a more aggressive tumor phenotype.

J. Howe, MD

Computed tomographic colonography versus colonoscopy for investigation of patients with symptoms suggestive of colorectal cancer (SIGGAR): a multicentre randomised trial

Atkin W, for the SIGGAR investigators (Imperial College London, UK; et al)

Lancet 381:1194-1202, 2013

Background.—Colonoscopy is the gold-standard test for investigation of symptoms suggestive of colorectal cancer; computed tomographic colonography (CTC) is an alternative, less invasive test. However, additional investigation after CTC is needed to confirm suspected colonic lesions, and this is an important factor in establishing the feasibility of CTC as an alternative to colonoscopy. We aimed to compare rates of additional colonic investigation after CTC or colonoscopy for detection of colorectal cancer or large (≥10 mm) polyps in symptomatic patients in clinical practice.

Methods.—This pragmatic multicentre randomised trial recruited patients with symptoms suggestive of colorectal cancer from 21 UK hospitals. Eligible patients were aged 55 years or older and regarded by their referring clinician as suitable for colonoscopy. Patients were randomly assigned (2:1) to colonoscopy or CTC by computer-generated random numbers, in blocks of six, stratified by trial centre and sex. We analysed the primary outcome—the rate of additional colonic investigation—by intention to treat. The trial is an International Standard Randomised Controlled Trial, number 95152621.

Findings.—1610 patients were randomly assigned to receive either colonoscopy (n = 1072) or CTC (n = 538). 30 patients withdrew consent, leaving for analysis 1047 assigned to colonoscopy and 533 assigned to CTC.

160 (30.0%) patients in the CTC group had additional colonic investigation compared with 86 (8·2%) in the colonoscopy group (relative risk 3·65, 95% CI 2.87–4.65; $p < 0.0001$). Almost half the referrals after CTC were for small (<10 mm) polyps or clinical uncertainty, with low predictive value for large polyps or cancer. Detection rates of colorectal cancer or large polyps in the trial cohort were 11% for both procedures. CTC missed 1 of 29 colorectal cancers and colonoscopy missed none (of 55). Serious adverse events were rare.

Interpretation.—Guidelines are needed to reduce the referral rate after CTC. For most patients, however, CTC provides a similarly sensitive, less invasive alternative to colonoscopy.

▶ Screening for colon cancer can take many forms, but perhaps the most effective is colonoscopy. However, a less-invasive form of screening, computed tomographic colonography (CTC) has been studied for the last decade as a potential alternative. These 2 modalities had not been compared previously in a randomized, controlled trial. This report discusses a trial with 2:1 randomization in favor of colonoscopy vs CTC at 21 hospitals in the United Kingdom between 2004 and 2007. There were 610 patients in the study, and the most important finding was that both tests were equally useful for discovering colon cancers and larger polyps. This incidence was 11.4% in the colonoscopy group vs 10.7% in the CTC group. One of the problems in the CTC group was that 30% required additional diagnostic tests, which was 3 times the rate of incomplete colonoscopy in the other group. Sixteen percent of patients having CTC had an extracolonic finding reported, and 10% of the entire group having CTC required referral for additional investigation; 9 of 48 of these patients ended up having an extracolonic malignancy. In the colonoscopy group, 5.7% of patients were found with colorectal cancer vs 5.6% in the CTC group. However, in the CTC group, when cancer was suspected, these patients needed a colonoscopy to confirm this. Patients were followed up for 3 years, and 1 patient in the CTC group had a missed colon cancer (the patient developed this within the first 3 years of follow-up). This did not occur in the colonoscopy group. A similar number of extracolonic cancers were diagnosed within 3 years of follow-up in the 2 groups. Patients who had colonoscopies had more adverse effects than patients who had CTC. The authors conclude from this study that the rate of detection of colorectal cancer or large polyps is similar in the 2 groups, but CTC has a disadvantage of requiring an additional procedure to make the diagnosis. Additionally, CTC resulted in 30% getting further colonic investigation, and 60% were found to have extracolonic lesions, most of which were thought to be unimportant but 10% of which required further work up. Patients felt that CTC was more convenient than colonoscopy, however, and in patients who cannot tolerate sedation, CTC is a good alternative to colonoscopy.

J. Howe, MD

Epithelial Barriers, Microbiota, and Colorectal Cancer

Gallimore AM, Godkin A (Cardiff Univ, Wales, UK)

N Engl J Med 368:282-284, 2013

Background.—Colorectal cancer is much more prevalent in developed countries than in developing countries, which indicates that environmental factors such as diet and lifestyle are contributory. Colorectal cancer and other diseases are already associated with Western diets low in fiber but high in red meat, saturated fats, and processed sugars. Strong evidence indicates that aspirin and other nonsteroidal anti-inflammatory drugs (NSAIDs) help prevent the growth of polyps and cancer in the colon, which implicates inflammation in the pathogenesis of this disease. Persons who have inflammatory bowel disease are more likely than those without this disease to develop colorectal cancer. Microbiota are now being considered as another factor associated with colorectal cancer.

Inflammation.—Human colorectal cancer evidences an "inflammatory" molecular signature, with a type 17 helper T-cell (Th17) response found to be more influential than a type 1 helper T-cell (Th1) response in patients with a poorer prognosis, even during early stages of the disease. Why some persons express Th17 in response to interleukin-23 and others produce Th1, with its better prognostic association is unknown, but may reflect the individual's background microbiota. Human and mouse models have been shown to secrete greater levels of interleukin-23 and interleukin-17. Interleukin-23 is produced when the toll-like receptors (TLRs) of myeloid cells in mucosa are stimulated by bacterial products from commensal microbiota. Downstream cells are altered by interleukin-23 and contribute to the inflammatory signature, along with other cytokines.

Epithelial Cell Barriers.—Epithelial cells with genetic mutations lead to loss of adenomatous polyposis coli (APC) function and activate β-catenin through the loss of epithelial barrier function. The development of colonic adenomas and carcinomas is associated with loss of this barrier. As a result, luminal bacteria can more readily translocate into the lamina propria and activate myeloid cells, a process that leads to the production of interleukin-23. This then promotes interleukin-17 production and progresses to epithelial cell proliferation, gradual loss of function, and growth of tumors.

Conclusions.—Future research is needed, but inflammation, epithelial barrier failure, and microbiota appear to interact in ways that facilitate the development of colorectal cancer. It would be interesting to know if certain constituent bacteria in the microbiota are beneficial and can be encouraged, whereas less helpful ones could be discouraged.

▶ Much has been made of the progression of genetic mutations resulting in colorectal cancer, leading to the acceptance of the classic Vogelgram as our main model for colorectal carcinogenesis. A recent article by Grivennikov et al[1] now provides evidence for the possibility of the breakdown of epithelial integrity giving rise to cancer caused by microbial invasion. In a mouse model, they showed that epithelial cell transformation, which led to loss of adenomatous polyposis coli function and activation of β-catenin, could lead to the loss of proteins joining cells together as well as mucin (Fig 1 in the original article). This enhanced the invasion of bacteria into the lamina propria, where these bacteria would activate myeloid cells. These myeloid cells would then produce interleukin 23, which then would generate responses from T cells to produce interleukin 17, which activates STAT3 and causes epithelial cell proliferation, invasion, and increased survival. This model suggests that the specific microbes in the intestine may influence the inflammatory response, which can be mediated through either a type 17 helper T cell response (which would then lead to cancer) vs a type 1 helper T cell response (where cytotoxic interferon-γ is produced). It is unclear whether the production of interleukin 17 over interferon-γ is influenced by the specific type of bacteria present or whether these are responses intrinsic to the host. In animal models, treatment with broad-spectrum antibiotics or interleukin 23 deficiency did appear to reduce colorectal cancers. This review article nicely summarizes and illustrates this process, which represents a new way of thinking about colorectal carcinogenesis.

J. Howe, MD

Reference

1. Grivennikov SI, Wang K, Mucida D, et al. Adenoma-linked barrier defects and microbial products drive IL-23/IL-17-mediated tumour growth. *Nature*. 2012; 491:254-258.

Independent Validation of a Prognostic Genomic Signature (ColoPrint) for Patients With Stage II Colon Cancer

Maak M, Simon I, Nitsche U, et al (Technische Universität München, Germany; Agendia NV, Amsterdam, The Netherlands; et al)
Ann Surg 257:1053-1058, 2013

Objectives.—The aim of this study was to independently validate a genomic signature developed both to assess recurrence risk in stage II patients and to assist in treatment decisions.

Background.—Adjuvant therapy is recommended for high-risk patients with stage II colon cancer, but better tools to assess the patients' prognosis accurately are still required.

Methods.—Previously, an 18-gene signature had been developed and validated on an independent cohort, using full genome microarrays. In this study, the gene signature was translated and validated as a robust diagnostic test (ColoPrint), using customized 8-pack arrays. In addition, clinical validation of the diagnostic ColoPrint assay was performed on 135 patients who underwent curative resection (R0) for colon cancer stage II in Munich. Fresh-frozen tissue, microsatellite instability status, clinical parameters, and follow-up data for all patients were available. The diagnostic ColoPrint readout was determined blindly from the clinical data.

Results.—ColoPrint identified most stage II patients (73.3%) as at low risk. The 5-year distant-metastasis free survival was 94.9% for low-risk patients and 80.6% for high-risk patients. In multivariable analysis, ColoPrint was the only significant parameter to predict the development of distant metastasis with a hazard ratio of 4.28 (95% confidence interval, 1.36−13.50; $P = 0.013$). Clinical risk parameters from the American Society of Clinical Oncology (ASCO) recommendation did not add power to the ColoPrint classification. Technical validation of ColoPrint confirmed stability and reproducibility of the diagnostic platform.

Conclusions.—ColoPrint is able to predict the development of distant metastasis of patients with stage II colon cancer and facilitates the identification of patients who may be safely managed without chemotherapy.

▶ The promise of gene-based testing for risk stratification for multiple cancers has been a long time in coming and has been shown to be useful in breast cancer. One group of patients in whom this would be useful would be those with stage 2 colon cancer where previous studies of adjuvant chemotherapy have shown little survival benefit; however, a small subset of these patients, approximately 10%, will develop distant metastases and could potentially benefit from adjuvant chemotherapy if these high-risk patients could be identified. Previous variables identified by the American Society of Clinical Oncology and the National Comprehensive Cancer Network include clinicopathologic factors such as less than 12 lymph nodes being examined, T4 tumors, the presence of invasion (perineural, vascular, lymphatic), obstruction or perforation, high-grade tumors, and positive resection margins. In addition to this, having high microsatellite instability (MSI) is a factor that portends good prognosis in these patients, and no benefit has been shown for chemotherapy with this group. In this study, a previously validated 18 gene test called ColoPrint was used to evaluate 188 stage 2 colorectal cancer patients. This test had previously been developed using whole genome microarrays, and these 18 genes were selected as being prognostic. RNA was extracted from tumors frozen in liquid nitrogen and then assayed using this platform. Overall, the rate of distant metastases in this group of stage 2 patients was 8.9%, and of all the previously mentioned factors, the only factor that was significantly associated with risk of metastasis was the ColoPrint assay, in which patients were stratified into high-risk (26.7%) versus low-risk (73.3%) groups. In those groups there was a hazard ratio of 4.28 for the high-risk group versus the low-risk group, and 5-year disease-free survival of the low-risk group was 95% versus 81% for the high-risk group. This assay was very reproducible and, therefore, appears to be of clinical value for determining those patients who might benefit from adjuvant chemotherapy. The only other predictor of these clinicopathologic factors that might also be useful is MSI; therefore, some combination of the ColoPrint assay and MSI may ultimately be the most useful test for selecting these patients in the future.

J. Howe, MD

Risk Factors for Survival after Lung Metastasectomy in Colorectal Cancer Patients: A Systematic Review and Meta-Analysis

Gonzalez M, Poncet A, Combescure C, et al (Centre Hospitalier Vaudois (CHUV), Lausanne, Switzerland; Univ Hosp Geneva, Switzerland; et al)

Ann Surg Oncol 20:572-579, 2013

Background.—Resection of lung metastases (LM) from colorectal cancer (CRC) is increasingly performed with a curative intent. It is currently not possible to identify those CRC patients who may benefit the most from this surgical strategy. The aim of this study was to perform a systematic review of risk factors for survival after lung metastasectomy for CRC.

Methods.—We performed a meta-analysis of series published between 2000 and 2011, which focused on surgical management of LM from CRC and included more than 40 patients each. Pooled hazard ratios (HR) were calculated by using random effects model for parameters considered as potential prognostic factors.

Results.—Twenty-five studies including a total of 2925 patients were considered in this analysis. Four parameters were associated with poor survival: (1) a short disease-free interval between primary tumor resection and development of LM (HR 1.59, 95 % confidence interval [CI] 1.27–1.98); (2) multiple LM (HR 2.04, 95 % CI 1.72–2.41); (3) positive hilar and/or mediastinal lymph nodes (HR 1.65, 95 % CI 1.35–2.02); and (4) elevated prethoracotomy carcinoembryonic antigen (HR 1.91, 95 % CI 1.57–2.32). By comparison, a history of resected liver metastases (HR 1.22, 95 % CI 0.91–1.64) did not achieve statistical significance.

Conclusions.—Clinical variables associated with prolonged survival after surgery for LM in CRC patients include prolonged disease-free interval between primary tumor and metastatic spread, normal prethoracotomy carcinoembryonic antigen, absence of thoracic node involvement, and a single pulmonary lesion.

► Approximately 5% to 15% of patients with colorectal cancer (CRC) will develop pulmonary metastases. Resection of these pulmonary metastases can potentially lead to long-term survival in these patients. The current indications for pulmonary metastasectomy recommended by the National Comprehensive Cancer Network are that the lesions should be technically resectable, the patient is fit for pulmonary resection, there are no extrathoracic lesions (with the exception of liver metastases), and the primary tumor be resected. Factors that predict increased risk of death from CRC in patients with lung metastases have not been well defined, however. This study is a meta-analysis of series published between 2000 and 2011 that had greater than 40 patients. This included 25 reports for a total of 2925 patients. Seventy-five percent had 1 lung metastasis, whereas the other 25% had multiple lung metastases, and the 5 year survival after metastasectomy was reported to be between 27% and 68%. These studies were inconsistent in the factors that they examined, but ultimately there were 5 different factors that appeared to be most important, and these were the focus of the study. They found that a shorter disease-free interval was associated with increased risk, for a hazard ratio of 1.59, but the interval was not defined. Patients with multiple lung metastases had a hazard ratio of 2.04 versus those with single metastases. Patients who had mediastinal or hilar lymph node involvement had a hazard ratio of 1.65 versus those who did not. Those with preoperative carcinoembryonic antigen (CEA) elevation had a hazard ratio of 1.91 relative to those with normal levels. One factor that was not significant for increased risk was a previous history of liver metastases. This article does not define the criteria for patients who may benefit from pulmonary metastasectomy, but it does suggest the factors that place them at a higher risk of death from colorectal cancer. Those factors include short disease-free interval, which may be associated with more aggressive cancers; multiple pulmonary lesions; involved hilar or mediastinal nodes (although in most studies these nodes were not dissected out, and the report does recommend the use of positron emission tomography scans before resection to sort this issue out); they would recommend that patients with suspicious nodes have mediastinoscopy, and if those nodes are positive, to not undergo resection, but rather palliative therapy; and CEA level, which should not be used to exclude patients from resection but should be a useful marker to follow after resection. For general surgeons working below the diaphragm, it is important to note that the presence of liver and pulmonary metastases do not contraindicate resection of both sites to achieve long-term survival.

J. Howe, MD

Gastric

Treatment Trends and Predictors of Adjuvant and Neoadjuvant Therapy for Gastric Adenocarcinoma in the United States

Sherman KL, Merkow RP, Bilimoria KY, et al (Northwestern Univ, Chicago, IL; et al)
Ann Surg Oncol 20:362-370, 2013

Purpose.—Over the last decade, evidence suggesting the benefits of adjuvant therapy in the treatment of stage IB-III gastric adenocarcinoma has emerged, though the influence of these clinical trials and current treatment patterns is unknown. Our objectives were (1) to assess changes in gastric adenocarcinoma treatment over time, (2) to identify predictors of neoadjuvant or postoperative adjuvant therapy use, and (3) to identify factors associated with neoadjuvant therapy use.

Methods.—Patients with stage IB–III gastric adenocarcinoma diagnosed between 1998 and 2007 in the National Cancer Data Base who underwent surgical resection were selected. Models were developed to identify factors associated with treatment.

Results.—We identified 30,448 patients diagnosed with stage IB–III gastric adenocarcinoma who underwent surgical resection. Rates of systemic therapy receipt (either before or after surgery) increased by 71 % from 1998 to 2007 ($p < 0.001$). Receipt of neoadjuvant therapy receipt increased by 237 % over 10 years ($p < 0.001$), with the highest rate of increase seen at high-volume academic centers. American Joint Committee on Cancer

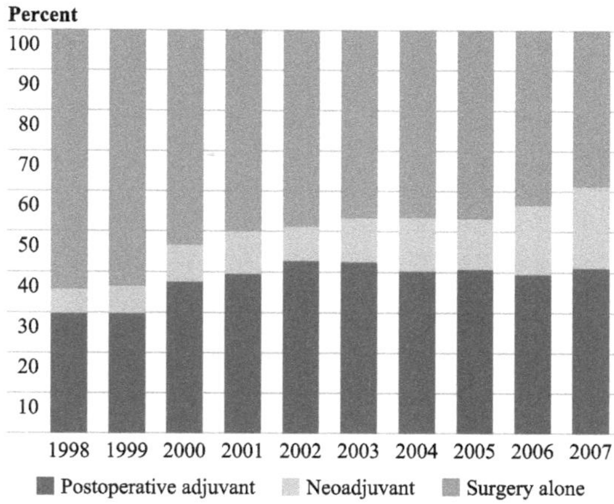

FIGURE 1.—Treatment trends in stage IB–III gastric adenocarcinoma. (With kind permission from Springer Science+Business Media. Sherman KL, Merkow RP, Bilimoria KY, et al. Treatment trends and predictors of adjuvant and neoadjuvant therapy for gastric adenocarcinoma in the United States. *Ann Surg Oncol.* 2013;20:362-370, with permission from Society of Surgical Oncology.)

(AJCC) stage and age were the strongest predictors of pre- or postoperative systemic therapy among surgical patients. Neoadjuvant therapy receipt was most strongly predicted by tumor location in the gastric cardia.

Conclusions.—Treatment trends over the past decade reflect rapid adoption of evidence from randomized controlled trials by increased receipt of pre- and postoperative systemic therapy in the treatment of stage IB–III gastric adenocarcinoma. Although age and AJCC stage are strongly associated with receiving systemic adjuvant therapy, tumor location is the most significant predictor of neoadjuvant therapy (Fig 1).

▶ There have been 2 landmark studies in gastric cancer in the last decade showing the advantages of adjuvant or neoadjuvant treatment in gastric cancer. In 2001, the Intergroup 0116 trial was published, which showed that there was a survival advantage to following surgery with chemoradiation in gastroesophageal cancer. In 2006, the MAGIC trial found an advantage with pre- and postoperative epirubicin, cisplatin, and fluorouracil therapy in gastroesophageal junction tumors in terms of both overall and progression-free survival. The objective of this study was to review the National Cancer Data Base for trends in adjuvant and neoadjuvant treatment in gastric cancer. They reviewed the database for cases between 1998 and 2007 and found 30 448 for comparison. They also divided individual hospitals into academic or research centers and comprehensive community cancer centers of high and low volumes and specifically looked at cardia versus noncardia lesions. The most significant findings of this study are that the use of systemic chemotherapy increased 71% over the period of the study, from 36% to 61% of patients. The use of neoadjuvant therapy increased 237% over the time of the study, from 6% to 20% (Fig 1). Factors that were most significant for the selection of systemic therapy were younger age, male sex, and reduced comorbidities, with the strongest predictor being American Joint Committee on Cancer

(AJCC) stage. Patients with stage 2 cancer received adjuvant therapy 3 times more commonly than those with stage 1B cancer, and for stage 3 patients, 3.5 times more than stage 1B. Hospital type did not seem to influence adjuvant therapy in multivariable analyses. Looking at the subgroup of patients who underwent neoadjuvant therapy, it was clear that patients with tumors at the gastric cardia received this more commonly than those with cancer at other sites, and this factor remained significant on multivariable analyses. Patients older than 75 years were less likely to receive neoadjuvant treatment as well as were those who were treated at high-volume centers. This study confirmed that there was increased utilization of adjuvant and neoadjuvant treatment in US centers after the publications of the Intergroup and MAGIC trials and defined AJCC stage as one of the most important predictors for adjuvant treatment, and tumor location for neoadjuvant treatment. The reason for the latter was thought to be the increased complexity and morbidity of cases involving the gastric cardia. Interestingly, despite the increased use of adjuvant or neoadjuvant therapy over the study, even in the group treated between 2005 and 2007, 34% of patients with stage 3 gastric adenocarcinomas were not treated with adjuvant or neoadjuvant treatment. Therefore, we still have a way to go to satisfy the current National Comprehensive Cancer Network guidelines that patients with stage 1B-3 gastric cancers should have systemic therapy either pre- or postoperatively.

J. Howe, MD

Conditional Probability of Survival Nomogram for 1-, 2-, and 3-Year Survivors After an R0 Resection for Gastric Cancer

Dikken JL, Baser RE, Gonen M, et al (Memorial Sloan-Kettering Cancer Ctr, NY; et al)

Ann Surg Oncol 20:1623-1630, 2013

Background.—Survival estimates after curative surgery for gastric cancer are based on AJCC staging, or on more accurate multivariable nomograms. However, the risk of dying of gastric cancer is not constant over time, with most deaths occurring in the first 2 years after resection. Therefore, the prognosis for a patient who survives this critical period improves. This improvement over time is termed conditional probability of survival (CPS). Objectives of this study were to develop a CPS nomogram predicting 5-year disease-specific survival (DSS) from the day of surgery for patients surviving a specified period of time after a curative gastrectomy and to explore whether variables available with follow-up improve the nomogram in the follow-up setting.

Methods.—A CPS nomogram was developed from a combined US-Dutch dataset, containing 1,642 patients who underwent an R0 resection with or without chemotherapy/radiotherapy for gastric cancer. Weight loss, performance status, hemoglobin, and albumin 1 year after resection were added to the baseline variables of this nomogram.

Results.—The CPS nomogram was highly discriminating (concordance index: 0.772). Surviving 1, 2, or 3 years gives a median improvement of

5-year DSS from surgery of 7.2, 19.1, and 31.6 %, compared with the baseline prediction directly after surgery. Introduction of variables available at 1-year follow-up did not improve the nomogram.

Conclusions.—A robust gastric cancer nomogram was developed to predict survival for patients alive at time points after surgery. Introduction of additional variables available after 1 year of follow-up did not further improve this nomogram.

▶ Nomograms for the prediction of cancer mortality have become popular over the last decades. These look at a variety of clinicopathologic factors and assign points to different categories, which, in their aggregate, can help predict the likelihood of survival. For gastric cancer, a highly effective nomogram has been developed combining data from one large US center and another in the Netherlands. The objective of this study was to determine whether this nomogram could be improved over long-term follow-up by including factors might influence a general improvement in prognosis in patients who survive to various time points after surgery. The previous nomogram looked only at the probability of survival after the time of surgery. The current nomogram added factors at 1 year after surgery, such as weight loss, albumin, performance status, and hemoglobin. Much of the report is a complicated description of the algorithm, but the results are interesting and represent an improvement over the previous nomogram in some ways. First, the factors that were previously included were not improved upon by the new model or by the addition of new features over time. However, the conditional probability of survival was an important factor that would impact patients as they continued to survive after surgery. For example, in Fig 3 of the original article, we see that from the time of surgery, somebody's probability of 5-year disease-specific survival would be 40%. However, if they live for 1 year after surgery, their chance of 5-year survival now becomes 45%, if they live for 2 years after surgery their chance of living 5 years is 57%, and if they live for 3 years this percentage increases to 70%. The value of this nomogram is its incorporation of something people who treat cancer have known for a long time—the further out a patients survives from time of surgery, the more likely they will enjoy long-term survival.

J. Howe, MD

Hepatic Colorectal

Surgical Management of Patients with Synchronous Colorectal Liver Metastasis: A Multicenter International Analysis

Mayo SC, Pulitano C, Marques H, et al (Johns Hopkins Univ School of Medicine, Baltimore, MD; Scientific Inst San Raffaele, Milan, Italy; Unit of Hepato-Biliary-Pancreatic Surgery, Lisbon, Portugal; et al)

J Am Coll Surg 216:707-718, 2013

Background.—The goal of this study was to investigate the surgical management and outcomes of patients with primary colorectal cancer (CRC) and synchronous liver metastasis (sCRLM).

Study Design.—Using a multi-institutional database, we identified 1,004 patients treated for sCRLM between 1982 and 2011. Clinicopathologic and outcomes data were evaluated with uni- and multivariable analyses.

Results.—A simultaneous CRC and liver operation was performed in 329 (33%) patients; 675 (67%) underwent a staged approach ("classic" staged approach, n = 647; liver-first strategy, n = 28). Patients managed with the liver-first approach had more hepatic lesions and were more likely to have bilateral disease than those in the other 2 groups ($p < 0.05$). The use of staged operative strategies increased over the time of the study from 58% to 75% ($p < 0.001$). Liver-directed therapy included hepatectomy (90%) or combined resection + ablation (10%). A major resection (>3 segments) was more common with a staged approach (39% vs 24%; $p < 0.001$). Overall, 509 patients (50%) received chemotherapy in either the preoperative (22%) or adjuvant (28%) settings, with 11% of patients having both. There were 197 patients (20%) who had a complication in the postoperative period, with no difference in morbidity between staged and simultaneous groups or major vs minor hepatectomies ($p > 0.05$). Ninety-day postoperative mortality was 3.0%, with no difference between simultaneous and staged approaches ($p = 0.94$). The overall median and 5-year survivals were 50.9 months and 44%, respectively; long-term survival was the same regardless of the operative approach ($p > 0.05$).

Conclusions.—Simultaneous and staged resections for sCRLM can be performed with comparable morbidity, mortality, and long-term oncologic outcomes.

▶ Twenty-five to 30% of patients with colorectal cancer will present with synchronous liver metastases. The classic means of treating these patients would be a staged resection of the primary colorectal tumor followed by liver resection as a later procedure. However, there are other options available, which include simultaneous resection of both sites of tumors, and, more recently, some have been performing resection of the liver lesions first, followed by the colorectal tumor at the second procedure. This study reviewed patients with synchronous colorectal cancer and liver metastases from a multi-institutional database between 1982 and 2011 and evaluated the order in which these were treated as well as complications and survival rates. They found that 64% of patients had the colorectal tumor removed first followed by a liver operation later. The liver operation was performed first in 2.8%, and in 33% simultaneous resection was performed. There was a trend toward more staged procedures over the period of the study. Complications and mortality rates were similar among all groups, with a 90-day mortality rate of 3%, and an overall complication rate of 19.6%. The median overall survival was 50.9 months with a 44% 5-year survival rate, and there were no significant differences according to the sequence in which the colorectal and liver lesions were addressed. Factors associated with decreased survival included male sex, the presence of a rectal primary, and having a combined resection and ablation technique performed. The overall message of this study is that all 3 of these options are reasonable and result in similar complication and similar survival rates.

J. Howe, MD

Use of Bioresorbable Membranes to Reduce Abdominal and Perihepatic Adhesions in 2-Stage Hepatectomy of Liver Metastases From Colorectal Cancer: Results of a Prospective, Randomized Controlled Phase II Trial

Dupré A, Lefranc A, Buc E, et al (Léon Bérard Cancer Ctr, Lyon, France; D'estaing Univ Hosp, Clermont-Ferrand, France; et al)

Ann Surg 258:30-36, 2013

Objective.—To assess by prospective randomized controlled trial the feasibility and efficacy of using a bioresorbable hyaluronic acid/carboxymethylcellulose membrane (HA membrane) to prevent abdominal and perihepatic adhesions in metastatic colorectal cancer patients requiring 2-stage hepatectomy.

Background.—Two-stage hepatectomy offers the possibility of long-term survival to selected patients whose liver metastases cannot be removed in a single procedure. However, the second operation is made more difficult by adhesions arising from the first. HA membrane reduces adhesions in gynecologic and abdominal surgery but this is the first trial in hepatectomy.

Methods.—Fifty-four candidates for 2-stage hepatectomy were randomized at the end of the first procedure to implantation of HA membrane ($n = 41$) or standard management ($n = 13$). Thirty patients from the membrane arm and 11 well-matched controls underwent the planned second hepatectomy.

Results.—Positioning of the HA membranes was feasible in all but one patient and did not increase complications associated with the first hepatectomy. At second hepatectomy, patients in the HA membrane arm required 33% less time than controls to achieve complete liver mobilization (median: 50 vs 75 minutes; primary endpoint). The risk of extensive adhesions was reduced in the HA membrane group (31% had grade 3–4 adhesions vs 55% in controls), as was adhesion severity (17% thick and hypervascular adhesions vs 46%). The proportion of patients with complications at second hepatectomy was higher in the control group (55% vs 23% in the HA membrane group, $P = 0.07$).

Conclusion.—Use of 4 HA membranes at the end of first hepatectomy reduced the extent and severity of adhesions and facilitated the second hepatectomy in patients with liver metastases who required a 2-stage hepatectomy. A larger study to confirm these findings is warranted. (NCT01262417).

► A new approach for patients with bilobar colorectal liver metastases is a 2-stage hepatectomy, in which one side of the liver is cleared at the first operation, possibly in conjunction with removing the primary tumor, and in a later-stage operation the other liver lobe is cleared of tumors. One problem with this approach is that significant adhesions can form between the liver and the abdominal wall during the time between the stages, which can lead to increased complication rates. For this reason, a prospective, randomized trial was carried out randomly assigning patients to receive Seprafilm, a hyaluronic acid (HA) and carboxymethyl cellulose membrane, over and under the liver as well as under the incision after the first procedure. This product has been found to reduce the rate of adhesions in patients after abdominal surgery but not necessarily the rate of small bowel obstruction. Patients were randomly assigned 3:1 to receive the HA after the first hepatectomy. The patients were treated with preoperative chemotherapy before the first operation and with chemotherapy in between the first and second operations. A total of 41 patients were assigned to the HA arm and 13 patients to the control arm, and eventually, 30 patients were evaluable who received HA and second-stage hepatectomy, whereas 11 were evaluable in the control group. The primary endpoint of this study was the time involved in mobilization of the liver, which was found to be significantly lessened in patients who had received the HA (50 minutes vs 75 minutes in the control group, a 33% reduction). Secondary endpoints in this study were to look at the extent and severity of adhesions, blood loss, and perioperative morbidity. This study found that grade 3 to 4 adhesions were reduced in the HA group versus the control group, bleeding was slightly less in the HA group, and the proportion of patients having at least one complication was reduced in the HA group (23% vs 55% of controls, $P = .07$). This study found that using HA membranes after first hepatectomy improved the time to mobilization of the liver and reduced the rate of complications as well as the severity of adhesions. The authors conclude that this treatment was both safe and feasible and that the use of HA is justified in patients having 2-stage liver surgery. This was a relatively small trial, and many endpoints did not reach statistical significance; therefore, a larger trial would need to be carried out to confirm these findings.

J. Howe, MD

Fast-track surgery improves postoperative recovery in patients undergoing partial hepatectomy for primary liver cancer: A prospective randomized controlled trial

Ni CY, Yang Y, Chang YQ, et al (Second Military Med Univ, Shanghai, China; et al)
Eur J Surg Oncol 39:542-547, 2013

Background and Aim.—Fast-track surgery (FTS), combining several techniques with evidence-based adjustments, has shown its effectiveness to accelerate recovery, reduce morbidity and shorten hospital stay in many operations. This randomized controlled study was carried out aiming to compare the short-term outcomes of partial hepatectomy for liver cancer managed with FTS or with conventional surgery (CS).

Methods.—To compare the short-term effects between FTS and CS, a randomized controlled trial was carried out for liver cancer patients undergoing partial hepatectomy from September 2010 to June 2012.

Results.—Patients with liver cancers before receiving partial hepatectomy were randomized into the FTS group ($n = 80$) and the CS group ($n = 80$). Compared with the CS group, the FTS group had significantly less complications ($P < 0.05$), shorter durations of nausea/vomiting, paralytic ileus and hospital stay, higher general comfort questionnaire measures (*GCQ*) by *Kolcaba Line* (all $P < 0.05$), and lower serum levels of C-reactive protein on postoperative days 1, 3, and 5.

Conclusions.—FTS was safe and efficacious. It lessened postoperative stress reactions and accelerated recovery for patients undergoing partial hepatectomy for liver cancer.

▶ Major hepatectomy is a procedure associated with significant operative risk, postoperative complications, and extended length of stay. Is it possible to reduce the length of stay after these complicated procedures? This study randomized patients to a fast-track postoperative course vs conventional care. Fast-track surgery (FTS) includes removing the nasogastric tube as soon as possible after surgery, restricting intravenous fluid, minimizing the length of time with an abdominal drain, drinking liquids starting on postoperative day 1, removing the catheter on day 2, discontinuing the epidural on day 3, and advancing to a normal diet. Conventional care included nothing by mouth until postoperative day 3, removing the urinary catheter on day 3, and removing epidural catheters later. The criteria for discharge included the ability to take food by mouth, having control using by mouth pain medications, tolerating solid food, and being able to ambulate independently. The authors randomized 160 hepatectomy patients over a 2.5-year period from a single hospital into these 2 categories. They found that overall complications and grade 1 complications in conventional care versus FTS group were 25% and 13%, respectively. The nasogastric tube and abdominal drains were removed earlier in the FTS group, and there was a significant difference in length of stay between groups, with the FTS group staying a mean of 6.9 days vs 8.0 days for the conventional care group. The authors concluded that using this fast-track protocol results in quicker postoperative recovery with earlier discharge and that they actually have fewer complications. They believed that this could be further improved by additional measures in the future, one perhaps being the greater use of laparoscopic liver surgery.

J. Howe, MD

Is There a Possibility of a Cure in Patients With Colorectal Peritoneal Carcinomatosis Amenable to Complete Cytoreductive Surgery and Intraperitoneal Chemotherapy?

Goéré D, Malka D, Tzanis D, et al (Institut Gustave Roussy, Villejuif Cedex, France)

Ann Surg 257:1065-1071, 2013

Background.—Although a randomized trial demonstrated a survival benefit of cytoreductive surgery (CRS) and intraperitoneal chemotherapy

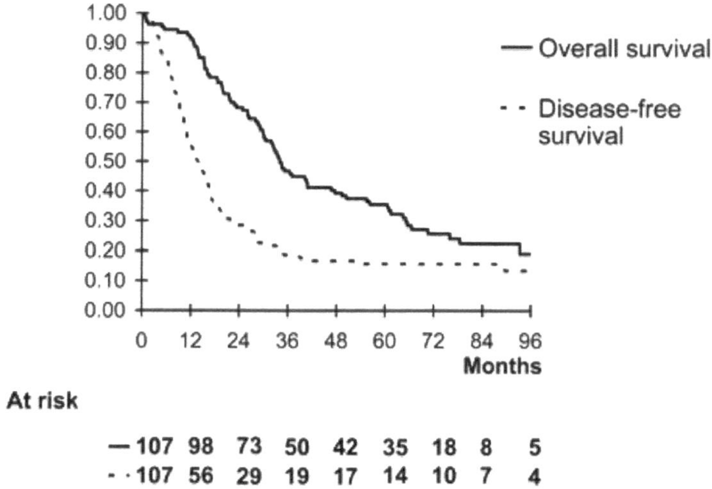

FIGURE 1.—Overall survival and disease-free survival in 107 patients who underwent complete CRS with IPC. (Reprinted from Goéré D, Malka D, Tzanis D, et al. Is there a possibility of a cure in patients with colorectal peritoneal carcinomatosis amenable to complete cytoreductive surgery and intraperitoneal chemotherapy?. *Ann Surg*. 2013;257:1065-1071, Copyright 2013, with permission from Southeastern Surgical Congress.)

(IPC) over systemic chemotherapy alone, the treatment of peritoneal carcinomatosis from colorectal cancer (CRPC) is still a matter of debate. The aims of this study were to evaluate long-term outcome after CRS and IPC and to identify the prognostic factors associated with a cure.

Methods.—Patients were considered cured if the disease-free survival interval lasted at least 5 years after the treatment of CRPC or its last recurrence. Patients who had died postoperatively, or from non–cancer-related deaths, or patients with a follow-up of less than 5 years since the last curative treatment were excluded from the analysis.

Results.—From 1995 to 2006, 107 patients (median age, 48 years; range, 19–67 years) underwent complete CRS, followed by IPC. Postoperative complications occurred in 50 patients (53%), including 4 postoperative deaths. After a median follow-up of 77 months (range, 60–144 months), 5-year and 10-year overall survival rates were 35% and 15%, respectively. Seventeen patients (16%) were considered cured after a disease-free interval of at least 5 years, of whom 14 never developed a recurrence. Cured patients had a significantly lower median peritoneal cancer index than noncured patients, respectively 4 (3–16) and 12 (2–36) ($P = 0.0002$). In multivariate analysis, a peritoneal cancer index of 10 or less was the only independent factor predicting cure.

Conclusions.—The cure rate (16%) after complete CRS of colorectal peritoneal carcinomatosis, followed by IPC, in selected patients is close to that obtained after resection of colorectal liver metastases (Fig 1).

► The treatment of peritoneal carcinomatosis caused by colorectal cancer has come a long way in the last few decades. Often thought to be an incurable disease, patients can benefit greatly from cytoreductive surgery followed by intraperitoneal chemotherapy. An important question that comes up is whether these patients can actually be cured of their disease and whether these results warrant the high complication rates associated with these procedures. This study from a single center in France evaluated 107 patients treated between 1995 and 2005 who had cytoreductive surgery and either postoperative intraperitoneal chemotherapy or intraoperative heated chemotherapy. It excluded 41 patients who had unresectable peritoneal carcinomatosis seen over the same interval at their center. They compared factors in patients who had no evidence of disease recurrence at 5 years versus those who did develop recurrence. Overall, they had 17 patients with no evidence of recurrence at 5 years for a total of 16%. Of the overall cohort of 107 patients, the 5-year overall survival rate was 35% and 10-year survival rate was 15%, whereas the disease-free survival rate was 16% at 5 years and 13% at 10 years (Fig 1). When comparing the groups with recurrence and without, 4 factors emerged on univariate analysis as being significantly different. The mean peritoneal cancer index was 4 in the cured group versus 12 in the noncured group; the operating time was less in the cured group; postoperative stay was slightly less at 19 days versus 21 days in the cured group versus the noncured group; operative blood loss was less in the cured group. Overall postoperative complications were seen at 53%, and cured patients had an incidence of 24% versus 61% in the noncured patients. On multivariate analysis, the only factor that emerged as being independently significant was the peritoneal cancer index, where the hazard ratio was 9 for those with an index greater than 10. This study showed that patients with peritoneal carcinomatosis can be cured of their disease with cytoreductive surgery and intraperitoneal chemotherapy, and long-term results are similar to that obtained after resection of liver metastases for colorectal cancer. Even though only about one-third of patients with peritoneal carcinomatosis cause by colorectal cancer will be eligible for such therapy, it is clear that a subset of these patients can be cured, and, therefore, it should be offered in the discussion of therapeutic modalities. The alternative of chemotherapy alone has resulted in much lower 5-year survival rates of anywhere from 0% to 13%.

J. Howe, MD

Rectal

Impact of Robotic Surgery on Sexual and Urinary Functions After Fully Robotic Nerve-Sparing Total Mesorectal Excision for Rectal Cancer

Luca F, Valvo M, Ghezzi TL, et al (European Inst of Oncology, Milano, Italy; Moinhos de Vento Hosp, Porto Alegre, Brazil)

Ann Surg 257:672-678, 2013

Background.—Urinary and sexual dysfunctions are recognized complications of rectal cancer surgery. Their incidence after robotic surgery is as yet unknown. The aim of this study was to prospectively evaluate the impact of robotic surgery for rectal cancer on sexual and urinary functions in male and female patients.

Methods and Procedures.—From April 2008 to December 2010, 74 patients undergoing fully robotic resection for rectal cancer were prospectively included in the study. Urinary and sexual dysfunctions affecting quality of life were assessed with specific self-administered questionnaires in all patients undergoing robotic total mesorectal excision (RTME). Results were calculated with validated scoring systems and statistically analyzed.

Results.—The analyses of the questionnaires completed by the 74 patients who underwent RTME showed that sexual function and general sexual satisfaction decreased significantly 1 month after intervention: 19.1 ± 8.7 versus 11.9 ± 10.2 ($P < 0.05$) for erectile function and 6.9 ± 2.4 versus 5.3 ± 2.5 ($P < 0.05$) for general satisfaction in men; 2.6 ± 3.3 versus 0.8 ± 1.4 ($P < 0.05$) and 2.4 ± 2.5 versus 0.7 ± 1.6 ($P < 0.05$) for arousal and general satisfaction, respectively, in women. Subsequently, both parameters increased progressively, and 1 year after surgery, the values were comparable to those measured before surgery. Concerning urinary function, the grade of incontinence measured 1 year after the intervention was unchanged for both sexes.

Conclusions.—RTME allows for preservation of urinary and sexual functions. This is probably due to the superior movements of the wristed instruments that facilitate fine dissection, coupled with a stable and magnified view that helps in recognizing the inferior hypogastric plexus.

▶ Multiple advances have been made in the treatment of rectal cancer over the years, beginning with the introduction of total mesorectal excision by Heald in 1982, neoadjuvant chemotherapy and radiation, and, more recently, minimally invasive techniques to treat rectal cancer. Laparoscopic colorectal resections have been performed for approximately 2 decades, but it is not clear that the laparoscopic approach has resulted in decreased rates of sexual or urinary dysfunction. Two studies published in 2009 suggest that the rate of sexual dysfunction is similar after laparoscopic procedures vs the open procedure. In this study, a group from Milan looked at the impact on sexual and urinary function in male and female patients after robotic, nerve-sparing, total mesorectal excision for rectal caner. They used well-described questionnaires, and patients filled these out preoperatively, then at 1 month, 6 months, 1 year, and 2 years postoperatively. Patients with T3 or T4 lesions were treated with radiation and chemotherapy preoperatively. They had 74 total patients and found that sexual and urinary dysfunction occurred at 1 and 6 months after surgery with significant decreases in both male and female scores on questionnaires, but that by 1 year after surgery, these values became comparable with preoperative values. This was not affected by preoperative neoadjuvant chemoradiation. The presence of a temporary diverting stoma did not appear to have an independent negative effect in men, but it did in women. The authors found that they could perform a good mesorectal excision robotically in which 88% of patients had complete mesorectal excision; excision was near complete in the other 12%, with no incomplete resections. The authors concluded that the improvement over time of sexual and urinary function was probably related to resolution of postoperative inflammation and recovery of nerve dysfunction caused by intraoperative tension on the structures. They also concluded that the robotic technique allowed for better preservation of function as opposed to either open or laparoscopic methods, and this was probably due to the improved articulation of dissection in the narrow confines of the pelvis. Furthermore, improved visualization allows for better delineation of tissue planes and preservation of the inferior hypogastric plexus.

J. Howe, MD

Hepatocellular

Revisiting Liver Anatomy and Terminology of Hepatectomies

Bismuth H (Hôpital Paul Brousse, Villejuif, France)
Ann Surg 257:383-386, 2013

Background.—Since the development of liver surgery, several descriptions of liver anatomical division and hepatectomies have been made, causing some confusion among surgeons.

Methods.—The initial anatomical description according to Couinaud is reviewed and corrected taking into account the descriptions made in the following decades.

Results.—It seems that by reviewing the description of the different authors, a precise anatomical division of the liver may be achieved and a simple terminology of hepatectomies may be proposed.

Conclusions.—It is hoped that the proposal of this anatomical description and this terminology of hepatectomies may find a consensus among the liver surgical community from America, Asia, and Europe (Fig 9).

▶ The anatomic delineation of different liver segments was nicely elucidated by Couinaud in 1954. However, since that time, there have been several different classification schemes for liver anatomy, which has made the nomenclature for liver resections somewhat confusing. This article reviews these different classifications and proposes a uniform naming scheme for surgeons to describe their hepatectomies. Bismuth himself introduced a classification scheme in 1982, in which he corrected Couinaud by dividing the liver into anterior and posterior right sectors rather than into medial and posterolateral sectors and one sector on the left. He proposes 6 segments: the right posterior segments 6 and 7 in the right posterior sector, segments 5 and 8 in the right anterior sector, and segments 3 and 4 in the left sector as one segment and segment 2 as the other one; plus the caudate lobe (segment 1). Other classification schemes described in this article are that of Takasaki, which divides the liver into 3 main territories, and that of Brisbane, where the terminology *section* is used instead of *sector*. The latter terminology has not been embraced by hepatic surgeons. It is acknowledged that the most difficult naming of the anatomy of the liver results in the lateral left liver, which Bismuth points out is neither a segment nor a sector. The presence of the umbilical fissure would define the left lateral aspect as a lobe but clearly when we discuss left lobectomy, most would also include segment 4. He urged that the word *lobectomy* should not be used, using instead, *hepatectomy*. This article gives a

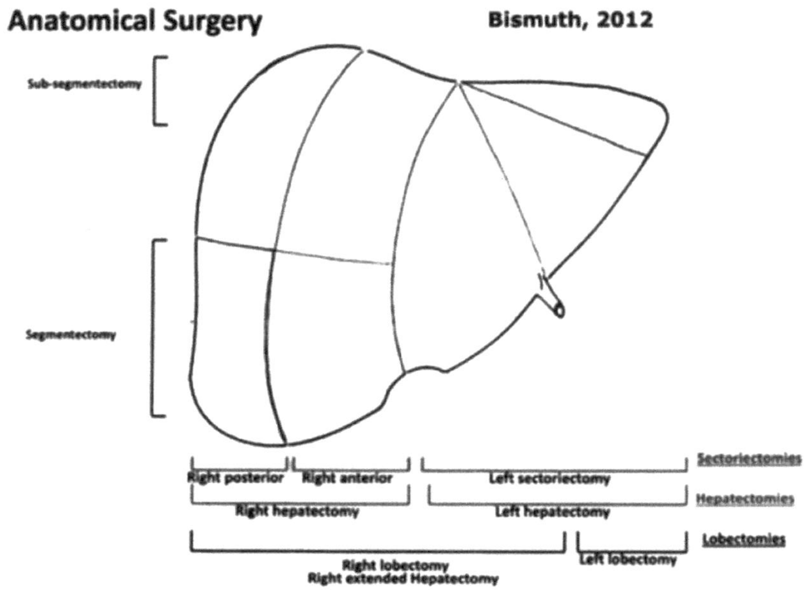

FIGURE 9.—Anatomical surgery of the liver with definition of segmentectomies, sectorectomies, hepatectomies, and lobectomies. (Reprinted from Bismuth H. Revisiting liver anatomy and terminology of hepatectomies. *Ann Surg*. 2013;257:383-386, Copyright 2013, with permission from Southeastern Surgical Congress.)

nice overview of the different anatomic controversies and nomenclature with multiple different systems in an attempt to clarify it so that hepatectomies performed in North America, Asia, and Europe will have uniform naming (Fig 9). It is not clear whether Bismuth actually achieves this in this article, however, because the anatomic classification of the left hemiliver remains somewhat confusing.

J. Howe, MD

Radiofrequency Ablation With or Without Transcatheter Arterial Chemoembolization in the Treatment of Hepatocellular Carcinoma: A Prospective Randomized Trial

Peng Z-W, Zhang Y-J, Chen M-S, et al (Sun Yat-sen Univ, Guangzhou, PR China, et al)

J Clin Oncol 31:426-432, 2013

Purpose.—To compare radiofrequency ablation (RFA) with or without transcatheter arterial chemoembolization (TACE) in the treatment of hepatocellular carcinoma (HCC).

Patients and Methods.—A randomized controlled trial was conducted on 189 patients with HCC less than 7 cm at a single tertiary referral center between October 2006 and June 2009. Patients were randomly asssigned to receive TACE combined with RFA (TACE-RFA; n = 94) or RFA alone (n = 95). The primary end point was overall survival. The secondary end point was recurrence-free survival, and the tertiary end point was adverse effects.

Results.—At a follow-up of 7 to 62 months, 34 patients in the TACE-RFA group and 48 patients in the RFA group had died. Thirty-three patients and 52 patients had developed recurrence in the TACE-RFA group and RFA group, respectively. The 1-, 3-, and 4-year overall survivals for the TACE-RFA group and the RFA group were 92.6%, 66.6%, and 61.8% and 85.3%, 59%, and 45.0%, respectively. The corresponding recurrence-free survivals were 79.4%, 60.6%, and 54.8% and 66.7%, 44.2%, and 38.9%, respectively. Patients in the TACE-RFA group had better overall survival and recurrence-free survival than patients in the RFA group (hazard ratio, 0.525; 95% CI, 0.335 to 0.822; $P = .002$; hazard ratio, 0.575; 95% CI, 0.374 to 0.897; $P = .009$, respectively). There were no treatment-related deaths. On logistic regression analyses, treatment allocation, tumor size, and tumor number were significant prognostic factors for overall survival, whereas treatment allocation and tumor number were significant prognostic factors for recurrence-free survival.

Conclusion.—TACE-RFA was superior to RFA alone in improving survival for patients with HCC less than 7 cm.

▶ Hepatocellular cancer (HCC) is the third leading cause of cancer death globally and the sixth most common cancer overall. Several treatment modalities for HCC exist, including resection, radiofrequency ablation (RFA), transarterial catheter embolization (TACE), and liver transplantation. TACE is commonly used for intermediate-stage HCC, and RFA has become a reasonable alternative to partial hepatectomy, especially in patients who are suboptimal surgical candidates. This is a prospective, randomized trial from China that compared the efficacy of RFA plus TACE versus RFA alone. One hundred eighty-nine patients with tumors less than 7 cm in diameter or multiple HCC lesions each less than 3 cm in diameter were randomized to either arm. The combination of TACE/RFA was performed at 1 procedure; TACE included installation of carboplatin, epirubicin, and mitomycin with lipiodol into the territory of the tumor. This was followed by RFA of the lesion. RFA was performed using a 3.5-cm electrode, and larger tumors were ablated via multiple overlapping ablations. Patients were followed up with computed tomography scans at 4 weeks and then at various intervals thereafter. The groups were essentially equal in terms of clinicopathologic factors, and technical success was achieved in the vast majority of patients. Twice as many patients in the RFA-alone group had progression of tumor, defined by local or distant recurrences within the liver, which was highly statistically significant; the rates were 54.7% for the RFA group versus 35.1% for the TACE RFA group. When recurrence was identified, patients were treated again with either TACE or RFA depending on their previous treatment, and some were also given chemotherapy. Patients who underwent TACE/RFA also had improved overall survival and disease-free survival relative to the RFA alone group, with a hazard ratio of 0.525 for overall survival and 0.575 for recurrence-free survival. Evaluation of both groups by multivariate analysis revealed that the significant independent risk factors were which treatment the patients received, the tumor size, and tumor number. Complications from both treatments were generally minimal, although more than half the patients had pain in both groups. There were no mortalities. This study showed the superiority of TACE/RFA over RFA alone for tumors less than 7 cm or multiple tumors less than 3 cm. The explanation for improved efficacy of TACE/RFA is that TACE before RFA could reduce the vascularity, and therefore the cooling effects within the lesion, which might compromise the efficacy of RFA. In addition, patterns of recurrence suggest that multiple micrometastases will develop around the primary tumor and pretreatment with TACE will increase the efficacy of RFA to kill these smaller tumors in the region of the original tumor. Therefore, patients who are to undergo nonoperative therapy for HCC will likely be better served by the combination of TACE/RFA versus RFA alone.

J. Howe, MD

Pancreatic

Pancreatic Ductal Adenocarcinoma: Is There a Survival Difference for R1 Resections Versus Locally Advanced Unresectable Tumors? What Is a "True" R0 Resection?

Konstantinidis IT, Warshaw AL, Allen JN, et al (Massachusetts General Hosp, Boston)

Ann Surg 257:731-736, 2013

Objective.—Patients who undergo an R0 resection of their pancreatic ductal adenocarcinoma (PDAC) have an improved survival compared with patients who undergo an R1 resection. It is unclear whether an R1 resection confers a survival benefit over locally advanced (LA) unresectable tumors. Our aim was to compare the survival of patients undergoing an R1 resection with those having LA tumors and to explore the prognostic significance of a 1-mm surgical margin.

Methods.—Clinicopathologic data from a pancreatic cancer database between January 1993 and July 2008 were reviewed. Locally advanced tumors had no evidence of metastatic disease at exploration.

Results.—A total of 1705 patients were evaluated for PDAC in the Department of Surgery. Of the 1084 (64%) patients who were surgically explored, 530 (49%) were considered unresectable (286 locally unresectable, 244 with distant metastasis). One hundred fifty-seven (28%) of the resected PDACs had an R1 resection. Patients undergoing an R1 resection had a slightly longer survival compared with those who had locally advanced unresectable cancers (14 vs 11 months; $P < 0.001$). Patients with R0 resections had a favorable survival compared with those with R1 resections (23 vs 14 months; $P < 0.001$), but survival after resections with 1-mm margin or less (R0-close) were similar to R1 resections: both groups had a significantly shorter median survival than patients with a margin of greater than 1 mm (R0-wide) (16 vs 14 vs 35 months, respectively; $P < 0.001$).

Conclusions.—Patients undergoing an R1 resection still have an improved survival compared with patients with locally advanced unresectable pancreatic adenocarcinoma. R0 resections have an improved survival compared with R1 resections, but this survival benefit is lost when the tumor is within 1 mm of the resection margin.

▶ The overall survival rate for pancreatic adenocarcinoma remains dismal in the United States, with an overall 5-year survival rate of approximately 4%. Most patients present with either locally advanced or metastatic disease, with just 15% presenting with resectable disease. It has been definitively shown that patients who have an R1 resection do significantly worse than patients who have an R0 resection performed. However, what constitutes an R0 resection is not consistent among studies. Some studies have reported R1 resections in 17% to 30% of cases, whereas others have reported that the incidence is 70% to 85%, but in those latter cases, tumor within 1 mm of the margins was considered positive. The objective of this study was to look at patients' margin status and determine whether there were differences in survival between those with close and wider margins. Patients with pancreatic adenocarcinoma treated at one academic hospital between 1993 and 2008 were studied. Two-thirds of 1705 patients were explored surgically, and half of these were considered to be unresectable (approximately half locally unresectable and half with metastatic disease). A total of 554 patients underwent pancreaticoduodenectomy or distal pancreatectomy, and 28% had R1 resections. Of the patients who had R0 resection, half had margins within 1 mm and half had margins greater than 1 mm. The important findings in this study were that patients who had an R1 resection had slightly improved survival over patients who had locally unresectable tumors (with a median survival of 14 vs 11 months), which was statistically significant. The survival rate of patients with R0 resections with tumor within 1 mm of the margin was very similar to that of patients with R1 resections (median survival of 16 vs 14 months, with the difference not statistically significant). However, when the margin was greater than 1 mm, the median survival was 35 months (vs 16 months for the less-than-1-mm group, which was statistically significant). Most commonly, the retroperitoneal margin was the one that was involved in R1 resections as well as when the margins were within 1 mm. Also of interest was that patients were divided into 3 different cohorts by years of treatment, and the percentage of patients who underwent exploration for locally advanced and metastatic disease decreased over the period of the study, possibly reflecting improved imaging. The question raised by this study and others is whether tumor within 1 mm of the margin should be considered R1 disease. The Royal College of Pathologists considers this to be a positive margin, and this study found that survival was markedly different in those with close versus wider margins.

J. Howe, MD

Re-resection for Isolated Local Recurrence of Pancreatic Cancer is Feasible, Safe, and Associated with Encouraging Survival

Strobel O, Hartwig W, Hackert T, et al (Univ Hosp Heidelberg, Germany)

Ann Surg Oncol 20:964-972, 2013

Background.—Local recurrence of pancreatic cancer occurs in 80% of patients within 2 years after potentially curative resections. Around 30% of patients have isolated local recurrence (ILR) without evidence of metastases. In spite of localized disease these patients usually only receive palliative chemotherapy and have a short survival.

Purpose.—To evaluate the outcome of surgery as part of a multimodal treatment for ILR of pancreatic cancer.

Methods.—All consecutive operations performed for suspected ILR in our institution between October 2001 and October 2009 were identified from a prospective database. Perioperative outcome, survival, and prognostic parameters were assessed.

Results.—Of 97 patients with histologically proven recurrence, 57 (59%) had ILR. In 40 (41%) patients surgical exploration revealed metastases distant to the local recurrence. Resection was performed in 41 (72%) patients with ILR, while 16 (28%) ILR were locally unresectable. Morbidity and mortality were 25 and 1.8% after resections and 10 and 0% after explorations, respectively. Median postoperative survival was 16.4 months in ILR versus 9.4 months in metastatic disease ($p < 0.0001$). In ILR median survival was significantly longer after resection (26.0 months) compared with exploration without resection (10.8 months, $p = 0.0104$). R0 resection was achieved in 18 patients and resulted in 30.5 months median survival. Presence of metastases, incomplete resection, and high preoperative CA 19-9 serum values were associated with lesser survival.

Conclusions.—Resection for isolated local recurrence of pancreatic cancer is feasible, safe, and associated with favorable survival outcome. This concept warrants further evaluation in other institutions and in randomized controlled trials.

▶ Surgical cure of patients with pancreatic adenocarcinoma remains elusive, and most patients will have recurrence or die from recurrent or metastatic disease within 2 to 5 years after resection. An interesting clinical problem is what to do with patients who appear to have isolated recurrence in the area of the pancreas or in the adjacent lymph nodes. This large series from Germany looked at 97 such patients who had undergone pancreaticoduodenectomy but then in follow-up had a recurrence. In 59% of cases, an isolated local recurrence was found, and in 41% of cases, distant metastases were found. Their strategy in patients with isolated local recurrence was to resect if possible, with some patients receiving intraoperative radiation therapy as well. Seventy-two percent of patients could have resection, whereas 28% of patients had no resection by virtue of invasion around the celiac or superior mesenteric artery. Some patients who had involvement of the base of these arteries did have the tumor peeled off; however, 10 patients also underwent a second operation for recurrence later on. Patients who had resection of the local recurrence did significantly better than patients whose recurrence could not be resected due to local invasion, and the overall median survival was 26 months with 20% of patients living 5 or more years. The effect of intraoperative radiation therapy vs no intraoperative radiation therapy did not appear to be significant, whereas in patients who were explored and could not be resected, those who received radiation therapy did better than those who were explored and not resected without radiation therapy. The group looked for factors that might help predict who might be a candidate for resection and found that preoperative CA19-9 levels greater than 400 were associated with a shorter survival, but not carcinoembryonic antigen (CEA), disease-free interval, or patient age. Sixty-three percent of patients resected had R0 or R1 resections. Because of lack of efficacy for systemic therapy, resection of isolated local recurrences should be performed and could result in resection in 72% of patients. Some of these patients had isolated paracaval lymph node recurrences, which were easier to treat, as opposed to recurrence in the pancreas or mesentery, which were more complex. Because 42% of patients had metastases found at exploration, and therefore were not resected, the author suggests that perhaps the high CA19-9 level could be useful, although they still would not recommend not exploring those patients. This study suggests that some patients can have prolonged survival after resection for isolated recurrence but that many patients will be found to have metastatic disease, and a significant subset will be found to be unresectable locally. Therefore, it appears that this procedure may be warranted if truly isolated disease is present but not if there is metastatic disease or involvement of the mesenteric vessels.

J. Howe, MD

Adjuvant Chemotherapy With Gemcitabine and Long-term Outcomes Among Patients With Resected Pancreatic Cancer: The CONKO-001 Randomized Trial

Oettle H, Neuhaus P, Hochhaus A, et al (Charité-Universitätsmedizin Berlin, Germany; Universitätsklinikum Jena, Germany; et al)

JAMA 310:1473-1481, 2013

Importance.—The prognosis for patients with pancreatic cancer is poor, even after resection with curative intent. Gemcitabine-based chemotherapy is standard treatment for advanced pancreatic cancer, but its effect on survival in the adjuvant setting has not been demonstrated.

Objective.—To analyze whether previously reported improvement in disease-free survival with adjuvant gemcitabine therapy translates into improved overall survival.

Design, Setting, and Patients.—CONKO-001 (Charité Onkologie 001), a multicenter, open-label, phase 3 randomized trial to evaluate the efficacy and toxicity of gemcitabine in patients with pancreatic cancer after complete tumor resection. Patients with macroscopically completely removed pancreatic cancer entered the study between July 1998 and

December 2004 in 88 hospitals in Germany and Austria. Follow-up ended in September 2012.

Interventions.—After stratification for tumor stage, nodal status, and resection status, patients were randomly assigned to either adjuvant gemcitabine treatment (1 g/m^2 d 1, 8, 15, q 4 weeks) for 6 months or to observation alone.

Main Outcomes and Measures.—The primary end point was disease-free survival. Secondary end points included treatment safety and overall survival, with overall survival defined as the time from date of randomization to death. Patients lost to follow-up were censored on the date of their last follow-up.

Results.—A total of 368 patients were randomized, and 354 were eligible for intention-to-treat-analysis. By September 2012, 308 patients (87.0%[95% CI, 83.1%-90.1%]) had relapsed and 316 patients (89.3% [95% CI, 85.6%-92.1%]) had died. The median follow-up time was 136 months. The median disease-free survival was 13.4 (95% CI, 11.6-15.3) months in the treatment group compared with 6.7 (95% CI, 6.0-7.5) months in the observation group (hazard ratio, 0.55 [95% CI, 0.44-0.69]; $P < .001$). Patients randomized to adjuvant gemcitabine treatment had prolonged overall survival compared with those randomized to observation alone (hazard ratio, 0.76 [95% CI, 0.61-0.95]; $P = .01$), with 5-year overall survival of 20.7% (95% CI, 14.7%-26.6%) vs 10.4% (95% CI, 5.9%-15.0%), respectively, and 10-year overall survival of 12.2% (95% CI, 7.3%-17.2%) vs 7.7% (95% CI, 3.6%-11.8%).

Conclusions and Relevance.—Among patients with macroscopic complete removal of pancreatic cancer, the use of adjuvant gemcitabine for 6 months compared with observation alone resulted in increased overall survival as well as disease-free survival. These findings provide strong support for the use of gemcitabine in this setting.

Trial Registration.—isrctn.org Identifier: ISRCTN34802808.

▶ The poor survival of patients with surgically resected pancreatic cancer has led to multiple clinical trials looking at the benefits of adjuvant treatment with chemotherapy. One of the most important of these was the CONKO-001 trial. This report represents an update after a median follow-up of 136 months. This trial was opened between 1998 and 2004 in 88 German and Austrian hospitals and accrued 368 patients. These patients had T1 to T3, N0 to N1 pancreatic cancers, which had either R0 or R1 resections performed. The patients were then randomly divided to receive gemcitabine (6 cycles over 6 months) versus observation after resection. The salient findings were that there was improved disease-free and overall survival in patients who received gemcitabine chemotherapy (Fig 2 in the original article). The overall 5-year survival rate was 20.7% at 5 years and 12.2% at 10 years for the gemcitabine group versus 10.4% at 5 years and 7.7% at 10 years in the observation group. These differences were statistically significant, and the overall hazard ratio in the patients receiving gemcitabine was 0.55. This therapy was generally tolerable, where 62% of patients received all 6 cycles and 87% received at least 1 cycle. Many of the patients in the observation group who had recurrence later received gemcitabine chemotherapy, and the authors point out that some might characterize this trial as comparing immediate versus delayed therapy with gemcitabine after resection. The study is significant, because it shows that if patients are treated in an adjuvant fashion with 6 months of gemcitabine, it led to a 24% improvement in overall survival, 10.3% improvement in 5-year overall survival, and 4.5% improvement in 10-year survival compared with observation. Other adjuvant trials have looked at various combinations, such as 5-fluorouracil/leucovorin (ESPAC-1) and cisplatin/fluorouracil (JSAP), with varying results. Clearly, gemcitabine is an agent with activity in the adjuvant treatment of pancreatic cancer and should be the standard by which other agents are measured.

J. Howe, MD

A prospective, randomized trial of Roux-en-Y reconstruction with isolated pancreatic drainage versus conventional loop reconstruction after pancreaticoduodenectomy

Ke S, Ding X-M, Gao J, et al (Beijing Chao-yang Hosp Affiliated to Capital Med Univ, China)
Surgery 153:743-752, 2013

Background.—Postoperative pancreatic fistula (POPF) is a major and serious complication after pancreaticoduodenectomy (PD). There have been no prospective randomized trials evaluating POPF rates in Roux-en-Y reconstruction (RYR) with isolated pancreatic drainage versus conventional loop reconstruction (CLR). The authors hypothesized that RYR decreases the incidence and severity of POPF in patients after PD.

Methods.—Between January 2006 and April 2012, the findings for 216 patients were analyzed in this multicenter, prospective trial in China. After providing appropriate preoperative informed consent, patients were randomly assigned to either RYR or CLR after completion of pancreaticoduodenal resection. We referred to the Johns Hopkins fistula definition and classified POPF as grade A, B, or C according to the International Study Group of Pancreatic Fistula classification.

Results.—The incidence of POPF was similar in the RYR (15.7%, 17/107) and CLR (17.6%, 19/109) groups. Both univariate and multivariate logistic regression analyses revealed that the factor most highly associated with POPF was ampullary or duodenal disease ($P < .05$). The incidence of type B POPF was higher in the CLR than in the RYR group. Furthermore, patients with POPF in the CLR group had a significantly longer postoperative hospital stay (31.9 ± 6.9 days) and higher total hospital costs than did the patients in the RYR group ($P < .05$).

Conclusion.—These data do not support the hypothesis that RYR is associated with a lower incidence of POPF than is CLR. However, they do indicate that RYR may contribute to decreasing fistula severity, duration of stay, and hospital expense.

▶ Although mortality rates have improved for pancreaticoduodenectomy performed for periampullary tumors, the rate of postoperative complications remains high, with the most significant being that of postoperative pancreatic fistula (POPF). This is reported to occur in somewhere between 5% and 25% of patients undergoing pancreaticoduodenectomy. This study sought to compare whether conventional loop pancreaticojejunostomy construction (CLR) could be improved by performing diversion of the pancreas by a separate Roux-en-Y anastomosis. The hypothetical benefits to performing Roux-En-Y would be diversion of the pancreatic secretions, which might result in less activation and erosion by pancreatic enzymes. The authors performed a prospective, randomized trial comparing these 2 reconstruction techniques in patients from 6 different centers in China. They ultimately randomly selected 216 patients between 2006 and 2012, in whom a single surgeon performed all of the resections and anastomoses to minimize the effect of surgeon experience on the results. All procedures included distal gastrectomy, and the pancreatic anastomoses were duct-to-mucosa, end-to-side with 2 layers. Duct stents were used in all patients as well as feeding jejunostomies distal to the gastrojejunal anastomosis. The Roux-en-Y was performed by bringing up a separate loop to the pancreas and a second loop to the biliary tree, which was connected to the gastrojejunostomy 30 cm distal to the hepaticojejunostomy, and the pancreaticojejunal Roux was sutured 20 cm downstream from the gastrojejunostomy. Two suction drains were used in each patient. Postoperative fistula was defined as greater than 50 mL/d of drainage on postoperative day 10 with an amylase level greater than 3 times normal, or radiographic demonstration of anastomotic disruption. Grade A fistulas were defined as just moderately elevated amylase in the drain with no changes in management; grade B, those that required diagnostic evaluation and possible therapeutic management; and grade C were severe fistulas that required major deviations from clinical management. There were no differences in the patient populations nor the incidence of malignant disease in the 2 groups There were no differences in postoperative complications in either of the 2 groups, including pancreatic fistula (16% in the Roux-en-Y group vs 18% in the CLR group), wound infection, and delayed gastric emptying (23% to 25% of these patients). A variety of clinicopathologic factors were examined to see whether there was an association with pancreatic fistula, and the only preoperative factor that correlated with this was low albumin levels. Associated intraoperative factors were operating time and blood loss, pancreatic texture being soft relative to intermediate or hard, and tumors of the ampulla or duodenum had a higher risk of fistula formation (2.0 and 8.0 hazard ratio, respectively). On multivariate analysis, the only significant factors for POPF were tumors of the ampulla or duodenum, and all the other factors on univariate analysis dropped out. Although the rates of POPF were the same in the 2 groups, there was a much higher incidence of grade A fistula in the Roux-en-Y group (65%) versus the CLR group (21%), and grade B and C complications were less (35% vs 79%). This was a well-conducted study because it was a randomized trial and addressed the issue of whether Roux-en-Y—isolated pancreatic reconstruction will decrease the rate of fistula formation by preventing activation of pancreatic enzymes by low pH or enterokinase. It showed that this did not reduce the rate of fistula formation; however, it may have decreased the severity of the fistulas that did occur. A problem with the technique was that it requires an additional anastomosis, but this did not appear to increase operating time. It also could increase the risk of marginal ulcers, but these can be avoided with use of proton pump inhibitors, and none of the patients in this series developed them.

J. Howe, MD

Pylorus resection in partial pancreaticoduodenectomy: impact on delayed gastric emptying

Hackert T, Hinz U, Hartwig W, et al (Univ of Heidelberg, Germany)
Am J Surg 206:296-299, 2013

Background.—Partial pancreaticoduodenectomy (PD) is complicated by postoperative delayed gastric emptying (DGE) in up to 45% of patients. The aim of this study was to evaluate the impact of pylorus resection on DGE following PD.

Methods.—Forty PD patients underwent pylorus resection with complete stomach preservation (prPD). They were compared with a pair-matched group of PD patients with pylorus preservation (ppPD) in a 1:1 ratio (age, sex, histopathology). The objectives were operative parameters, DGE incidence, morbidity, and length of hospital stay.

Results.—DGE incidence was significantly lower after prPD (15.0% vs 42.5%; $P = .0066$). Operative parameters and surgical morbidity (other than DGE) were not different (27.5% prPD vs 30.0% ppPD). There was a trend toward a shorter hospital stay in the prPD group.

Conclusions.—Resection of the pylorus with stomach preservation significantly reduces the frequency of DGE after PD without showing any disadvantage when compared with standard ppPD. This finding could be of high relevance for the clinical practice in routine PD and should consequently be investigated in a large randomized multicenter trial to create further evidence.

► A previous meta-analysis found that the classical Whipple procedure vs pylorus-preserving pancreaticoduodenectomy (PPD) showed no significant differences in terms of in-hospital mortality, morbidity, or survival but that the PPD resulted in shorter operating time and decreased intraoperative blood loss. With respect to delayed gastric emptying (DGE), more studies have favored reduced DGE in the classical Whipple procedure vs PPD. An argument for improved DGE in PPD vs the classic Whipple is the maintenance of vagal fibers to the distal stomach. Tani et al[1] found that antecolic duodenojejunostomy in PPD resulted in less DGE than retrocolic in a randomized study with a rate of DGE of 5% in the antecolic vs 50% for the retrocolic. The same group looked at the incidence of DGE in pylorus resecting pancreaticoduodenectomy

(PRPD) vs PPD in a randomized trial and found that the incidence of DGE was only 4.5% in the PRPD group vs 17% in the PPD group. This study by Hackert et al looked at their population from Germany in a prospective, matched-pair analysis in 40 PPD vs 40 PRPD patients. The 2 groups were evenly matched in terms of age and sex as well as indications for operation. They found that postoperative surgical morbidity was similar between groups in terms of operating time, blood loss, hospital mortality, reoperation rate, and intensive care unit stay. The exception was the rate of DGE. The incidence of DGE in the PRPD group was 15% vs 42.5% in the PPD group. They also looked at severity of DGE, which is graded as A thru C (A = 4–7 days of nasogastric tube [NGT] or reinsertion after postoperative day 3; B = 8–14 days of NGT or reinsertion after 7 days; C = > 14 days of NGT or reinsertion after postoperative day 14), where the numbers of each subtype were too small to show significant differences, but there was a significant difference in DGE overall between the 2 operations. The long-term effects of PRPD is that removing the pylorus could increase the risk of jejunogastric reflux as seen with antrectomy; however, Kawai et al[2] found that there was no significant difference in postgastrectomy syndromes in PPD vs PRPD. This study helped confirm the finding that DGE may be improved by resection of the pylorus, although there was no follow-up more than 30 days in this study; therefore, the possibility of increased incidence of reflux and dumping syndrome would need to be studied over a longer period.

J. Howe, MD

References

1. Tani M, Terasawa H, Kawai M, et al. Improvement of delayed gastric emptying in pylorus-preserving pancreaticoduodenectomy: results of a prospective, randomized, controlled trial. *Ann Surg.* 2006;243:316-320.
2. Kawai M, Tani M, Hirono S, et al. Pylorus ring resection reduces delayed gastric emptying in patients undergoing pancreatoduodenectomy: a prospective, randomized, controlled trial of pylorus-resecting versus pylorus-preserving pancreatoduodenectomy. *Ann Surg.* 2011;253:495-501.

Population-Level Analysis of Pancreatic Neuroendocrine Tumors 2 cm or Less in Size

Kuo EJ, Salem RR (Yale Univ School of Medicine, New Haven, CT)
Ann Surg Oncol 20:2815-2821, 2013

Background.—There is a paucity of evidence regarding incidence and predictors of survival in pancreatic neuroendocrine tumors (PNETs) ≤2 cm in size.

Methods.—Patients having undergone resection for nonfunctioning PNETs were selected from the SEER database (1988–2009) and an institutional pathology database (1996–2012). PNETs ≤2 cm were compared with PNETs >2 cm. Data were analyzed with χ^2 tests, ANOVA, the Kaplan–Meier method, log rank tests, and Cox proportional hazard, and binary logistic regression.

Results.—The incidence of PNETs ≤2 cm in the United States has increased by 710.4 % over the last 22 years. Rates of extrapancreatic extension, nodal metastasis, and distant metastasis in PNETs ≤2 cm in the SEER database were 17.9, 27.3, and 9.1%, respectively. The rate of nodal metastasis in our institutional series was 5.7%. Disease-specific survival at 5, 10, and 15 years for PNETs ≤2 cm was 91.5, 84.0, and 76.8%. Decreased disease-specific survival was not associated with nodal metastasis, but rather with high grade [moderately differentiated, hazard ratio (HR) 37.2, 95% confidence interval (CI) 2.7–518.8; poorly differentiated, HR 94.2, 95% CI 4.9–1,794.4; reference, well differentiated], and minority race (Asian, HR 30.2, 95% CI 3.1–291.7; Black, HR 60.1, 95% CI 2.1–1,027.9; reference, White).

Conclusions.—Pancreatic neuroendocrine tumors ≤2 cm are increasingly common, and the most significant predictors of disease-specific survival are grade and race. The SEER database excludes PNETs considered to be benign, and rates of extrapancreatic extension, nodal metastasis, and distant metastasis are overestimated. Small size, however, does not preclude malignant behavior.

▶ A common clinical problem encountered by surgical oncologists is what to do with the enhancing pancreatic lesion less than 2 cm in size after workup suggests that this is a neuroendocrine tumor. Is the incidence of lymph node metastases or distant metastases significant enough to recommend that all these tumors be resected? Are there certain preoperative factors that would predict for worse prognosis? In this study, the Surveillance, Epidemiology, and End Results (SEER) database was queried from 1988 to 2009 to look for tumors less than 2 cm vs greater than 2 cm that were found to be neuroendocrine in origin. Functional tumors were excluded, and it should be noted that the SEER database excluded tumors considered to be benign, which may have affected the inclusion of patients in earlier decades (while in the past 2 decades there has been increasing recognition that even smaller tumors might be malignant, and these have been included more frequently). One interesting finding was that the proportion of small tumors doubled over the study period for an overall increase of 710%. This may have been not only owing to more frequent inclusion of smaller tumors in SEER but also the increasing sensitivity of imaging techniques, specifically for computed tomography and endoscopic ultrasound scan. The most significant finding in this study was that the incidence of nodal metastases was 27.3% for tumors less than 2 cm. This study also divided tumors into 5-mm increments less than 2 cm in size and found the incidence of nodal metastases to be 25% in 1- to 5-mm tumors, increasing to 36% in 1.6- to 2.0-cm tumors. Furthermore, this study found that the overall incidence of distant metastases was 9.1% for tumors less than 2 cm and that the disease-specific survival was 90% at 5 years and 80% at 10 years. Factors that appeared to be associated with lower survival were high-grade or poorly differentiated tumors and Asian or Black race, which could reflect disparities in treatment. Interestingly, the presence of nodal metastases did not correlate with survival, which could potentially have been related to inadequate nodal sampling in the database. The significance of this study was it showed that there was a high incidence of lymph node metastases even in these small tumors; however, this did not seem to correlate with survival. Therefore, it is still unclear what the optimal treatment of these tumors is, especially because the patients in this study all underwent resection. Whether observation is a viable option for patients with these tumors is still not known, especially because nodal involvement did not appear to correlate with survival, and the rate of distant metastases was generally low.

J. Howe, MD

Neuroendocrine

Resection of At-Risk Mesenteric Lymph Nodes Is Associated with Improved Survival in Patients with Small Bowel Neuroendocrine Tumors

Landry CS, Lin HY, Phan A, et al (Baylor Univ Med Ctr, Dallas, TX; The Univ of Texas M. D. Anderson Cancer Ctr, Houston)

World J Surg 37:1695-1700, 2013

Background.—Neuroendocrine tumors of the small intestine commonly metastasize to regional lymph nodes (LNs). Single-institution reports suggest that removal of LNs improves outcome, but comprehensive data are lacking. We hypothesized that the extent of lymphadenectomy reported in a large administrative database would be associated with overall survival for jejunal and ileal neuroendocrine tumors.

Methods.—A search of the Surveillance Epidemiology and End Results database was performed for patients with jejunal and ileal neuroendocrine tumors from 1977 to 2004. Descriptive patient characteristics were collected to include age at diagnosis, sex, race, grade, primary tumor size, LN status, number of LNs resected, presence of distant metastasis, and the type of operation. Statistical analyses were limited to patients with only one primary tumor to exclude patients with other malignancies. Univariate and multivariate analyses were performed to analyze the number of LNs resected and the LN ratio (number of positive LNs/total number of LNs removed) to determine the effect on cancer-specific survival.

Results.—Altogether, 1,364 patients were included in this analysis. Removal of any LNs was associated with improved cancer-specific survival when compared to patients with no LN removal reported ($p = 0.0027$) on univariate analysis. Among those who had any LNs removed, a median of eight LNs were identified in resection specimens with a median LN ratio of 0.29 (range 0–1). On multivariate analysis (adjusting for age and tumor size), patients with >7 LNs removed experienced better cancer-specific survival than those with ≤7 LNs removed (median survival not reached vs. 140 months): hazard ratio and 95 % confidence interval were 0.573 (0.402, 0.817) ($p = 0.002$).

Conclusions.—This review of a large number of surgical patients demonstrates that regional mesenteric lymphadenectomy in conjunction with

resection of the primary tumor is associated with improved survival of patients with small bowel neuroendocrine tumors.

▶ Neuroendocrine tumors of the small bowel (SBNETs) are the most common type of small bowel tumor, and their incidence has been increasing over the past few decades. The optimal treatment for these tumors per National Comprehensive Cancer Network guidelines is resection of the primary tumor with regional lymphadenectomy, and it has been shown that this results in a survival benefit. However, what is not clear is how many lymph nodes need to be removed at the time of surgery to improve survival. The authors of this study attempted to determine this number and thereby derive an idea of what might be an adequate lymphadenectomy for patients with SBNETs. They reviewed patients who had resection between 1997 and 2004 and were recorded in the Surveillance, Epidemiology, and End Results program database. A total of 1364 patients were included, after excluding patients with multiple tumors, unknown interventions, missing data, or deaths from noncancerous causes. A variety of clinicopathologic factors were examined for their influence on survival, but again the focus of this study was to look at the number of lymph nodes removed, the lymph node ratio, and how these correlated with survival. Of these 1364 patients, 221 (16%) had no lymph nodes removed. The median number of lymph nodes removed was 8, and the median lymph node ratio of positive to total nodes removed was 0.29. Furthermore, survival was significantly improved in patients who had 8 or more lymph nodes removed vs those with less (hazard ratio 0.66), and lymph node ratio of less than .29 (hazard of 1.5 if >0.29); these factors remained significant on multivariable analysis. The study also found that patients who had lymph nodes removed were more likely to be young, with larger tumors, and with ileal rather than jejunal tumors. The authors conclude that removing at least 8 lymph nodes at the time of surgery results in improved survival and that this would be a reasonable target number. It should also be recognized that some patients have encasement of the mesenteric vasculature by enlarged lymph nodes and a severe fibrotic reaction, which makes this removal difficult and even potentially harmful. It is hard to know how to use this information because many patients at exploration have large calcified mesenteric masses that are actually a conglomeration of lymph nodes but may be counted as only 1 large lymph node by the pathologist. Generally, one should strive for an anatomically adequate lymphadenectomy—in other words, one should take the mesenteric vessels with lymph nodes near their origins from the superior mesenteric artery/vein. The suggestion of improved survival with 8 lymph nodes is a good guide for performing an adequate lymphadenectomy; however, multiple other factors in SBNETs confound the use of this number.

J. Howe, MD

Prognostic Validity of the American Joint Committee on Cancer Staging Classification for Midgut Neuroendocrine Tumors

Strosberg JR, Weber JM, Feldman M, et al (H. Lee Moffitt Cancer Ctr and Res Inst, Tampa, FL; Univ of South Florida, Tampa)

J Clin Oncol 31:420-425, 2013

Purpose.—The American Joint Committee on Cancer (AJCC) staging manual has introduced a TNM staging classification for jejunal-ileal (midgut) neuroendocrine tumors (NETs). This classification has not been validated in a population consisting solely of midgut NETs. The purpose of this study was to test the prognostic validity of the classification in such a population.

Methods.—Patients with jejunal and ileocecal NETs who were treated at the Moffitt Cancer Center between 2000 and 2010 were assigned stages (I through IV). Kaplan-Meier analyses for overall survival (OS) were performed on the basis of TNM stage and pathologic grade. Multivariate modeling was performed using Cox proportional hazards regression.

Results.—We identified 691 patients with jejunal-ileocecal NETs. The AJCC classification in aggregate was highly prognostic for OS ($P < .001$). Five-year OS rates for stages I through IV were 100%, 100%, 91%, and 72%, respectively. The survival difference between stages III and IV was significant ($P < .001$); the difference between stages I/II versus III was not statistically significant ($P = .1$). Among patients with stage IIIB tumors, 5-year survival rates were 95% for resectable tumors versus 78% for unresectable mesenteric tumors ($P = .02$). A proliferative threshold of five mitoses per 10 high-power fields (HPF) was of greater prognostic value than a threshold of two mitoses per 10 HPF for discriminating between low- and intermediate-grade tumors.

Conclusion.—Stage I and II midgut NETs are associated with identical survival rates. Stage IIIB tumors are heterogeneous, with significant differences in survival observed between resectable mesenteric lymph nodes versus unresectable masses in the root of the mesentery. A higher mitotic cutoff of five per 10 HPF may lead to improved prognostic differentiation between low- and intermediate-grade tumors. Revisions to the current AJCC staging and grading classification may be warranted.

► Neuroendocrine tumors of the jejunum and ileum, otherwise known as *midgut carcinoid tumors*, often present with advanced disease, yet patients have prolonged survival. Up until recently, there was no American Joint Committee on Cancer (AJCC) staging system for midgut carcinoid tumors. In the seventh edition of the AJCC staging manual, the European Neuroendocrine Tumor Society staging system was adopted. This study proposed to look at a single institutional series of 691 patients to determine the utility of this staging system. Several interesting things were found in this large series. More than 80% of patients were diagnosed with symptoms, at least 22% had multifocal tumors, and 68% presented with stage 4 disease. The most common symptoms were abdominal pain in 41%, followed by diarrhea in 32%, flushing in 25%, and bowel obstruction in 24%. It found that stage 1 and 2 localized tumors had identical survival rate of 100% over 5 years, which decreased to 91% for stage 3 and 72% for stage 4 tumors. Furthermore, they divided patients with stage 3B tumors, those with involved lymph nodes, into resectable and unresectable mesenteric deposits. There was a clear survival difference between patients having resectable disease with 95% 5-year survival rate vs 78% when lymph nodes involving the root of the mesentery were unresectable. They also found that a cutoff of less than 2 mitoses per high power field was not as good a discriminator as less than 5 mitoses for low-grade tumors. There was a low incidence of symptomatic carcinoid heart disease, which was only 8% vs published series of 25% to 50%, which they thought could be related to the use of somatostatin analogues. The authors propose that stage 1 and 2 tumors (ie, localized tumors) be combined into a single category and that stage 3 should be separated into resectable and unresectable nodal metastases, and that the mitotic rate distinguishing between low and intermediate grade tumors should be raised to 5 per high powered field. The strengths of this study were its large numbers from a single institution, and implementation of their recommendations would likely result in better discriminatory ability of the staging system.

J. Howe, MD

Melanoma

Evidence for a Better Nodal Staging System for Melanoma: The Clinical Relevance of Metastatic Disease Confined to the Sentinel Lymph Nodes

Reintgen M, Murray L, Akman K, et al (Univ of South Florida, Tampa, FL)

Ann Surg Oncol 20:668-674, 2013

Background.—The hypothesis tested in this study was whether patients with stage III metastatic melanoma confined to their sentinel lymph nodes (SLNs) had a more favorable prognosis than patients who had SLN and non-SLN (NSLN) metastases.

Methods.—Patients were identified who were clinically negative in their regional basins but with lymphatic mapping were found to have positive SLNs (331 patients). All patients subsequently underwent a complete lymph node dissection of the lymphatic basin involved, and the total number of metastatic SLNs and NSLNs were documented.

Results.—As the regional metastatic disease involves NSLNs, disease-free survival (DFS) and overall survival (OS) decreases. For patients with a total of 2 nodes positive, those with disease confined to the SLNs had a significant better prognosis (DFS and OS: $P < .00001$) than those in whom 1 SLN and 1 non-SLN was involved. This difference was apparent for those patients with N2 and N3 disease (2 or more nodes positive in their regional basin). A multivariate regression analysis that included Breslow thickness, ulceration, number of positive nodes, and NSLN positivity showed that NSLN positivity ($P = .0019$) was the most powerful predictor of DFS and OS.

Conclusions.—When metastatic melanoma overwhelms the SLN and involves NSLNs, the biologic behavior changes to portend a worse survival, regardless of the total node count positive. These data make the argument that the current N staging system should be changed to incorporate SLN vs NSLN involvement.

▶ The current American Joint Committee on Cancer (AJCC) staging system for melanoma classifies nodal status as N0, N1 (where 1 node is involved), N2 (where 2–3 nodes are involved), or N3 (with 4 or more metastatic nodes). Several studies have previously shown that the absolute number of nodes is not the only important factor in melanoma and that the presence of involved nonsentinel lymph nodes (NSLN) may also relate to prognosis. In this study, Reintgen et al from Moffitt Cancer Center looked at their database for patients who had invasive melanoma with a positive sentinel lymph node who then went on to have completion lymph node dissection. The question they ask is whether involvement of NSLNs at the completion of node dissection would affect the patients' overall survival or recurrence. They compared groups that had NSLNs that were negative vs positive; the groups were fairly evenly matched, except those with positive NSLNs had thicker melanomas and higher rates of ulceration. In both groups, the median number of NSLNs removed was 15, and they found that there was decreased disease-free survival in the NSLN-positive group and that patients with metastases confined to sentinel lymph nodes (SLNs) had better disease-free survival (regardless of the total number of positive nodes) than those patients with positive NSLNs. In a multivariable analysis that also incorporated tumor thickness and ulceration, the most powerful predictive factor for disease-free survival was the involvement of NSLNs. The number of positive nodes was also a significant factor, but ulceration and tumor thickness were not. This study is important because it shows that it's not the absolute number of lymph nodes that are involved but whether the lymph nodes move on from the SLNs to the NSLNs, which may be important in survival. The mechanism for this may be that SLNs are effective barriers for metastases, but that when these are overwhelmed, cells go to other regional nodes, and this is a bad prognostic sign. Other studies have found similar results, including the Sunbelt Melanoma Trial and studies in SLN mapping of the breast. This study also highlights that perhaps the AJCC staging system could be improved by incorporating this factor into the nodal status rather than just using the absolute number of positive nodes.

J. Howe, MD

Sentinel Lymph Node Biopsy for Melanoma in Pregnant Women

Andtbacka RHI, Donaldson MR, Bowles TL, et al (Univ of Utah and Intermountain Health Care, Salt Lake City)

Ann Surg Oncol 20:689-696, 2013

Background.—The incidence of melanoma is rising in young women of childbearing age. Melanoma diagnosed during pregnancy presents unique challenges. This study was conducted to determine the effect of sentinel lymph node biopsy (SLNB) for melanoma on maternal and fetal outcomes in pregnant women.

Methods.—A prospective melanoma database was retrospectively queried for women diagnosed with melanoma during or immediately before pregnancy as well as SLNB in pregnant women. The outcomes of SLNB for the mothers and fetuses were evaluated.

Results.—Fifteen pregnant women underwent wide local excision (WLE) and SLNB for melanoma from 1997 to 2012. The median gestational age was 20 weeks. More than half of the women noticed changes in the primary melanoma lesion during the pregnancy. The median Breslow thickness was 1.00 mm. Lymphatic mapping and SLNB were performed with some combination of radiocolloid or vital blue dye without adverse effects. Three patients had micrometastatic disease and underwent a completion lymphadenectomy. Sixteen children were born at a median gestational age of 39 weeks. The median 1- and 5-minute Apgar scores were 8 and 9, respectively. At a median follow-up of 54.4, months none of the patients had experienced recurrence, and all children were healthy and free of melanoma.

Conclusions.—In this series of pregnant women with melanoma, SLNB was performed safely during pregnancy without adverse effects to the mothers and fetuses. We recommend that clinicians explain the risks and benefits of the SLNB procedure to pregnant women so an informed decision can be made about the procedure.

▶ Sentinel lymph node biopsy (SNLB) has become standard practice for staging of regional lymph node basins in patients with melanoma and breast cancer. Limited studies have examined the safety of this procedure in pregnant women. In breast cancer, it appears that it is safe, but limited studies have been done in melanoma. This study used a prospectively collected melanoma database to identify patients who underwent SNLB during pregnancy. Over a 15-year period, 15 women had undergone wide local excision and SNLB for melanoma. The median Breslow depth was 1.00 mm, the median gestational age was 19 weeks of pregnancy at the time of diagnosis, and 9 of 15 had changes in the melanoma/lesion during pregnancy. The most commonly seen features were increasing size in 7 of the 9, one had ulceration, and the other became exophytic. Fourteen of 15 women underwent lymphoscintigraphy and injection of Technetium-99 sulfur colloid for lymphatic mapping, and 10 of 15 had injection of blue dye (8 isosulfan blue and 2 methylene blue). Three patients had microscopic metastases in their sentinel nodes and underwent completion lymph node dissection of the involved basin, and in all cases no additional lymph nodes were found; no adverse effects were noted in the mother or the baby. The placentas were examined in all cases, and none of these had melanoma. The important points raised by this article are that SNLB is safe in pregnancy and that radioisotope-based mapping is preferable to blue dye mapping because the latter has a small risk of anaphylaxis, which could potentially compromise pregnancy. Available literature does not suggest that pregnancy increases one's risk for melanoma, and there is no clear indication that the course of melanoma is adversely affected by pregnancy. However, many of the women in the series did have changes in their lesions during pregnancy, which raises some questions. The authors also suggest that if lymph node dissection is necessary, it may be able to wait until after the completion of the pregnancy.

J. Howe, MD

Other

Quantification of harms in cancer screening trials: literature review

Heleno B, Thomsen MF, Rodrigues DS, et al (Univ of Copenhagen, Denmark; Nova Med School, Lisbon, Portugal; et al)

BMJ 347:f5334, 2013

Objectives.—To assess how often harm is quantified in randomised trials of cancer screening.

Design.—Two authors independently extracted data on harms from randomised cancer screening trials. Binary outcomes were described as proportions and continuous outcomes with medians and interquartile ranges.

Data Sources.—For cancer screening previously assessed in a Cochrane review, we identified trials from their reference lists and updated the search in CENTRAL. For cancer screening not assessed in a Cochrane review, we searched CENTRAL, Medline, and Embase.

Eligibility Criteria for Selecting Studies.—Randomised trials that assessed the efficacy of cancer screening for reducing incidence of cancer, cancer specific mortality, and/or all cause mortality.

Data Extraction.—Two reviewers independently assessed articles for eligibility. Two reviewers, who were blinded to the identity of the study's authors, assessed whether absolute numbers or incidence rates of outcomes related to harm were provided separately for the screening and control groups. The outcomes were false positive findings, overdiagnosis, negative psychosocial consequences, somatic complications, invasive follow-up procedures, all cause mortality, and withdrawals because of adverse events.

Results.—Out of 4590 articles assessed, 198 (57 trials, 10 screening technologies) matched the inclusion criteria. False positive findings were quantified in two of 57 trials (4%, 95% confidence interval 0% to 12%), overdiagnosis in four (7%, 2% to 18%), negative psychosocial consequences in five (9%, 3% to 20%), somatic complications in 11 (19%, 10% to 32%), use of invasive follow-up procedures in 27 (47%, 34% to 61%), all cause mortality in 34 (60%, 46% to 72%), and withdrawals because of adverse effects in one trial (2%, 0% to 11%). The median percentage of space in the results section that reported harms was 12% (interquartile range 2-19%).

Conclusions.—Cancer screening trials seldom quantify the harms of screening. Of the 57 cancer screening trials examined, the most important harms of screening–overdiagnosis and false positive findings–were quantified in only 7% and 4%, respectively.

▶ In recent decades, a large number of individuals have been screened for a variety of cancer types in an attempt at early diagnosis, offering the potential for early intervention and reduced cancer-related mortality. One thing lacking from many clinical screening trials of this sort is a quantification of the risks of the screening procedures. These primarily involve the risk of the screening test itself, such as colonoscopy or radiation from CT, and the potential harm that comes from false-positive findings, which may lead to unnecessary interventions, overdiagnosis, and psychosocial effects. The reason this is important in trials that screen potentially healthy individuals is that the reduction of cancer mortality, although meaningful in its own right, needs to be counterbalanced with the risk to the population as a whole on which these screening interventions are performed. This study reviewed randomized trials of cancer screening to include breast, colorectal, liver, lung, ovarian, prostate, and testicular cancers. The authors reviewed the Cochrane Systematic Reviews as well as Medline for these trials, which had to in some way address the issue of cancer screening efficacy and reduction in cancer incidence and cancer mortality. Of more than 4000 articles, 57 screening trials (which equated to 242 articles) were selected for further analysis. The authors found that harmful effects of screening were infrequently reported. Overdiagnosis was addressed in only 7% of trials, and only 4% of trials looked at the incidence of false-positive results. Only 1 of the 57 trials looked at the number of patients who withdrew from screening because of harmful events. Some trials did report these results, but only in the screened rather than the nonscreened arms. If these trials were included as having been reported, then perhaps one-third of trials would have information on the harms of screening. The conclusions of this article were that only a minority of cancer screening trials provide evidence of the harm of screening, and therefore it is often difficult to determine the benefits from the majority of screening trials vs their potential for harm.

J. Howe, MD

Management of Patients with Abdominal Malignancy after Remote Jejunoileal Bypass: Surgical Considerations Decades Later

Kamiński JP, Maker VK, Maker AV (Univ of Illinois Metropolitan Groups Hosps, Chicago)
J Am Coll Surg 217:929-939, 2013

Background.—In the 1960s jejunoileal bypass (JIB) surgery was introduced as a treatment for morbid obesity. Short- and long-term follow-up, however, found multiple metabolic complications, such as diarrhea, acute liver failure, cirrhosis, renal lithiasis, and renal insufficiency, along with considerable mortality and morbidity rates. Safer bariatric surgical methods were developed, and up to a third of the patients who underwent JIB chose to have a reversal procedure to manage conditions such as life-threatening malnutrition, immune complex disease, renal oxalate stones, osteomalacia, and severe electrolyte disturbance. Quality of life issues also prompted some to choose reversal. After 40 years, these patients are aging and come to a generation of surgeons who never performed JIB or reversal procedures, often with abdominal malignancies. The preoperative,

operative, and postoperative management of JIB and reversed JIB patients were detailed.

Preoperative Care.—Many former JIB patients have severely altered gastrointestinal (GI) physiology, causing metabolic and electrolyte imbalances, micronutrient deficiencies, hepatic insufficiency, biliary and renal stone disease, osteomalacia, autoimmune diseases, gout, and renal insufficiency. The patient's ability to undergo major surgery must be assessed. Search for the cause of a colon malignancy is also advised. JIB is sometimes considered a risk factor for colorectal cancer.

Intraoperative Issues.—Factors that determine operative success include having an intact ileocecal valve, the length of functional small bowel, and the amount of functional colon. Intraoperatively it is important to assess anatomic abnormalities of the GI tract, including large-caliber, substantially thickened areas of the proximal jejunum and distal ileum and highly atrophic, thin, pliable bypassed small intestine. The colon can be massive, more than 7 feet long, hypervascular, and have an abnormally thick wall. The length of the jejunal and ileal segments help estimate the length of functional small bowel. Patients with an intestinal malignancy should undergo appropriate oncologic operations without considering decreased nodal sampling or suboptimal margins. JOB reversal may not be necessary if the combined length of functional small bowel is 50 to 70 cm and the colon is intact; if the 50- to 70-cm functional bowel has an intact ileocecal valve; or if 100 to 150 cm of functional small bowel is present with no colon or intact ileocecal valve. Reversal can be done at the same time as oncologic surgery. During reversal the functional jejunal limb is divided at the jejunoileal anastomosis. The proximal end of the defunctionalized jejunum, or its most proximal loop that can be moved when severe scarring is present, is anastomosed to the functional, hypertrophic jejunal limb. The size mismatch requires care to establish a patulous anastomosis. If staples are used, the common enterotomy channel should be triangulated with the GIA staple line to ensure closure of the common enterotomy channel does not partially obstruct flow into the smaller defunctionalized limb.

If liver dysfunction is present, bypass reversal is required. With hepatic malignancy or a need for liver resection, parenchymal-sparing procedures are advised. Cross-sectional imaging and a liver biopsy can identify the extent of liver disease, which, combined with calculations of the proposed future liver remnant from three-dimensional cross-sectional imaging and volumetrics, helps predict the risk of liver failure postoperatively and aids in surgical planning. An indocyanine green clearance test is advised for high-risk cirrhotic patients to estimate hepatic functional reserve.

Postoperative Considerations.—Nutritional support is critical postoperatively because the patient cannot tolerate extended periods of negative protein caloric balance. Their increased metabolic needs must be met while aggressively providing support for existing metabolic, electrolyte, hepatic, bone, and renal imbalances. Early total parenteral nutrition (TPN) can be considered, with a transition to enteral feeding after bowel function is restored. An elemental formula via the nasogastric tube, which is efficiently

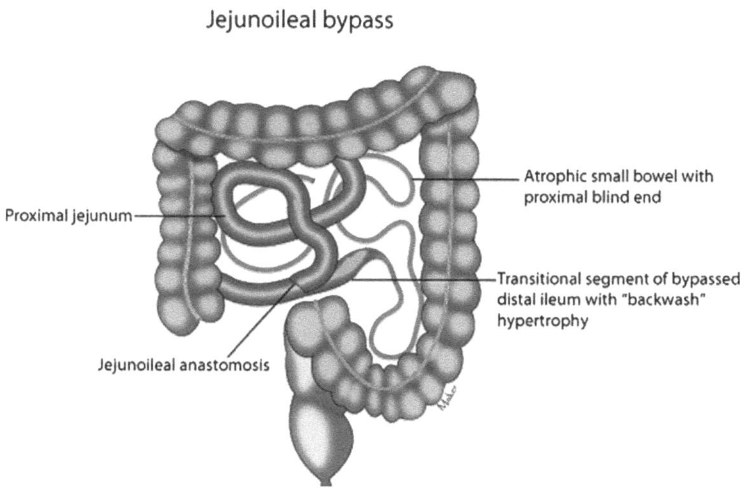

FIGURE 1.—Anatomy of the jejunoileal bypass (JIB) and surgical considerations. Scott's end-to-end operation involved 30 cm of jejunum anastomosed to the last 30, 20, or 15 cm of ileum and the 90% bypassed small bowel was drained into the colon. The classic JIB anatomy (shown) consisted of 15 inches of jejunum anastomosed side-to-side to the distal 10 inches of ileum. During a period of several years post JIB, the proximal jejunum and terminal ileum distal to the anastomosis become longer, thickened, and dilated due to adaptive hyperplasia and hypertrophy. The bypassed proximal bowel develops 2 zones; a proximal longer segment that atrophies in length and diameter, and a second zone of terminal ileum just proximal to the jejunoileal anastomosis. We have found that this second transitional zone has the same anatomical and physiological characteristics as the distal "in-line" terminal ileum due to backwash reflux and, as a result, plays a role in the functional adaptive response of the small bowel. (Reprinted from Kamiński JP, Maker VK, Maker AV. Management of patients with abdominal malignancy after remote jejunoileal bypass: surgical considerations decades later. *J Am Coll Surg*. 2013;217:929-939, Copyright 2013, with permission from the American College of Surgeons.)

absorbed by the proximal intestine and helps preserve intestinal mass in the proximal small bowel, augments oral intake. Transitioning to a regular diet includes a focus on constipating foods (boiled milk, rice, toast, peanut butter, etc) to help normalize evacuation times. Bananas and apples act as natural binding agents. Specific supplements can also be used to support atrophied bowel. Native colonic bacteria normally present in the small bowel also inhabit the excluded loop of small bowel, but *Clostridium difficile* can be found in higher concentrations than in normal bowel. Even after a total colectomy, patients who had a JIB are at higher risk for infection with *C difficile* and should be tested for its pathogenic presence and treated appropriately.

Conclusions.—Most current GI and oncologic surgeons have no personal experience with JIB patients, but with aging, these individuals will be seen in surgical practices. The complications attending this surgery and its reversal produce surgical challenges that must be addressed (Fig 1).

▶ Jejunoileal (JI) bypass operations were performed for morbid obesity from the early 1960s to the 1980s. It is estimated that as many of 25 000 persons in the United States may have undergone this procedure. This article chronicles the history and the metabolic complications seen with this procedure so that surgeons currently who are unfamiliar with JI bypass will be knowledgeable when they treat these patients for malignancies. It is unclear from this article whether the patients are at higher risk for malignancy, with the argument that there is increased proliferation in the small bowel and the large intestine in compensation; at least in animal models, there is increased risk of colon carcinoma. However, a long-term surveillance study in patients who had undergone JI bypass found that there was no increased risk of cancer. Several physiologic adaptations occur after these procedures, in which the jejunum is typically divided approximately 15 inches distal to the ligament of Treitz and then sutured to the distal 15 to 30 cm of ileum with a side-to-side anastomosis (Fig 1). This includes hypertrophy of the distal small bowel to increase its absorptive capacity, which extends into the colon as well. There is also a segment of ileum just proximal to the anastomosis that will become hypertrophied because of backwash of contents into this area, again in an attempt to increase absorption. This article summarizes nicely the complications of JI bypass, including the electrolyte imbalances, vitamin deficiencies, hepatic insufficiency, predisposition to gallstones and kidney stones, bone disease, and potential for renal insufficiency. When patients are operated on for intestinal malignancy, reversal may sometimes be necessary if the following is not observed: (1) small bowel length of 50 to 70 cm with an intact colon, (2) 50 to 70 cm of small bowel with an intact ileocecal valve, (3) 100 to150 cm of functional small bowel without any colon or an ileocecal valve. If the small bowel segment is short, and a significant amount of colon or the ileocecal valve is going to be removed for cancer, then a reversal of the JI bypass by anastomosing the jejunum from the site of the anastomosis near the site of the previous division of the proximal jejunum would be indicated. Preoperative and postoperative considerations are addressed, including poor nutrition, liver dysfunction, and the need to manage diarrhea. This is an excellent overview for younger surgeons who have probably not seen this procedure, and it will make them aware of the significant associated problems that go with this territory.

J. Howe, MD

12 Vascular Surgery

Aneurysm

Observations from the IMPROVE trial concerning the clinical care of patients with ruptured abdominal aortic aneurysm

IMPROVE trial investigators (Imperial College, London, UK; St George's Hosp, London, UK; et al)

Br J Surg 101:216-224, 2014

Background.—Single-centre series of the management of patients with ruptured abdominal aortic aneurysm (AAA) are usually too small to identify clinical factors that could improve patient outcomes.

Methods.—IMPROVE is a pragmatic, multicentre randomized clinical trial in which eligible patients with a clinical diagnosis of ruptured aneurysm were allocated to a strategy of endovascular aneurysm repair (EVAR) or to open repair. The influences of time and manner of hospital presentation, fluid volume status, type of anaesthesia, type of endovascular repair and time to aneurysm repair on 30-day mortality were investigated according to a prespecified plan, for the subgroup of patients with a proven diagnosis of ruptured or symptomatic AAA. Adjustment was made for potential confounding factors.

Results.—Some 558 of 613 randomized patients had a symptomatic or ruptured aneurysm: diagnostic accuracy was 91·0 per cent. Patients randomized outside routine working hours had higher operative mortality (adjusted odds ratio (OR) 1·47, 95 per cent confidence interval 1·00 to 2·17). Mortality rates after primary and secondary presentation were similar. Lowest systolic blood pressure was strongly and independently associated with 30-day mortality (51 per cent among those with pressure below 70 mm Hg). Patients who received EVAR under local anaesthesia alone had greatly reduced 30-day mortality compared with those who had general anaesthesia (adjusted OR 0·27, 0·10 to 0·70).

Conclusion.—These findings suggest that the outcome of ruptured AAA might be improved by wider use of local anaesthesia for EVAR and that a minimum blood pressure of 70 mm Hg is too low a threshold for permissive hypotension.

► The authors performed an elegant randomized, controlled trial to examine the optimal treatment (endovascular aneurysm repair [EVAR] vs open) for ruptured abdominal aortic aneurysms. Similar to the other randomized trial included in this year's selections, the authors found no difference in the 30-day mortality rate based on the technique (EVAR, 35.7% vs open, 39.3%). These findings are particularly noteworthy given the sample size (N = 558) but must be interpreted with some caution because the study centers were largely "centers of excellence" that were required to satisfy specific baseline requirements for their volume of elective aneurysm repairs, both EVAR and open. Furthermore, the study included both symptomatic (ie, intact) and ruptured aneurysms, although the overall number of symptomatic aneurysms (N = 22) was small and likely had little impact on the outcomes. The multivariate analysis identified several predictors associated with mortality, including lowest systolic blood pressure, the use of local anesthesia (odds ratio [OR], 0.27) and time of randomization (after hours OR, 1.4). Despite this relationship with the lowest systolic blood pressure and outcome, the volume of fluid replacement was not found to be predictive of mortality, thereby, questioning the concept of permissive hypotension for ruptured aneurysms with a systolic target of 70 to 80 mm Hg supported in another retrospective study included with this year's readings. The improved outcomes associated with the anesthetic time and the time of randomization suggest best-practice protocols and seem to justify the concentration of ruptured aneurysm in high-volume centers of excellence that have experienced teams (eg, surgeons, anesthesiologists, endovascular technicians) available at all times (ie, 24/7) with the ability to provide the full spectrum of care in terms of the various techniques and approaches. It is interesting that the outcomes in this study were not different between patients presenting to the treating hospital initially when compared with those transferred from other centers, although it is conceivable that unstable patients were not transferred. Interestingly, 10% of the study patients with a presumed diagnosis of a ruptured aneurysm were found to have another cause for their abdominal pain at the time of laparotomy or definitive cross-sectional imaging even though most had an incidental aneurysm. This seems to further justify the widespread approach of obtaining a computed tomography scan in patients with a presumed ruptured aneurysm, including those with abdominal pain and a known aneurysm. Furthermore, the study suggested that the mortality rate for the aortouni-iliac configuration may be higher in the setting or ruptured aneurysms, consistent with the findings in a recent meta-analysis. The overall study results are largely consistent with those of the smaller Amsterdam trial noted above and seem to dispel the widespread bias that EVAR is superior to open repair for ruptured aneurysms in high-volume, experienced centers.

T. S. Huber, MD, PhD

Endovascular Repair Versus Open Repair of Ruptured Abdominal Aortic Aneurysms: A Multicenter Randomized Controlled Trial

Reimerink JJ, on behalf of the Amsterdam Acute Aneurysm Trial Collaborators (Academic Med Ctr, Amsterdam; et al)

Ann Surg 258:248-256, 2013

Objective.—Randomized comparison of endovascular repair (EVAR) with open repair (OR) in patients with a ruptured abdominal aortic aneurysm (RAAA).

Background.—Despite advances in operative technique and perioperative management RAAA remains fraught with a high rate of death and complications. Outcome may improve with a minimally invasive surgical technique: EVAR.

Methods.—All patients with a RAAA in the larger Amsterdam area were identified. Logistics for RAAA patients was changed with centralization of care in 3 trial centers. Patients both fit for EVAR and for OR were randomized to either of the treatments. Nonrandomized patients were followed in a prospective cohort. Primary endpoint of the study was the composite of death and severe complications at 30 days.

Results.—Between April 2004 and February 2011, we identified 520 patients with a RAAA of which 116 could be randomized. The primary endpoint rate for EVAR was 42% and for OR was 47% [absolute risk reduction (ARR) = 5.4%; 95% confidence interval (CI): −13% to +23%]. The 30-day mortality was 21% in patients assigned to EVAR compared with 25% for OR (ARR = 4.4% 95% CI: −11% to +20%). The mortality of all surgically treated patients in the nonrandomized cohort was 30% (95% CI: 26%–35%) and 26% (95% CI: 20% to 32%) in patients with unfavorable anatomy for EVAR, treated by OR at trial centers.

Conclusions.—This trial did not show a significant difference in combined death and severe complications between EVAR and OR. Mortality for OR both in randomized patients and in cohort patients was lower than anticipated, which may be explained by optimization of logistics, preoperative CT imaging, and centralization of care in centers of expertise.

► The authors report an interesting randomized, controlled trial (N = 116) comparing endovascular (EVAR) with open repair (OR) for ruptured abdominal aortic aneurysms. They had hypothesized that EVAR was associated with reduced mortality and severe complications based on the published experienced that has touted the benefit for EVAR in this setting and the 50% mortality rate for OR reported historically. Somewhat surprisingly, they found that there were no differences in the primary endpoint (ie, death and severe complications at 30 days) or 30-day mortality rates (EVAR, 21% vs OR, 25%). Furthermore, there were no differences in the survival curves out as far as 6 years as estimated by the Kaplan-Meier technique. These equivocal outcomes were largely attributed to the fact that the mortality rate for OR was lower than estimated based on the historical data. Interestingly, there did not appear to be much of a difference among the softer endpoints that largely favor EVAR for intact aneurysm repairs with the exception that the EVAR group had a lower intraoperative blood loss (although there was no difference in total blood products throughout the index hospitalization). Analysis of the patients with ruptured aneurysms that were not randomized found that the primary outcome and mortality rates were comparable to the study patients, defusing the potential argument that better-risk patients (ie, those that were EVAR candidates) underwent OR in the trial, thereby reducing the mortality rate and diluting any potential difference from the endovascular approach. The endovascular techniques and, perhaps more importantly, the available devices, have continued to evolve since the initiation of the study, but the aorto-uni-iliac graft and femorofemoral crossover approach utilized in the study remain both current and effective. The endovascular inclusion criteria were fairly liberal given the instructions for use for most endovascular devices, although unsuitable anatomy accounted for the major exclusion criteria, largely because of the length or diameter of the infrarenal neck. The excellent results for both EVAR and OR suggest that factors other than the operative technique may be contributory or responsible, including the centralization of care for patients with ruptured aneurysms. There appears to be a favorable association between volume and outcome for almost every major surgical procedure, and, thus, it is not surprising that this may have an important factor in the current study. These results suggest that the greatest opportunities to reduce the mortality associated with ruptured aneurysms may be to optimize the care delivery systems and potentially concentrate the experience in centers of excellence.

T. S. Huber, MD, PhD

Comparison of fenestrated endovascular and open repair of abdominal aortic aneurysms not suitable for standard endovascular repair

Canavati R, Millen A, Brennan J, et al (Royal Liverpool Univ Hosp, UK)
J Vasc Surg 57:362-367, 2013

Background.—Abdominal aortic aneurysms that are unsuitable for a standard endovascular repair (EVAR) could be considered for fenestrated endovascular repair (f-EVAR). The aim of this study was to conduct a risk-adjusted retrospective concurrent cohort comparison of f-EVAR and open repair for such aneurysms.

Methods.—All patients who underwent repair of an abdominal aortic aneurysm that was unsuitable for a standard EVAR due to inadequate neck within one institution between January 2006 and December 2010 were identified. Case notes were retrieved for clinical data, Vascular Physiological and Operative Severity Score for enUmeration of Mortality and Morbidity (V-POSSUM) score, and aneurysm morphology. Computed tomography scans were reviewed to establish aneurysm morphology.

Results.—A total of 107 patients were identified. The open surgery cohort included 54 patients (35 men) who were a median age of 72 years (interquartile range [IQR], 9.5; range, 60-86 years). The aortic cross-clamp was infrarenal in 20 patients, suprarenal or above in 21, and inter-renal in eight. Postoperatively, 63 major complications were noted in 30 patients, nine of whom required 16 reinterventions. Cumulative hospital stay of the cohort was 1170 days (median, 12; IQR, 13; range, 1-205 days) of which 234 days (median, 28; IQR, 36; range, 1-77 days) were in the intensive therapy unit (ITU). Perioperative mortality was 9.2% (n = 5), exactly as estimated by V-POSSUM. The f-EVAR cohort included 53 patients (47 men) who were a median age of 76 years (IQR, 11.50; range, 55-87 years). Two fenestrations and one scallop was the most frequent configuration (n = 31). Postoperatively, 37 major complications were noted in 18 patients, six requiring reintervention. Hospital stay was 559 days (median, 7; IQR, 4.5; range, 4-64 days), of which 31 days (median, 4; IQR, 10.5; range, 1-15 days) were in the ITU. Two patients died perioperatively (3.7%), resulting in an observed crude absolute risk reduction of 5.5% compared with open repair. The V-POSSUM estimated perioperative death in five patients (9.4%) in the f-EVAR cohort. In a hypothetic scenario of the f-EVAR cohort undergoing open repair, V-POSSUM estimated seven deaths (13.2%), resulting in an estimated risk-adjusted absolute risk reduction due to f-EVAR of 9.5%.

Conclusions.—In this group of patients, f-EVAR reduced mortality and morbidity substantially compared with open repair and also reduced total hospital stay and ITU utilization.

▶ The authors report a retrospective, risk-adjusted, cohort comparison of patients undergoing fenestrated endovascular aneurysm repair (f-EVAR) and open repair for aneurysms not amenable to the standard EVAR approach. The authors generally recommended open repair for younger, healthier patients and f-EVAR for older patients with more advanced comorbidities even though there were no significant differences in the comorbidities between the groups. The report is distinctly different from those detailing outcome after f-EVAR in patients deemed physiologically too high risk for open repair. Furthermore, it is worth emphasizing that the endovascular devices were commercially available and, presumably, within the manufacturer's instructions for use (IFU). Similar to the seminal randomized trials comparing EVAR with open repair, the perioperative morbidity, mortality, and hospital length of stay were all lower in the f-EVAR group. Furthermore, the magnitude of the remedial interventions also appeared to be lower. The perioperative morality rate in the open group (9.2%) was predictably higher than those associated with infrarenal repair but identical to that predicted using the V-POSSUM model and likely consistent with clinical practice across the country despite select reports from centers of excellence reporting better outcomes. Importantly, the study focused on the perioperative outcome; thus, the longer-term outcomes were not available. It is likely that the f-EVAR will be associated with a whole new host of complications including target vessel thrombosis. The initial reports from the randomized EVAR trials reported similar mortality advantages, although this was not maintained in the midterm reports. Admittedly, the scenario with f-EVAR may be somewhat different given the higher perioperative mortality associated with open repair of perirenal aneurysms. The questions that these data pose are whether f-EVAR should replace open repair in this setting and whether there is sufficient equipoise for a randomized trial. Our clinical practice has been similar to that of the authors, and we have recommended open repair for good-risk patients with perirenal aneurysms while reserving f-EVAR for those deemed higher risk. However, our approach continues to evolve with a lower threshold for f-EVAR in good-risk patients based on our own experience and data such as these. The lack of longer-term data is somewhat unsettling in terms of both our own clinical practice and any generic recommendations for f-EVAR, but I would echo the authors' comments that "a lack of a survival benefit sustained over many years does not equate with no survival benefit of all." There appears to be sufficient equipoise for a randomized trial, although the experimental design and implementation will likely be challenging given the heterogeneous group of perirenal aneurysms and the perceived advantages, both morbidity and mortality, attributed to the f-EVAR approach.

T. S. Huber, MD, PhD

Endovascular Repair of Type B Aortic Dissection: Long-term Results of the Randomized Investigation of Stent Grafts in Aortic Dissection Trial

Nienaber CA, for the INSTEAD-XL trial (Univ of Rostock, Germany; et al)

Circ Cardiovasc Interv 6:407-416, 2013

Background.—Thoracic endovascular aortic repair (TEVAR) represents a therapeutic concept for type B aortic dissection. Long-term outcomes and morphology after TEVAR for uncomplicated dissection are unknown.

Methods and Results.—A total of 140 patients with stable type B aortic dissection previously randomized to optimal medical treatment and TEVAR ($n = 72$) versus optimal medical treatment alone ($n = 68$) were analyzed retrospectively for aorta-specific, all-cause outcomes, and disease progression using landmark statistical analysis of years 2 to 5 after index procedure. Cox regression was used to compare outcomes between groups; all analyses are based on intention to treat. The risk of all-cause mortality (11.1% versus 19.3%; $P = 0.13$), aorta-specific mortality (6.9% versus 19.3%; $P = 0.04$), and progression (27.0% versus 46.1%; $P = 0.04$) after 5 years was lower with TEVAR than with optimal medical treatment alone. Landmark analysis suggested a benefit of TEVAR for all end points between 2 and 5 years; for example, for all-cause mortality (0% versus 16.9%; $P = 0.0003$), aorta-specific mortality (0% versus 16.9%; $P = 0.0005$), and for progression (4.1% versus 28.1%; $P = 0.004$); Landmarking at 1 year and 1 month revealed consistent findings. Both improved survival and less progression of disease at 5 years after elective TEVAR were associated with stent graft induced false lumen thrombosis in 90.6% of cases ($P < 0.0001$).

Conclusions.—In this study of survivors of type B aortic dissection, TEVAR in addition to optimal medical treatment is associated with improved 5-year aorta-specific survival and delayed disease progression. In stable type B dissection with suitable anatomy, preemptive TEVAR should be considered to improve late outcome.

Clinical Trial Registration.—URL: http://www.clinicaltrials.gov. Unique identifier: NCT01415804.

▶ The INSTEAD-XL trial reports the longer-term outcomes from the original INSTEAD trial comparing optimal medical therapy with thoracic endovascular aortic repair (TEVAR; plus optimal medical therapy) for patients with uncomplicated type B dissections presenting between 2 and 52 weeks of their initial symptoms. In contrast to the early publication, there was a decrease in aortic-related mortality (7% vs 19%, $P = .04$), a decrease in aortic progression (4% vs 28%, $P = .004$) and a trend toward a reduction in all-cause mortality (11% vs 19%, $P = .13$). Statistical analysis found that the observed benefits for TEVAR occurred between 2 and 5 years. TEVAR was associated with thrombosis of the false lumen in 91% of the cases with the true lumen diameter increasing (19.4 + 8.2 to 32.6 + 5.5 mm) and the false lumen diameter decreasing significantly (29.3 + 12.4 to 8.6 + 13.4 mm) at 5 years. In contrast, medical therapy alone did not result in any real true lumen recovery or false lumen shrinkage, although it was associated with a significant increase in maximal aortic diameter (43.6 + 9.2 to 56.4 + 6.8 mm) at the 5-year time point. The authors appropriately point out in their discussion that the term *uncomplicated* is likely a misnomer given the longer-term associated adverse events. These potential seminal results suggest that TEVAR may be superior to medical management alone in select, uncomplicated dissections by inducing false lumen thrombosis and preventing aneurysmal degeneration. The benefit associated with TEVAR was seen after 2 years, thereby underscoring the importance of proper patient selection in terms assuring that the patient's life expectancy is sufficient to derive the benefit of the intervention (and offset the procedural risks). These findings have the potential to significantly change practice patterns, but it is important to re-emphasize that the study population included only uncomplicated patients (eg, no evidence of rupture, no malperfusion, aortic diameter 5.5 cm) that were identified between 2 and 52 weeks of their symptoms. Furthermore, the results may not be applicable outside of a clinical trial setting given the facts that the study was performed at experienced centers, compliance and effectiveness of the medical therapies were excellent, and the patient follow-up was 100%.

T. S. Huber, MD, PhD

Surveillance Intervals for Small Abdominal Aortic Aneurysms: A Meta-analysis

The RESCAN Collaborators (Univ of Leicester, England, UK; Med Res Council (MRC) Biostatistics Unit, Cambridge, England, UK; MRC Clinical Trials Unit, London, England, UK; et al)

JAMA 309:806-813, 2013

Importance.—Small abdominal aortic aneurysms (AAAs [3.0 cm-5.4 cm in diameter]) are monitored by ultrasound surveillance. The intervals between surveillance scans should be chosen to detect an expanding aneurysm prior to rupture.

Objective.—To limit risk of aneurysm rupture or excessive growth by optimizing ultrasound surveillance intervals.

Data Sources and Study Selection.—Individual patient data from studies of small AAA growth and rupture were assessed. Studies were identified for inclusion through a systematic literature search through December 2010. Study authors were contacted, which yielded 18 data sets providing repeated ultrasound measurements of AAA diameter over time in 15 471 patients.

Data Extraction.—AAA diameters were analyzed using a random-effects model that allowed for between-patient variability in size and growth rate. Rupture rates were analyzed by proportional hazards regression using the modeled AAA diameter as a time-varying covariate. Predictions of the risks of exceeding 5.5-cm diameter and of rupture within given time intervals were estimated and pooled across studies by random effects meta-analysis.

Results.—AAA growth and rupture rates varied considerably across studies. For each 0.5-cm increase in AAA diameter, growth rates increased on average by 0.59 mm per year (95% CI, 0.51-0.66) and rupture rates increased by a factor of 1.91 (95% CI, 1.61-2.25). For example, to control the AAA growth risk in men of exceeding 5.5 cm to below 10%, on average, a 7.4-year surveillance interval (95% CI, 6.7-8.1) is sufficient for a 3.0-cm AAA, while an 8-month interval (95% CI, 7-10) is necessary for a 5.0-cm AAA. To control the risk of rupture in men to below 1%, the corresponding estimated surveillance intervals are 8.5 years (95% CI, 7.0-10.5) and 17 months (95% CI, 14-22).

Conclusion and Relevance.—In contrast to the commonly adopted surveillance intervals in current AAA screening programs, surveillance intervals of several years may be clinically acceptable for the majority of patients with small AAA (Table 1).

▶ The authors have performed an elegant meta-analysis to determine the growth rate of small abdominal aortic aneurysms (3.0—5.4 cm) to define the most appropriate surveillance intervals. The study is quite timely given the recent publication of the 10-year data from the Multicentre Aneurysm Screening Study that documented a reduction in aneurysm-related deaths and the United States Preventative Services Task Force recommendation that men between 65 and 74 years of age with a smoking history undergo screening. In the current study, the actual ultrasound-based source data were obtained from 18 clinical trials encompassing more than 15 000 patients. The authors found that the annual growth rates of the small aneurysms varied by diameter and, somewhat predictably, the larger aneurysms had a larger annual growth rate (Table 1). The annual growth rates were similar for both men and women. Based on these growth rates, they were able to predict the interval until an aneurysm of a certain diameter reached the common surgical threshold of 5.5 cm, and these values ranged from 7.4 years from men with a 3.0-cm aneurysm to 0.7 year for both men and

TABLE 1.—Pooled (Meta-Analysis) Estimates of Abdominal Aortic Aneurysm Growth and Rupture for Men and Women

	AAA Diameter, cm									
	3.0		3.5		4.0		4.5		5.0	
	Mean (95% CI)	95% PI	Mean (95% CI)	95% PI	Mean (95% CI)	95% PI	Mean (95% CI)	95% PI	Mean (95% CI)	95% PI
Growth rate, mm/y										
Men	1.28 (1.03-1.53)	0.17-2.40	1.86 (1.64-2.08)	0.85-2.88	2.44 (2.22-2.65)	1.47-3.41	3.02 (2.79-3.25)	2.00-4.04	3.61 (3.34-3.88)	2.45-4.77
Women	1.46 (1.07-1.85)	0.03-2.89	1.98 (1.65-2.32)	0.75-3.22	2.51 (2.22-2.81)	1.47-3.56	3.06 (2.80-3.33)	2.18-3.95	3.62 (3.36-3.89)	2.79-4.45
Time to breach surgery threshold, y[a]										
Men	7.4 (6.7-8.1)	4.9-11.3	5.0 (4.6-5.4)	3.4-7.1	3.2 (3.0-3.4)	2.3-4.4	1.8 (1.7-2.0)	1.3-2.5	0.7 (0.6-0.8)	0.4-1.2
Women	6.9 (6.1-7.8)	4.5-10.6	4.8 (4.3-5.3)	3.3-6.8	3.1 (2.9-3.4)	2.3-4.3	1.8 (1.7-2.0)	1.3-2.5	0.7 (0.6-0.8)	0.4-1.3
Rate of rupture, per 1000 person-years										
Men	0.5 (0.3-0.7)	0.3-0.7	0.9 (0.6-1.3)	0.5-1.5	1.7 (1.1-2.4)	0.6-4.3	3.2 (2.2-4.6)	1.0-10.0	6.4 (4.3-9.5)	1.7-23.5
Women	2.2 (1.3-4.0)	0.9-5.7	4.5 (2.8-7.2)	2.1-9.7	7.9 (4.5-13.9)	1.7-36.1	14.7 (8.1-27.7)	2.3-95.1	29.7 (15.9-55.4)	3.9-222.9
Time to 1% chance of rupture, y[b]										
Men	8.5 (7.0-10.5)	5.1-14.2	5.5 (4.4-6.8)	2.8-10.7	3.5 (2.8-4.3)	1.8-6.9	2.2 (1.8-2.8)	1.1-4.4	1.4 (1.2-1.8)	0.7-2.8
Women	3.5 (1.9-6.4)	0.8-14.6	2.1 (1.2-3.6)	0.4-11.1	1.4 (0.9-2.1)	0.3-5.8	0.9 (0.6-1.4)	0.2-3.5	0.7 (0.5-1.1)	0.2-3.3

Abbreviation: AAA, aortic abdominal aneurysm; PI, prediction interval.
[a]Time taken to reach a 10% chance that the 5.5-cm threshold for surgery has been crossed.
[b]Time taken to reach a 1% chance of rupture.

women with a 5.0-cm aneurysm. The rate of aneurysm rupture was significantly greater for women when analyzed based on diameter, and the corresponding predicted times until the aneurysm reached a 1% chance of rupture were likewise shorter. Importantly, women had a 4-fold-greater risk of rupture for all aneurysm diameters. These valuable data should help refine surveillance protocols and the threshold for operative repair in women. There is currently a fair amount of variability in the recommended surveillance protocols from the various national and international societies. Using the most conservative estimates (ie, the lower 95% confidence intervals for rupture risk), the authors recommend surveillance in men every 2 years for aneurysms 3.0 to 3.9 cm, yearly for those 4.0 to 4.9 cm and every 6 months for those 5.0 to 5.4 cm. Interestingly, these intervals are quite similar to those recommended by the Society for Vascular Surgery. The dramatically increased risk of rupture for women suggests that a lower threshold than 5.5 cm should likely be used for recommending repair. Indeed, the rupture risk of a 4.5-cm aneurysm in women was found to be similar to a 5.5-cm aneurysm in men, suggesting that 4.5 cm may be the most appropriate threshold. However, it is important to remember that the decision to recommend operative repair is based not only on the rupture risk, but also the operative mortality, life expectancy, and patient preference. Notably, the operative mortality rate associated with aneurysm repair has consistently been found to be higher for women, thereby confounding the simple recommendation for a 4.5-cm threshold in women. The authors cite several limitations of their study, including the heterogeneity of the data (in terms of the growth rates and rupture risks) and the difficulty ensuring that all the aneurysm ruptures were captured, potentially leading to an underreporting of the rupture risk. I would also contend that the study is fundamentally limited by the ultrasound-based nature of the aneurysm measurements. Ultrasound scan is a wonderful screening tool for the infrarenal aorta but is less reliable for imaging the iliac arteries and the perirenal aorta. A computed tomography arteriogram (CTA) should likely be performed sometime during the surveillance period to assess the full extent of the aorta, including the thoracic component and the iliac vessels. In our own practice, we switch from ultrasound scan to CTA as our surveillance imaging study of choice at an aneurysm diameter of 4.0 cm.

T. S. Huber, MD, PhD

The current management of isolated degenerative femoral artery aneurysms is too aggressive for their natural history

Lawrence PF, for The Vascular Low-Frequency Disease Consortium (Univ of California Los Angeles; Mayo Clinic, Rochester, MN; et al)

J Vasc Surg 59:343-349, 2014

Background.—Previous studies have combined anastomotic, catheter-induced, and atherosclerotic isolated femoral artery aneurysms (FAAs) to achieve adequate numbers for analysis and have recommended repair of asymptomatic FAAs with diameters ≥2.5 cm and all symptomatic FAAs. This study evaluated the contemporary management of isolated FAAs.

Methods.—Patients with FAAs were evaluated using a standardized, prospectively maintained database by a research consortium.

Results.—From 2002 to 2012, 236 FAAs were identified in 182 patients (mean age, 72 years; male-to-female ratio, 16:1) at eight institutions. The mean nonoperative mean diameter was 2.8 ± 0.7 cm, and the operative diameter was 3.3 ± 1.5 cm. FAA location was the common femoral artery in 191, superficial femoral artery (SFA) in 34, and profunda femoris artery in 11. Synchronous aneurysms (mean, 1.7 per patient) occurred in the aorta (n = 113), in the iliac (n = 109), popliteal (n = 86), and hypogastric (n = 56) arteries, and in the contralateral common femoral artery (n = 34), SFA (n = 9), and profunda femoris artery (n = 2). Of the aneurysms repaired, 66% were asymptomatic; other indications for repair were claudication (18%), local pain (8%), nerve compression (3%), rupture (2%), acute thrombosis (1%), and rest pain (0.5%). Acute aneurysm-related complications (rupture, thrombosis, embolus) were associated ($P < .05$) with FAA diameter >4 cm and intraluminal thrombus, but not location. Mean diameter of asymptomatic aneurysms that developed acute complications was 5.7 ± 1.3 cm for rupture, 4 ± 1.1 cm for thrombosis, and 3.5 cm for embolus. Repair was by interposition or bypass graft in 177 FAAs and by endovascular repair in three SFA aneurysms. Two perioperative deaths, of myocardial infarction and multisystem organ failure, occurred at 30 days. Operative complications included wound infection (6%), seroma (3%), and bleeding (2%). No amputations occurred through 5 years in the operative or nonoperative groups. Survival in operated-on patients was 99% (n = 138) at 3 months, 92% at 1 year, and 81% (n = 20) at 5 years.

Conclusions.—This largest study of isolated FAAs demonstrates that (1) acute complications did not occur in FAAs ≤3.5 cm, repair criteria of asymptomatic FAAs should be changed to >3.5 cm, and chronic intraluminal thrombus should reduce the threshold for repair, and that (2) current indications for symptomatic FAA repair result in low morbidity and should remain unchanged.

▶ The authors have performed a multicenter, retrospective study to examine the natural history and operative indications for atherosclerotic or *nonspecific* femoral artery aneurysms (FAAs). Their overall approach is novel and affords the opportunity to examine similar outcomes for a host of rare vascular surgical conditions within the construct of their vascular low-frequency consortium. The authors justify their analysis based on the tenets that the natural history of FAAs is poorly defined and that our limited understanding is based on older studies that largely predated the current imaging technologies and endovascular therapies. The authors reported that 34% of the patients underwent initial operative repair with most of the procedures (89%) performed for symptoms (eg, thrombosis, emboli, rupture). Notably, the mean aneurysm diameters were larger among those treated operatively initially (3.6 + 1.9 cm vs 2.9 + .8 cm). Among those patients that were initially asymptomatic, 73 (64%) ultimately underwent operative repair because of the development of intraluminal thrombus (46), increase in size greater than 2.5 cm (35), acute complications (12), or rapid enlargement (7). Multivariate analysis demonstrated that patient age, aneurysm diameter, and the presence of intraluminal thrombus were associated with operative repair and the development of symptoms among those initially asymptomatic. The findings and resultant conclusions are limited by the retrospective nature of the study design and the inherent selection bias. Indeed, it is difficult to define the natural history and indication for operative treatment if all aneurysms over a certain threshold were repaired. However, none of the asymptomatic aneurysms that were initially managed expectantly developed symptoms until they were greater than 3.5 cm, suggesting that this is likely a better threshold for repair than the current 2.5-cm diameter with the caveat that the presence of intraluminal thrombus may lower the diameter criteria. The study also emphasizes several additional points. Notably, the perioperative morbidity (20%) and mortality (1.1%) associated with operative repair are quite low, whereas the 5-year survival rate for all patients with FAAs (61%) was similar to that of those with abdominal aortic aneurysms, and the risk of amputation is low (ie, no amputations in this study). Furthermore, FAAs are almost exclusively a disease process of men, they rarely rupture, and that the incidence of synchronous/metachronous aneurysms in the aortoiliac and femoropopliteal segments is significant, justifying additional imaging.

T. S. Huber, MD, PhD

Compliance with long-term surveillance recommendations following endovascular aneurysm repair or type B aortic dissection

Kret MR, Azarbal AF, Mitchell EL, et al (Oregon Health and Science Univ, Portland)

J Vasc Surg 58:25-32, 2013

Objective.—Lifelong surveillance is recommended for both endovascular aneurysm repair and acute, uncomplicated type B thoracic aortic dissection, though compliance remains a significant challenge. We sought to determine factors associated with failure to obtain recommended surveillance.

Methods.—Patients surviving to discharge who had endovascular repair of thoracic (thoracic endovascular aortic aneurysm repair [TEVAR]) or abdominal aortic aneurysms (endovascular aortic aneurysm repair [EVAR]) or medical management for type B dissections from 2004-2011 were reviewed. Primary end points were compliance with follow-up and need for reintervention. Comorbidities examined included coronary artery disease, congestive heart failure, hypertension, chronic obstructive pulmonary disease, diabetes, and chronic kidney disease. Socioeconomic factors examined were age, sex, distance from hospital, discharge destination (ie, home or skilled nursing facility), and insurance type. Endoleak and sac expansion were recorded, as were complications, including endograft migration, infection or thrombosis, and aneurysm degeneration.

Results.—Two hundred four patients, median age 71.9 years, were identified; 171 had EVAR and 33 had type B dissection. EVAR patients included

45 thoracic, 100 abdominal, and 12 thoracoabdominal endografts, as well as 7 iliac artery aneurysm repairs and 7 proximal/distal graft extensions. Median follow-up was 28 ± 10.5 months. Overall, 56% were lost to follow-up, whereas 11% never returned for surveillance after initial hospitalization. Follow-up was compared for each of the comorbidities and socioeconomic factors; none were found to significantly affect follow-up. The known complication rate was 9.3% (n = 19), with reintervention performed in 14% of EVAR/TEVAR patients. Thirty-eight percent of medically managed patients with type B dissections eventually required surgical intervention. All-cause 5-year mortality was 27% as determined by the Social Security Death Index.

Conclusions.—Despite a significant rate of reintervention following EVAR, TEVAR, and type B dissection, long-term compliance with surveillance is limited. In addition, predicting who is at risk of being lost to follow-up remains difficult. If current recommendations for lifelong surveillance are to be followed, coordinated protocols are required to capture EVAR, TEVAR, and type B dissection patients to ensure optimal follow-up for these patients. However, the lack of survival benefit in those with complete follow-up suggests that further study is needed with regard to ideal duration of long-term follow-up.

▶ The authors have examined the success of their follow-up surveillance protocols after endovascular aneurysm repair (both endovascular aortic aneurysm repair [EVAR] and thoracic endovascular aortic aneurysm repair [TEVAR]) and medical management for type B dissections at their tertiary care, academic medical center. Notably, national guidelines recommend surveillance in these settings given the risk of continued aneurysm growth and device malfunction in the case of both EVAR and TEVAR and aneurysmal degeneration in the setting of type B dissections. The authors' surveillance protocols included a computed tomography scan at 6 months after the index procedure and then yearly intervals thereafter. Patients were considered lost to follow-up if there was greater than 1 year between their last documented surveillance imaging and clinic visit. Overall, 14% of the patients required intervention after EVAR or TEVAR, and aneurysmal degeneration was detected in 38%. These numbers are largely consistent with those in the published literature but may actually underestimate the real incidences, given the fact that 56% of the patients were lost to follow-up per the study definition, including 84% of the patients that had a TEVAR for a traumatic injury. Unfortunately, the authors were unable to identify any real predictors in terms of being lost to follow-up other than the presence of complications. Indeed, I would have predicted that the travel distance from the medical center and the insurance status would have been important. From a practical standpoint, this makes it impossible to identify patients during the preoperative period that are unlikely to follow-up and may benefit from an alternative approach (ie, open repair) or a more intensive surveillance effort. The authors identified several potential solutions that are largely system-related issues rather than patient-related issues, including a dedicated health care provider tasked with monitoring follow-up, expanded options for local imaging (ie, closer to the patients' homes), or telemedicine networks. It was interesting that presence of a complication was associated with improved follow-up, and the survival of the patients lost to follow-up was improved. Taken together, these findings suggest that patients may seek additional medical help (ie, follow-up) if they are having problems; otherwise, no news is good news. It is unlikely that the observations are isolated to the authors' center. It has been our anecdotal impression that our own follow-up is less than ideal despite our aggressive efforts, and it seems that we have been encountering an increased number of patients with continued aneurysm growth after EVAR that requires open conversion, most without any evidence of continued surveillance. It is tempting to be more liberal with open repair of abdominal aortic aneurysms and recommend TEVAR for uncomplicated type B dissections given the poor compliance with follow-up. However, most patients (and providers) favor an endovascular-first approach and are reluctant to accept an open repair if they are an EVAR candidate. Furthermore, those patients who are noncompliant with their follow-up after medical management of their type B dissection are also not likely to be compliant with their recommended TEVAR surveillance.

T. S. Huber, MD, PhD

Pathogenesis and Management of Retrograde Type A Aortic Dissection After Thoracic Endovascular Aortic Repair

Khoynezhad A, White RA (Cedars-Sinai Med Ctr, Los Angeles, CA; Harbore–UCLA Med Ctr, Torrance, CA)

Ann Vasc Surg 27:1201-1206, 2013

Background.—Retrograde type A aortic dissection is a feared complication of thoracic aortic endografting. The aim of this study was to review the incidence, etiology, and management of this life-threatening complication.

Methods.—A retrospective analysis of the literature in the last 10 years was performed. Data on retrograde type A aortic dissection from this literature search, along with authors' ersonal experience, provided the basis for this review.

Results.—The incidence of retrograde type A aortic dissection ranges from 1.3% to 6.8%. In is most commonly associated with endografting of acute or chronic aortic dissection. Up to one third of patients will have this complication 3 months or later after the index procedure. Open surgical repair remains the "gold standard" for retrograde type A aortic dissection, although medical and endovascular approaches may be utilized in selected patients with prohibitive operative risk. Mortality remains high ranging from 20% to 57%. Potential etiologies of retrograde type A aortic dissection include aortic injury from catheter and wire or stent graft manipulation, poor perioperative antihypertensive control, inappropriate patient and device selection, aggressive balloon dilation, and stent graft oversizing.

Conclusions.—Retrograde type A aortic dissection remains a deadly complication of thoracic aortic endografting. The high incidence of delayed type A aortic dissection underscores the importance of imaging follow-up in patients undergoing a thoracic endograft procedure.

▶ The authors provide a nice review of retrograde type A aortic dissections associated with thoracic endovascular aortic repair (TEVAR). The review is very timely given the widespread application of TEVAR for the various aortic pathologies (ie, aneurysms, dissections, penetrating ulcers, traumatic disruption), the different surgeons/proceduralists implanting the devices, and the potential lethal nature of the complication. The authors estimate that the incidence ranges from 2% to 7% (ie, between 1 in 50 and 1 in 15 cases). The dissections can occur at the time of device implantation or later with a significant proportion (up to 25%) of the patients being asymptomatic. This delayed presentation and the potential absence of symptoms both underscore the importance of long-term follow-up and serial imaging. Several mechanisms are imputed to contribute to the dissections, including those related to technical conduct of the operation, the devices, and the patient's anatomy/medical conditions. Every attempt should be made to minimize the number of manipulations of the various catheters and wires within the aortic arch, and we try not to balloon dilate the thoracic endograft in the setting of a dissection. Similarly, the devices should be appropriately sized relative to the aortic diameter to avoid over dilation. There may be a role for dissection-specific devices with lower radial forces and no barbs or bare springs. TEVARs should generally be avoided in patients with Marfan's disease and other connective tissue defects given predisposition to dissections and the fragility of the aortic tissue. The natural history of retrograde type A dissections remains poorly defined, but it is likely comparable to the more common de novo type A dissections with a 1-year mortality rate of 90% with the same concerns related to rupture, cardiac tamponade, aortic insufficiency, and coronary dissection. The gold standard remains emergent operative repair with arch replacement, although a variety of hybrid approaches have been reported. In our own practice, retrograde dissections have not been too much of a problem, but we have been very proactive in terms of the potential strategies to reduce the adverse outcome as detailed above in addition to aggressive blood pressure control. Furthermore, we have an integrated team approach comprising both vascular and cardiothoracic surgeons with extensive experience in dissections and their open and endovascular treatment.

T. S. Huber, MD, PhD

Delayed volume resuscitation during initial management of ruptured abdominal aortic aneurysm

Dick F, Erdoes G, Opfermann P, et al (Univ Hosp Bern and Univ of Bern, Switzerland)

J Vasc Surg 57:943-950, 2013

Objective.—In acute traumatic bleeding, permissive arterial hypotension with delayed volume resuscitation is an established lifesaving concept as abridge to surgical control. This study investigated whether preoperatively administered volume also correlated inversely with survival after ruptured abdominal aortic aneurysm (rAAA).

Methods.—This retrospective study analyzed prospectively collected and validated data of a consecutive cohort of patients with rAAAs (January 2001 to December 2010). Generally, fluid resuscitation was guided clinically by the patient's blood pressure and consciousness. All intravenous fluids (crystalloids, colloids, and blood products) administered before aortic clamping or endovascular sealing were abstracted from paramedic and anesthesia documentation and normalized to speed of administration (liters per hour). Logistic regression modeling, adjusted for suspected confounding covariates, was used to investigate whether total volume was independently associated with risk of death within 30 days of rAAA repair.

Results.—A total of 248 patients with rAAAs were analyzed, of whom 237 (96%) underwent open repair. A median of 0.91 L of total volume per hour (interquartile range, 0.54-1.50 L/h) had been administered preoperatively to these patients. The postoperative 30-day mortality rate was 15.3% (38 deaths). The preoperative rate of fluid infusion correlated with 30-day mortality after adjustment for confounding factors, and the association persisted robustly through sensitivity analyses: each additional liter per hour increased the odds of perioperative death by 1.57-fold (95% confidence interval, 1.06-2.33; $P = .026$).

Conclusions.—Aggressive volume resuscitation of patients with rAAAs before proximal aortic control predicted an increased perioperative risk of death, which was independent of systolic blood pressure. Therefore, volume resuscitation should be delayed until surgical control of bleeding is achieved.

▶ The authors have attempted to examine the role of volume resuscitation for patients with ruptured abdominal aortic aneurysms (rAAA) to resolve the long-standing impression that permissive hypotension is associated with improved outcome. The concept is based on the perception that large fluid volumes increase arterial pressure leading to additional blood loss and hemodilution, creating a vicious cycle that leads to coagulopathy and release of any retroperitoneal tamponade. Although they did not have a formal written protocol, the general approach was to tolerate systolic blood pressures between 60 and 70 mm Hg while limiting the volume of resuscitation fluid until the bleeding was controlled. They retrospectively analyzed a total of 248 patients undergoing repair of rAAA at a tertiary care institution, responsible for approximately 25% of the rAAAs in Switzerland. They reported that the volume of fluid resuscitation (odds ratio [OR], 1.57) and the age (OR, 1.08) were the only independent predictors of mortality in their logistic regression model examining the predictors of perioperative mortality. Furthermore, it appeared that the volume of the colloid resuscitation (vs crystalloid) was responsible for the adverse outcome. These data help resolve the debate about the most appropriate preoperative fluid therapy for patients with rAAA and seem to justify a more widespread application of the approach to the emergency room and prehospital setting, albeit somewhat difficult, as the diagnosis of a ruptured aneurysm is not always clear in these settings. It is important to emphasize that the observed associations do not necessarily imply causality, but the findings are quite compelling given the limitations of the study design. The overall mortality rate for the rAAAs (15.3%) was impressively low and particularly noteworthy given that most of the repairs (96%) were performed using the open approach. Historically, the reported mortality rates for the open repair of rAAA have been approximately 50%, and this number has not changed much over the last 50 years.[1] The impressive mortality rates suggest a selection bias or "survival of the fittest" that may lessen the impact of the study's main conclusion, but the generic approach should likely be adopted (or continued).

T. S. Huber, MD, PhD

Reference

1. Bown MJ, Sutton AJ, Bell PR, Sayers RD. A meta-analysis of 50 years of ruptured abdominal aortic aneurysm repair. *Br J Surg*. 2002;89:714-730.

Statin therapy is associated with improved survival after endovascular and open aneurysm repair

de Bruin JL, for the DREAM Study Group (Vrije Universiteit Med Ctr, Amsterdam, The Netherlands; Univ Med Ctr Utrecht, The Netherlands)

J Vasc Surg 59:39-44.e1, 2014

Background.—The relationship between numerous risk factors and perioperative mortality after cardiovascular surgery has been studied extensively. While improved perioperative survival and fewer cardiovascular events have been related to statin therapy, its effect on long-term survival after aneurysm repair remains to be elucidated. The aim of this study is to determine the effect of statin therapy on long-term survival after open and endovascular aneurysm repair and to identify other cardiovascular and patient-related risk factors in this respect.

Methods.—A post-hoc analysis of a randomized trial comparing open and endovascular abdominal aortic aneurysm repair was performed. In this multicenter trial, 351 patients were randomly assigned to undergo either open abdominal aortic aneurysm repair or endovascular repair. Patients who were on lipid-lowering medication at their inclusion in the trial ($n = 135$) were compared with those who were not ($n = 216$).

Results.—During 6 years of follow-up, 118 (33.6%) patients died after randomization. Statin therapy, baseline characteristics, Society for Vascular Surgery/International Society for Cardiovascular Surgery risk factors, aneurysm size, reinterventions, antiplatelet or anticoagulant agents, and β-blockers were used to identify prognostic factors influencing survival. After identification of significant factors in a Kaplan-Meier analysis, a multivariable Cox regression analysis was applied. Statin therapy at inclusion in the trial was independently associated with better overall survival after open or endovascular aneurysm repair (hazard ratio [HR], 0.5; 95%

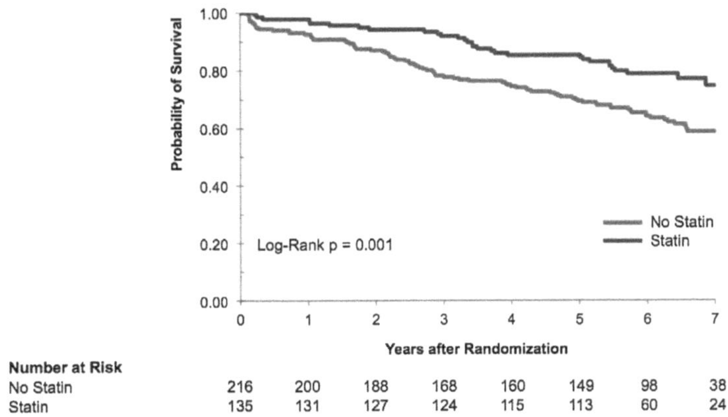

FIGURE 1.—Kaplan-Meier estimates of survival between patients with or without statins. The standard error of both survival estimates does not exceed 10%; the maximum standard errors are 5.5% and 4.5%, respectively, at the end of both curves. (Reprinted from the Journal of Vascular Surgery. de Bruin JL, for the DREAM Study Group. Statin therapy is associated with improved survival after endovascular and open aneurysm repair. *J Vasc Surg*. 2014;59:39-44.e1, Copyright 2014, with permission from the Society for Vascular Surgery.)

confidence interval [CI], 0.3-0.8; $P = .004$). Statins were especially associated with fewer cardiovascular deaths (HR, 0.4; 95% CI, 0.2-0.9; $P = .025$). Several risk factors were associated with poor survival after open and endovascular aneurysm repair: age >70 (HR, 3.4; 95% CI, 2.2-5.0; $P < .001$), a history of cardiac disease at baseline (HR, 1.9; 95% CI, 1.3-2.8; $P = .001$), and moderate/severe tobacco use (HR, 1.7; 95% CI, 1.2-2.5; $P = .004$). Gender, aneurysm size, the need for reintervention, pulmonary disease, renal disease, carotid disease, hypertension, diabetes mellitus, antiplatelet or anticoagulant agents, and β-blockers were not significantly associated with impaired long-term survival ($P > .05$).

Conclusions.—Despite the limitations of a post-hoc analysis of a prospectively maintained trial, we conclude that statin therapy at the beginning of the trial is independently associated with improved long-term survival after open or endovascular aneurysm repair, while age above 70 years, a history of cardiovascular disease, and tobacco use are associated with decreased long-term survival (Fig 1).

▶ The authors performed a post hoc analysis of the data from the DREAM trial, one of the pivotal randomized trials comparing open and endovascular repair, to examine the impact of statins on long-term mortality. Given the limitations of the trial and data, they were able to compare only the patients who were on statins at the time of study enrollment. Notably, no data were available in terms of the serum lipid levels or whether patients continued on the agents or complied with their prescribed regimen. Despite these concerns, they reported that taking statins at the time of study enrollment was associated with improved long-term survival by univariate analysis after both endovascular and open repair (Fig 1). In their multivariate analysis, they identified statin use (hazard ratio [HR] 0.53), age >70 years (HR 3.34), cardiac disease (HR 1.94), and tobacco use (HR 1.73) as predictors of survival. Most of these risk factors are not particularly surprising, but it was interesting that cardiovascular causes and cancer both accounted for the same number of deaths during follow-up (30.5% each) because cardiovascular causes are generally attributed to be the leading cause. The benefits of the statins on long-term survival may be even greater than reported in the trial because only 38% of the patients were actually on them at the time of study enrollment, and these patients had a higher incidence of cardiac disease. Furthermore, it is likely that a significant proportion of patients in the "no statin" group were started on the agents during study follow-up given their widespread adoption since the start of study enrollment in 2000, thereby potentially diluting their real benefit. The overall findings further underscore the importance of the statins as an effective strategy to reduce death from cardiovascular causes among our patients. Indeed, they seem to be the fluoride equivalent of our generation, and I have joked that they should be put in the water, particularly given that their safety profile is good and they have fairly minimal side effects. The statins have multiple effects beyond their impact on lipid levels including influencing the inflammatory response, plaque stabilization, thrombus formation, and endothelial function. In our own practice, we have tried to make sure that all our patients (in both the inpatient and outpatient settings) are on both aspirin and statins, consistent with the American Heart Association's recommendations for patients with peripheral vascular disease.

T. S. Huber, MD, PhD

Peripheral Arterial Occlusive Disease

Stent Placement Versus Balloon Angioplasty for the Treatment of Obstructive Lesions of the Popliteal Artery: A Prospective, Multicenter, Randomized Trial

Rastan A, Krankenberg H, Baumgartner I, et al (Universitäts-Herzzentrum Freiburg-Bad Krozingen, Germany; Universitäres Herz-und Gefäßzentrum Hamburg, Germany; Universität Bern, Switzerland; et al)
Circulation 127:2535-2541, 2013

Background.—Stenting has been shown to improve patency after femoral artery revascularization compared with balloon angioplasty. Limited data are available evaluating endovascular treatment for obstructive lesions of the popliteal artery.

Methods and Results.—This prospective, randomized, multicenter trial compared primary nitinol stent placement to percutaneous transluminal balloon angioplasty in patients with peripheral artery disease Rutherford-Becker class 2 to 5 who had a de novo lesion in the popliteal artery. The primary study end point was 1-year primary patency, defined as freedom from target-lesion restenosis (luminal narrowing of ≥50%) as detected by duplex ultrasound. Secondary end points included target-lesion revascularization rate and changes in Rutherford-Becker class. Provisional stent placement was considered target-lesion revascularization and loss of primary patency. Two hundred forty-six patients were included in this trial. The mean target-lesion length was 42.3 mm. One hundred ninety-seven patients were available for the1-year follow-up. The 1-year primary patency rate was significantly higher in the group with primary nitinol stent placement (67.4%) than in the percutaneous transluminal balloon angioplasty group (44.9%, $P = 0.002$). Target-lesion revascularization rates were 14.7% and 44.1%, respectively ($P = 0.0001$); however, when provisional nitinol stent placement was not considered target-lesion revascularization and loss in patency, no significant differences prevailed between the study groups (67.4% versus 65.7%, $P = 0.92$ for primary patency). Approximately 73% of patients in the percutaneous transluminal balloon angioplasty group and 77% in the nitinol stent group showed an improvement of ≥1 Rutherford-Becker class ($P = 0.31$).

Conclusions.—Primary nitinol stent placement for obstructive lesions of the popliteal artery achieves superior acute technical success and higher 1-year primary patency only if provisional stenting is considered target-lesion revascularization. Provisional stenting as part of a percutaneous transluminal balloon angioplasty strategy has equivalent 1-year patency and should be preferred over primary stenting.

Clinical Trial Registration.—URL: http://www.clinicaltrials.gov. Unique identifier: NCT00712309.

▶ The authors report the results of a randomized, controlled trial comparing balloon angioplasty alone with nitinol stents for isolated popliteal artery occlusive lesions. Patients classified as Rutherford 2–5 with a median popliteal lesion (stenosis > 70% or occlusion) of 42 mm were randomly divided ($N = 246$) between the 2 groups with the primary endpoint being target vessel restenosis (> 50%) at 1 year as defined by duplex ultrasound scan. Notably, placement of a provisional stent for a dissection or residual stenosis in the balloon angioplasty group was considered a target vessel restenosis and loss of patency. The authors reported that the primary patency rates at 1 year were significantly better for the stent group (67% vs 45%), albeit somewhat disingenuous. If the provisional stents at the time of balloon angioplasty were not considered target vessel restenosis but rather necessary remedial procedures (incidence, 25%), the 1-year patency rates were similar (67% vs 66%). Importantly, the overall technical success rate for both groups was 100%, the mean ankle/brachial indices increased significantly (baseline, 0.67 + 0.42 vs discharge, 0.98 + 035), the limb salvage rate was 100%, and the event-free survival rates were comparable. These findings corroborate other reports in the literature supporting the selective use of stents for balloon angioplasty failures in the iliac and femoral regions. Furthermore, they seem to attest to the safety of stenting the popliteal artery, often regarded as a "no stent" region because of the dynamic changes of the popliteal artery during walking, given the patency and low stent fracture rates (3.4%). Not surprisingly, the length of the lesion and the presence of an occlusion (rather than stenosis alone) correlated with target vessel restenosis on multivariate analysis. The data must be interpreted with some caution given the relatively short-term outcome, but they largely reinforce our own clinical practice with preferential use of balloon angioplasty for popliteal occlusive lesions, with stenting reserved for intraoperative technical failures.

T. S. Huber, MD, PhD

Predictors and outcomes of restenosis following tibial artery endovascular interventions for critical limb ischemia

Saqib NU, Domenick N, Cho JS, et al (Univ of Pittsburgh School of Medicine, PA)

J Vasc Surg 57:692-699, 2013

Objective.—Restenosis following tibial artery endovascular interventions (TAEIs) is thought to be benign but is not well characterized. This study examines the consequences and predictors of recurrent stenosis of TAEIs for critical limb ischemia.

Methods.—All TAEIs for critical limb ischemia performed between 2004 and 2010 were retrospectively reviewed. Restenosis was detected by noninvasive imaging and angiography when indicated. Restenoses were identified and the limb outcomes recorded. Tibial reinterventions were performed only for persistent, worsening, or recurrent tissue loss or rest pain with evidence of recurrence on duplex ultrasound or hemodynamic imaging. The χ^2 test and logistic regression were applied as indicated. One-year patency rates were calculated using the Kaplan-Meier method.

Results.—A total of 235 limbs in 210 patients were treated for critical limb ischemia (70% tissue loss, 30% rest pain). Tissue loss included gangrene (49%) and ulcers (51%), and involved the forefoot (80%), the heel (14%), or both (6%). Seventy-eight percent of limbs had Trans-Atlantic InterSociety Consensus C/D lesions, with mean preoperative runoff score of 12. Interventions were isolated tibial (45%) or multilevel (55%) (including tibial). Mean postoperative runoff score improved to 6.6, but restenosis occurred in 96 limbs (41%) at a mean of 4 months. The 1-year primary patency was 59% with a mean follow-up of 9 months. Restenosis presented with a persistent wound (32%), worsened wound (42%), rest pain (16%), or no symptoms (10%). A repeat TAEI was performed in 42 (44%), major amputation in 26 (27%), open bypass in 20 (21%), and observation in eight (8%). The overall amputation rate was 13%, but limb loss was significantly higher in patients with restenosis (n = 26 [27%]) than in patients with no restenosis (n = 5 [4%]; $P < .001$). Patients with restenosis and tissue loss were more likely to have presented with gangrene (63% vs 38%; $P = .0003$) but had comparable wound distribution ($P =$ NS). There was a trend toward a higher restenosis rate in patients with renal insufficiency (odds ratio, 5.57; $P = .08$), but this was unaffected by diabetes, statin therapy, or smoking ($P =$ NS). The rate of repeat intervention after the first reintervention was 36%, with an 87% overall limb salvage rate.

Conclusions.—TAEIs can be used successfully to treat patients with critical limb ischemia with acceptable limb salvage rates. Special attention should be given to patients with extensive tissue loss or gangrene because they are at risk for early restenosis and subsequent limb loss. Strict wound and hemodynamic surveillance, wound care, and timely reinterventions are crucial to achieve successful outcomes in this patient population. Amputation or alternative revascularization options, when feasible, should be considered in patients with restenosis and tissue loss given the high rate of limb loss with tibial reinterventions.

▶ The optimal treatment for patients with chronic limb ischemia (CLI) remains one of the most important, unanswered questions in our discipline. Many providers have evolved to an endovascular-first approach based on the impression that the endovascular failures (ie, restenosis or thrombosis) are benign and amenable to repeat intervention or open revascularization. The authors have examined the role of tibial artery angioplasty for patients with CLI. They have reported reasonable primary patency (59%) and limb salvage (87%) rates at 1 year, and, indeed, these rates rival those reported for open, surgical revascularization. However, the outcomes among the patients who had restenosis were not ideal, with 27% requiring major amputation. Notably, the presence of gangrene as an indication for intervention was the only significant predictor (odds ratio, 3.12) of restenosis. These results suggest that failure after tibial angioplasty is not particularly benign. Admittedly, many of the patients in the current series were not open revascularization candidates because they had a prohibitive medical risk or they lacked a suitable conduit or distal target. However, there was a subset of patients that were initially open, surgical candidates that progressed to a point that their limbs were not salvageable after the failed endovascular treatments. Clearly, it would be ideal to identify this subset of patients before their initial treatment. The authors' data suggest that patients with gangrene or those who can't comply with a longer-term follow-up program may be best treated with open, surgical revascularization, although it is important to emphasize that an open control group was not included in the study. In their discussion, the authors point out that the mean time to the detection of a recurrent stenosis was 5 months, whereas the mean time to wound healing was 11 months. Given these timelines, it is likely that many of the wounds deteriorated (potentially to point at which the foot was unsalvageable) after the failed endovascular procedure. In contrast, the data also suggest that multiple reinterventions are likely futile and that there is also a subset of patients with significant tissue loss best treated with primary amputation. In our own practice, we have recommended open, surgical revascularization for patients with significant tissue loss, provided that they are a reasonable surgical risk, based on our impression that the hemodynamic benefit and patency rates are superior to those of endovascular treatment, albeit based on limited data. Overall, the current study provides useful information that should help refine our collective clinical judgment for this difficult group of patients.

T. S. Huber, MD, PhD

Clinical consequence of bare metal stent and stent graft failure in femoropopliteal occlusive disease

Vartanian SM, Johnston PC, Walker JP, et al (Univ of California, San Francisco; Colorado Permanente Med Group, Denver)

J Vasc Surg 58:1525-1532, 2013

Objective.—The optimal role for bare metal stents (BMS) or stent grafts (SG) in femoropopliteal occlusive disease (FPOD) is as of yet undefined. Understanding the clinical consequences of failure can help guide initial treatment decisions. The goal of this study was to define the nature, frequency, and risk factors for adverse clinical events related to BMS and SG failure in FPOD.

Methods.—This is a single-institution retrospective review of primary endovascular interventions for FPOD using either a BMS or SG, from September 2007 through October 2011. Patients were excluded if they had any previous lower extremity interventions. Patient demographics, indications for intervention, anatomic characteristics, procedural details, clinical outcomes, and reintervention details were reviewed. Clinical outcomes included the composite end point of any reintervention, amputation, or stenosis, acute limb ischemia (ALI), and the composite end point of major adverse limb events, which included a need for bypass, thrombolysis, or major amputation.

Results.—Seventy-one limbs were treated with BMS and 63 with SG. Although patient demographics were largely similar between cohorts, key differences included indication for intervention (percent claudication BMS vs SG, 34/71 (48%) vs 42/63 (67%); $P < .05$) and the TransAtlantic Inter-Society Consensus II classification of lesions in the claudicant subgroup (TransAtlantic Inter-Society Consensus D BMS vs SG, 4/34 (12%) vs 17/42 (40%); $P < .01$). Freedom from reintervention at 1 year was better in the SG group (75% vs 64%; hazard ratio, 0.46; 95% confidence interval, 0.25-0.78; $P < .01$). Freedom from major adverse limb events was not different between groups; however, SG thrombosis resulted in a more frequent need for thrombolysis. On multivariate analysis, treating with a BMS vs SG was a significant predictor for freedom from thrombolysis (hazard ratio, 0.53; confidence interval, 0.37-0.76; $P < .01$). ALI during follow-up was seen only in the SG group (nine vs zero events, log- rank; $P < .02$).

Conclusions.—Failure modes of BMS and SG used to treat FPOD differ, and the clinical consequences may not be benign. Claudicants may not revert back to claudication with treatment failure. Although the overall reintervention rate at 1 year is lower for SG compared to BMS, we observed a higher rate of ALI and need for thrombolysis with SG failure. In light of these differential risks of treatment failure, we believe that the use of SG as initial therapy for FPOD should be carefully deliberated and mandates close postoperative surveillance.

▶ The authors report their experience with bare metal stents (BMS) and stent grafts (SG) for the treatment of femoropopliteal occlusive disease in an attempt to examine their adverse clinical event rates. The choice between BMS and SG was left to the discretion of the surgeon. Unfortunately, the procedural indications, the runoff scores, and the incidence of chronic total occlusions differed between the 2 groups, thereby, preventing their direct comparison. The reintervention rates at 1 year were higher in the BMS group (36% vs 25%) and are consistent with those in the published literature. However, these rates are somewhat arbitrary because a significant proportion of the interventions were performed based on abnormalities detected on routine surveillance. In our own practice, we have been more conservative and have only reintervened based on the recurrence of symptoms. Acute limb ischemia developed in 9 of 63 extremities undergoing SG but was not seen after BMS. Notably, all patients with acute limb ischemia were successfully revascularized, but the ischemic event was associated with the loss of infrageniculate vessels in 4 of 9 cases. When the analysis was limited to those patients presenting with claudication alone, 9% of the limbs treated with BMS developed critical limb ischemia, whereas 17% developed the same after SG ($P = .16$). Taken together, these results suggest that when the SGs thrombose, the patients may not return to their preintervention state (and are potentially much worse off). Indeed, this has been my nagging suspicion, although it has been difficult to extract or tease out from the literature. This is very reminiscent of the scenario after thrombosis of a prosthetic femoropopliteal bypass graft. These results seem to justify a conservative approach to femoropopliteal stenting (both BMS and SG), although the retrospective study design and the lack of noninterventional control limit the overall conclusions.

T. S. Huber, MD, PhD

The Risk of Major Elective Vascular Surgical Procedures in Patients With End-Stage Renal Disease

Gajdos C, Hawn MT, Kile D, et al (Univ of Colorado at Denver, Aurora; Univ of Alabama at Birmingham)

Ann Surg 257:766-773, 2013

Objective.—To examine the postoperative complications and death rate of major elective vascular surgery procedures in patients with end-stage renal disease (ESRD).

Background Data.—Patients with ESRD undergoing elective major vascular surgical procedures are thought to have a high rate of postoperative complications and death.

Methods.—The American College of Surgeons-National Surgical Quality Improvement Program database was used to select ESRD and non-ESRD patients who had elective major vascular surgical procedures between 2004 and 2008. Multivariable logistic regression analysis was used to examine the impact of ESRD on 30-day surgical outcomes adjusted for age, race, sex, work relative value units, American Society of Anesthesiology class, and recent operations (within the past 30 days).

Results.—ESRD patients undergoing elective major vascular surgery were significantly more likely than non-ESRD patients to develop surgical site infection, unplanned intubation, ventilator dependence, combined pulmonary outcome, and a need for reoperation within 30 days of surgery. Importantly, ESRD patients undergoing elective major vascular surgery were also at higher risk for composite outcome and death within 30 days from surgery. ESRD patients above age 65 years undergoing elective major vascular surgery had far worse 30-day outcomes when compared with the younger ESRD cohort. Examining these data by their anatomic site (carotid, aortic, and peripheral) demonstrated elevated rates of postoperative complications and death in patients with ESRD undergoing open abdominal aortic aneurysm repair, carotid endarterectomies, and peripheral vascular operations compared with the non-ESRD cohort. Endovascular abdominal aortic aneurysm repair in ESRD patients had complications and death rates comparable with non-ESRD patients.

Conclusions.—Patients with ESRD undergoing elective vascular surgery have a significantly elevated risk of postoperative complications and death after major vascular surgical operations—particularly in patients over age 65. These data, in combination with well-established reduced survival for the older ESRD population, call into question the utility of most carotid and aortic operations in these patients in the absence of symptoms or a rapidly enlarging aneurysm.

▶ The authors have used the American College of Surgeons National Surgical Quality Improvement Program database to examine the outcome of elective vascular surgical procedures in patients with end-stage renal disease (ESRD). The vascular surgical procedures were identified based on common procedure terminology codes and broken down into those corresponding to carotid, aortic, and peripheral vascular procedures. Notably, only open, surgical procedures were included among the carotid and peripheral codes. Patients with ESRD had a higher incidence of comorbidities, including diabetes, prior revascularization, gangrene, and reduced functional capacity. Importantly, they had a higher incidence of adverse postoperative outcomes, including death, and a composite measure of complications with the latter driven largely by pulmonary complications and surgical site infections. The higher incidence of adverse outcomes persisted after the analysis by the 3 vascular procedure types, but there was some difference in the specific adverse events found to be statistically significant. Not surprisingly, older patients with ESRD and those with critical limb ischemia had worse outcomes, although it was somewhat surprising that ESRD patients undergoing endovascular aneurysm repair only had a higher incidence of neurologic complications. The overall findings of the study are consistent with most surgeons' impressions that ESRD patients have a higher incidence of comorbid conditions and worse outcomes with almost every surgical procedure, not only just vascular procedures. The adverse outcomes associated with the vascular procedures underscore the importance of clinical judgment given the fact that the repair of intact aneurysms and carotid revascularization for stenoses are largely prophylactic operations. In these cases, the risk of the procedure must be offset by the natural history of the underlying condition, and the patients must live long enough to derive the benefit of the intervention. Unfortunately, the specific indications for the procedures in terms of presenting symptoms (eg, abdominal aortic aneurysm and abdominal pain, hemispheric stroke and carotid stenosis) and the diameters of the aneurysms were not available in the current analysis. It is certainly conceivable that a significant proportion of the aneurysm repairs were performed for smaller aneurysms (ie, < 5.5 cm), or a large percentage of the carotid endarterectomies were performed for asymptomatic lesions. However, the relatively small percentage of patients in the database with ESRD that underwent aortic (1.3%) or carotid (1%) procedures when expressed as a percentage of the total number of patients (both ESRD and non-ESRD) undergoing those procedures suggests that there was already a significant selection bias. The scenario for patients with ESRD and peripheral vascular disease is somewhat different, particularly for those with critical limb ischemia, as they require either revascularization or major amputation. Patients with ESRD, particularly those with diabetes, often have severe infrainguinal occlusive disease with limited revascularization options. Indeed, it has been debated whether revascularization should be attempted in this cohort of patients. The observation that patients with ESRD undergoing endovascular aneurysm repair only had a higher incidence of neurologic events provides some qualified support for the approach and raises the question whether the generic endovascular approach may also be better for carotid and peripheral occlusive disease.

T. S. Huber, MD, PhD

Vacuum-assisted wound closure versus alginate for the treatment of deep perivascular wound infections in the groin after vascular surgery

Monsen C, Wann-Hansson C, Wictorsson C, et al (Skåne Univ Hosp, Malmö, Sweden; Malmö Univ, Sweden)

J Vasc Surg 59:145-151, 2014

Background.—Vacuum-assisted wound closure (VAC) therapy may heal wounds faster than conventional dressings after surgical debridement of perivascular groin infections after vascular surgery.

Methods.—Patients with deep infected wounds (Szilagyi grade III) were surgically revised and left open for secondary healing, then randomized to either VAC or alginate (Sorbalgon) therapy, between February 2007 and November 2011. To test the hypothesis, it was calculated that 42 patients needed to be included (90% power, 5% level of significance). It was decided to perform an interim analysis after inclusion of 20 patients.

Results.—Among 66 patients undergoing groin revision, 20 patients were included in this study. Patients were randomized to VAC (n = 10) or alginate (n = 10). The two groups were comparable in patient and wound characteristics. Time to full skin epithelialization was significantly shorter in the VAC group (median, 57 days) compared with the alginate group (median, 104 days; $P = .026$). The number of positive wound cultures of bacteria and C-reactive protein values decreased equally in both groups between surgical revision and day 21. One femur amputation was performed in each group as a consequence of the groin infection, one patient died during the in-hospital stay in the alginate group, and none died in the VAC group.

Conclusions.—VAC achieves faster healing than alginate therapy after wound debridement for deep perivascular wound infections in the groin after vascular surgery. This finding does not allow further inclusion of patients from an ethical point of view, and this study was, therefore, stopped prematurely.

► The authors performed a small but elegant randomized controlled trial to examine the role of vacuum-assisted closure (VAC) devices for complex groin infections with the control group using alginate, presumably the best alternative treatment. All patients underwent operative debridement and then were randomly divided into the 2 groups. Notably, the wounds were extensive, with a mean depth between 4 cm (VAC) and 6 cm (alginate) for the groups and a surface area of 19 cm^2 and 22 cm^2, respectively. The wounds were classified as Szilagyi grade III (ie, infection involving the vascular graft), but it wasn't clear from the breakdown of the patients that a vascular graft was exposed in each case. Regardless, the VAC resulted in a shorter time to complete wound epithelialization when compared with the control group (57 vs 104 days). Indeed, the results were so dramatically better in the VAC group that the trial was stopped after the interval analysis because it was deemed unethical to continue. These findings provide some guidance for dealing with a very complex group of wounds (and patients) with the overall complexity reflected by the 10% transfemoral amputation in each group, a direct complication of the open wound. Unfortunately, the incidence of groin wound complications will likely increase with the epidemic of obesity in our society. Indeed, it is relatively easy to predict preoperatively which patients will have postoperative wound complications based on their body habitus alone. In our own practice, we have used a similar approach but have experienced somewhat mixed results. We have been particularly conservative in terms of keeping the patients in a closely monitored center (ie, intensive care unit or intermediate care) on blow-out precautions until the vessels or grafts are covered. Furthermore, we have been very aggressive about using autogenous material for the arterial reconstruction (interposition graft—femoral vein, patch—saphenous vein) and sartorius muscle flaps to cover the vessels with the VAC placed on top. There is no long-term follow-up in this study, but any underlying prosthetic material is likely at a high risk of ultimately causing infection, mandating long-term surveillance and potentially suppressive antibiotics.

T. S. Huber, MD, PhD

Platelet Responsiveness to Clopidogrel Treatment After Peripheral Endovascular Procedures: The PRECLOP Study: Clinical Impact and Optimal Cutoff Value of On-Treatment High Platelet Reactivity

Spiliopoulos S, Pastromas G, Katsanos K, et al (Patras Univ Hosp, Rio, Greece)

J Am Coll Cardiol 61:2428-2434, 2013

Objectives.—This study aimed to assess the clinical implications and optimal cutoff value of high platelet reactivity (HPR) in patients receiving clopidogrel for peripheral endovascular procedures.

Background.—As noted in coronary studies, HPR could be related to increased adverse events.

Methods.—This prospective trial included patients receiving clopidogrel 75 mg daily, before and after infrainguinal angioplasty or stenting. Platelet inhibition was assessed with the VerifyNow $P2Y_{12}$ point-of-care test. Primary endpoints were 1-year clinical events rate (composite endpoint of death, major stroke, major amputation, target vessel revascularization, and bypass) according to the $P2Y_{12}$ reaction units (PRU)-based quartile distribution, the estimation of the optimal PRU cutoff value for predicting clinical outcome, and the identification of independent predictors influencing event-free survival.

Results.—In total, 100 consecutive patients were enrolled. The 1-year cumulative events rate was 4% in the first quartile, 12% in the second, 52% in the third, and 84% in the fourth. Pairwise comparisons demonstrated a significant difference in the composite endpoint between successive quartiles (all $p < 0.05$ except for the first vs. second quartile). According to receiver-operating characteristic curve analysis, the optimal cutoff value for the composite endpoint was PRU ≥234 (area under the curve: 0.883; 95% confidence interval [CI]: 0.811 to 0.954; $p < 0.0001$; sensitivity: 92.1%; specificity: 84.2%). Cox multivariate regression analysis identified HPR (PRU ≥234) as the only independent predictor of an increased number of adverse events (hazard ratio: 16.9; 95% CI: 5 to 55; $p < 0.0001$).

Conclusions.—On-treatment HPR is associated with markedly increased adverse clinical events in patients undergoing peripheral endovascular procedures. Point-of-care clopidogrel assessment might be useful in individualizing antiplatelet therapy to attain superior clinical results. (High On-Treatment Platelet Reactivity Following Peripheral Endovascular Procedures [PRECLOP]; NCT01744613) (Fig 3).

▶ The authors report the results of a prospective study examining the impact of platelet responsiveness to clopidogrel after endovascular treatment of infrainguinal arterial occlusive disease. Notably, the antiplatelet regimen included 75 mg of clopidogrel (started 1 month before the procedure and continued indefinitely) and 100 mg of aspirin (started at the time of the operative procedure and continued for 6 months). The platelet responsiveness to clopidogrel was determined using the VerifyNow $P2Y_{12}$ point-of-care testing, and the results were stratified based on the quartiles of the responses. The authors found that the 1-year

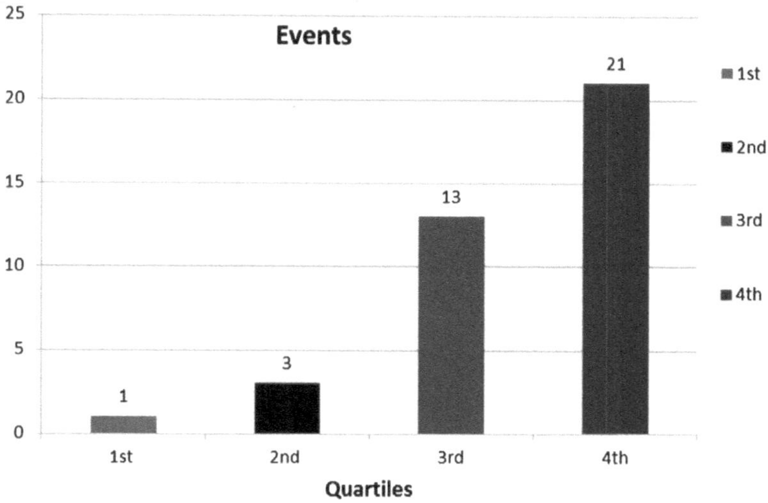

FIGURE 3.—Cumulative Adverse Events. Schematic representation of clinical adverse events according to quartile distribution of platelet ($P2Y_{12}$) reaction units (PRUs). (Reprinted from the Journal of the American College of Surgeons. Spiliopoulos S, Pastromas G, Katsanos K, et al. Platelet responsiveness to clopidogrel treatment after peripheral endovascular procedures: the PRECLOP study: clinical impact and optimal cutoff value of on-treatment high platelet reactivity. *J Am Coll Cardiol.* 2013;61: 2428-2434, Copyright 2013, with permission from the American College of Cardiology Foundation.)

composite endpoint (ie, death, bleeding, major amputation, target vessel revascularization) varied with the quartiles (Fig 3) although 95% of the clinical endpoints were due to target vessel revascularizations. Admittedly, target vessel revascularization is somewhat of a soft endpoint, but it likely serves as a surrogate marker for recurrent symptoms of claudication or ischemic rest pain. Multivariate logistic regression analysis found that a $P2Y_{12}$ reaction level greater than 234 was the only independent predictor of adverse clinical events. Notably, there were only 4 bleeding events (4%) with most related to access site complications. These data strongly suggest that the outcomes after infrainguinal endovascular procedures are partly related to platelet responsiveness to clopidogrel, and they are likely applicable to all percutaneous procedures, particularly carotid stenting given the adverse outcomes associated with stent thrombosis. The data further suggest that some type of point-of-care testing should be incorporated into clinical practice to identify patients at high risk for failure and to potentially help develop alternative, patient-specific, antiplatelet therapies. I do not have any experience with the VerifyNow $P2Y_{12}$ device used in the study, but the sensitivity, specificity, and predictive values generated by the receiver-operating curves are quite impressive. Notably, the negative predictive value was 94%, suggesting that patients with a value of less than 234 are unlikely to experience an adverse event at 1 year, whereas 67% (positive predictive value) of those with a value greater than 234 could (ie, experience an adverse event). The optimal alternative therapies remain to be determined, but potential strategies include higher doses of clopidogrel or alternative antiplatelet therapies (eg, prasugrel, ticagrelor).

T. S. Huber, MD, PhD

Venous

Outcomes of endovascular intervention for May-Thurner syndrome

Hager ES, Yuo T, Tahara R, et al (Univ of Pittsburgh Med Ctr, PA; Bradford Med Ctr, PA)

J Vasc Surg Venous Lymphat Disord 1:270-275, 2013

Background.—Endovascular interventions for May-Thurner syndrome (MTS) have become first-line therapy, often performed in a young patient population despite the lack of robust supportive data. This article reports on long-term outcomes from a large series of patients treated in the setting of de novo or postthrombotic presentation.

Methods.—A retrospective review of MTS patients treated between 2006 and 2010 was conducted at two institutions. Patients who presented with acute iliofemoral deep vein thrombosis (DVT) were treated with either catheter-directed thrombolysis (CDT) and/or pharmacomechanical thrombolysis and identified as having a venous stenosis by venogram or intravascular ultrasound (IVUS). Patients who presented with chronic venous insufficiency symptoms or recalcitrant ulceration but no DVT and evidence of MTS on duplex ultrasound, magnetic resonance venography, or computerized tomography venography were evaluated by venography. IVUS was selectively utilized. Stenting of the iliocaval junction was performed in all patients with a >50% diameter stenosis by IVUS or venogram.

Results.—Seventy patients with MTS underwent 77 lower extremity interventions. They were divided into two groups: postthrombotic (group 1) and de novo presentation of chronic swelling/pain or ulceration but no DVT (group 2). There were 56 extremities in group 1 and 21 extremities in group 2. Both groups were comparable in terms of gender distribution and comorbidities, but hypercoagulable state was more common in group 1 ($P = .014$), and average CEAP and Villalta scores on presentation were higher in group 2 ($P < .001$). There were left-sided symptoms in 40 (78%) patients in group 1 and 15 (79%) in group 2 ($P = 1.00$). Female patients were more likely to have left-sided symptoms compared with male patients (odds ratio, 4.88; 95% confidence interval, 1.49-15.89; $P = .014$). The average stent size was significantly different among the groups ($P < .027$), with different types used in each group. There was one patient in group 1 who had significant periprocedural bleeding (1 unit transfused) during the CDT portion of the procedure. Mean follow up was 29.7 months in group 1 (range, 18.4-58.3 months) and 22.4 months in group 2 (range, 17.1-42 months). Complete or partial symptom relief was reported for 52 (92.9%) extremities in group 1 and 20 (95.2%) extremities in group 2 ($P = 1.00$). The overall primary patency of group 1 at 36 months by life-table analysis was 91% with a secondary patency of 95%. The primary and secondary patency for group 2 was 91% at 36 months.

Conclusions.—Stenting of MTS has proven to be safe, efficacious, and durable for up to 36 months in both the postthrombotic patient as well as those treated for edema alone.

► There has been a widespread adaptation of the endovascular-based therapies for patients with iliofemoral deep venous thrombosis and chronic venous insufficiency. However, the longer-term outcomes in terms of symptomatic relief and vessel patency remain unresolved. Patients with the May-Thurner syndrome from compression of the common iliac vein by overlying common iliac artery (usually compression of the left common iliac vein by the right common iliac artery in women) represent an important subset of patients with iliofemoral deep venous thrombosis. Furthermore, the concerns about long-term durability are particularly germane in this group of patients because it is not clear whether the intraluminal stents are at risk of compression by the overlying artery. The authors have reported their experience with May-Thurner patients treated with catheter-directed thrombolysis or pharmacomechanical thrombolysis and have broken down their experience into 2 groups: patients with acute iliofemoral DVT (N = 56) and patients with chronic swelling/pain or ulceration but no DVT (N = 21). There is a nice description of their overall technique in the Methods section of the report that merits review for individuals interested in incorporating the approach into their practice. Regardless of the breakdown, the longer-term outcomes of both groups in terms of symptomatic relief (> 90%) and iliac stent patency (primary and secondary patency rates > 90% at 3 years) were excellent and attest to the effectiveness and safety of the approach. The relief of symptoms correlated with iliac vein stent patency, whereas, conversely, the recurrence of symptoms was associated with stent thrombosis. Interestingly, there were no instances of in-stent restenosis, suggesting that the radial forces of the stent are sufficient to overcome the compressive forces of the overlying common iliac artery throughout the midterm follow-up. However, it is important to emphasize that median patient age (< 53 years) was quite young, thereby mandating longer-term follow-up given the duration of their life expectancies. The failures in both groups were attributed to inadequate anticoagulation and undersizing of the iliac stents, thus, underscoring the importance of an aggressive anticoagulation regimen (particularly early) and the importance of accurately determining the iliac vein diameter. In our own practice, we have been impressed by the fact that venography alone often leads to undersizing of the stent, relying on intravascular ultrasound scan as an adjunct to determine the true vessel diameter. These results seem to support an aggressive approach to patients with the May-Thurner syndrome, but the results must be interpreted with some caution given the retrospective nature of the study and the lack of a control group treated with anticoagulation alone. The randomized, controlled trial examining catheter-directed thrombolysis for patients with iliofemoral DVT (CaVenT)[1] included in last year's selections found that the benefits of the technique were not quite as compelling as suggested by the nonrandomized trials in terms of symptomatic relief and vessel patency.

T. S. Huber, MD, PhD

Reference

1. Enden T, Haig Y, Kløw NE, et al. Long-term outcome after additional catheter-directed thrombolysis versus standard treatment for acute iliofemoral deep vein thrombosis (the CaVenT study): a randomised controlled trial. *Lancet*. 2012; 379:31-38.

Comparing endovenous laser ablation, foam sclerotherapy, and conventional surgery for great saphenous varicose veins

Biemans AAM, Kockaert M, Akkersdijk GP, et al (Erasmus Med Ctr, Rotterdam, The Netherlands; et al)

J Vasc Surg 58:727-734, 2013

Background.—Many case series have been published on treatments of varicose veins, but comparative randomized controlled trials remain sparse.

Objective.—To compare the anatomic success rate, frequency of major complications, and quality-of-life improvement of endovenous laser ablation (EVLA), ultrasound-guided foam sclerotherapy (UGFS), and conventional surgery (CS), after 1-year follow-up.

Methods.—A total of 240 consecutive patients with primary symptomatic great saphenous vein reflux were randomized to EVLA, UGFS, or CS, consisting of high ligation and short stripping. Primary outcome was anatomic success defined as obliteration or absence of the treated vein on ultrasound examination after 1 year. Secondary outcomes were complications, improvement of the "C" class of the CEAP classification, and improvement of disease-specific (Chronic Venous Insufficiency Quality-of-Life Questionnaire) and general (EuroQol 5) quality-of-life scores.

Results.—More than 80% of the study population was classified as C2 or C3 venous disease. After 1 year, the anatomic success rate was highest after EVLA (88.5%), followed by CS (88.2%) and UGFS (72.2%) ($P < .001$). The complication rate was low and comparable between treatment groups. All groups showed significant ($P < .001$) improvement of EuroQol 5 and Chronic Venous Insufficiency Quality-of-Life Questionnaire scores after therapy; 84.3% of all treated patients showed an improvement of the "C" of the CEAP classification.

Conclusions.—After 1-year follow-up, EVLA is as effective as CS and superior to UGFS according to occlusion on ultrasound duplex. Quality of life improves after treatment in all groups significantly.

▶ The authors report the 1-year results of a simple, randomized trial comparing conventional surgery (CS, stripping/high ligation) with endovascular laser ablation (EVLA) and foam sclerotherapy (UGFS) for the treatment of primary incompetence of the greater saphenous vein (GSV). The study is extremely timely and relevant given the widespread proliferation and adoption of these minimally invasive therapies and the overall prevalence of symptomatic varicose veins in the general population. The various surgical techniques were fairly standard and involved treatment of the GSV in the thigh to the level of the knee. The primary outcomes (ie, obliteration of the saphenous vein at 1 year as detected by ultrasound scan) were comparable for EVLA and CS (88.5% vs 88.2%, respectively) and significantly greater than that for UGFS (72.7%). However, the clinical improvement, complications, and overall quality-of-life assessments were comparable between the 3 groups. Notably, all 3 procedures were remarkably safe, and no deep venous thromboses, pulmonary emboli, or scotomas were detected among the 240 randomly assigned patients. Grade 1 neorevascularization was identified in the groin in 10% of the patients in the CS group, and the overall study enrollment was somewhat slow because of the reluctance of patients to undergo CS, with 10 of 17 study withdrawals occurring in patients assigned to CS. The results seem to favor the EVLA approach given the primary outcomes at 1 year and the minimally invasive approach. However, the results must be interpreted with some caution, because they are relatively early (ie, 1 year), and it is not certain whether they will translate into comparable or superior longer-term outcomes. Additionally, the primary endpoint or the obliteration of the GSV may not actually be the ideal endpoint, albeit objectively measured and quantifiable. It is important to emphasize that the patient-related outcome measures (ie, quality of life, clinical improvement, complications) were comparable among the 3 groups, suggesting that the UGFS is still a valid, effective approach. It is unfortunate that radiofrequency ablation (RFA), our group's preferred approach, was not included in the trial. The authors stated that they incorporated the most common treatment modalities across the Netherlands at the time of the study initiation (2007) in their study design. It is tempting to extend the results of the EVLA to patients treated with RFA, given the published experience that they are largely comparable, although this is not appropriate. The results largely support the findings in the literature and underscore the safety and effectiveness of the 3 approaches. I look forward to the longer-term results and further insights from the study.

T. S. Huber, MD, PhD

Managing iliofemoral deep venous thrombosis of pregnancy with a strategy of thrombus removal is safe and avoids post-thrombotic morbidity

Herrera S, Comerota AJ, Thakur S, et al (Toledo Hosp, OH)

J Vasc Surg 59:456-464, 2014

Background.—Extensive deep venous thrombosis (DVT) during pregnancy is usually treated with anticoagulation alone, risking significant post-thrombotic syndrome (PTS) in young patients. Catheter-directed thrombolysis (CDT) and operative venous thrombectomy have been safely and effectively used in nonpregnant patients, demonstrating significant reduction in post-thrombotic morbidity. This report reviews short- and long-term outcomes of 13 patients with extensive DVT of pregnancy treated with a strategy of thrombus removal.

Methods.—From 1999 to 2013, 13 patients with iliofemoral DVT during pregnancy were offered CDT, pharmacomechanical thrombolysis (PMT), and/or venous thrombectomy. Gestational age ranged from 8 to 34 weeks. Fetal monitoring was performed throughout hospitalization. Radiation exposure was minimized with pelvic lead shields, focal fluoroscopy, and limited angiographic runs. Follow-up included objective vein evaluation using venous duplex and PTS assessment using the Villalta scale.

Results.—CDT and/or PMT were used in 11 patients. Two patients underwent venous thrombectomy alone, and one patient had operative thrombectomy as an adjunct to CDT and PMT. Each patient had complete or near-complete thrombus resolution and rapid improvement in clinical symptoms. Eight of 11 having CDT or PMT underwent venoplasty and stenting of the involved iliac veins. Twelve of the 13 delivered healthy infants at term. One patient opted for termination of her pregnancy. Mean patient and gestational ages were 26 years and 26 weeks, respectively. Mean follow-up was 1.3 years, with only one recurrence. Duplex ultrasonography demonstrated patent veins in all but one patient and normal valve function in 10 patients. Eleven patients had Villalta scores <5 (considered normal), with a mean score of 0.7.

Conclusions.—Extensive DVT of pregnancy can be effectively and safely treated with a strategy of thrombus removal, resulting in a patent venous system, normal valve function in many, prevention of PTS, and reduction in recurrence.

▶ The authors report their experience with interventional treatment for iliofemoral deep venous thrombosis (DVT) in pregnant patients, including catheter-directed thrombolysis, pharmacomechanical thrombectomy, or open/surgical thrombectomy along with definitive endovascular treatment of the underlying venous stenosis. Although the series is somewhat small (N = 13) and spanned more than a decade (1999–2013), it likely represents the largest series reported in the literature. The overall results were impressive with all patients having a complete or near-complete thrombus removal and most having patent iliac veins and normal valve function as documented by ultrasound scan at mean follow-up of 1.3 years. Most importantly, 12 of 13 patients delivered healthy infants, with the other patient opting to terminate her pregnancy. Unfortunately, the incidence of DVT during pregnancy is relatively common, with an incidence of 1 to 2 per 1000 pregnancies, as highlighted by the authors, and, thus, most vascular surgeons will be confronted with this problem. Anticoagulation alone has been the traditional treatment, even in the presence of extensive clot. Notably, the current experience included only patients with phlegmasia cerulean dolens and persistent pain/edema lasting 2 to 14 days. The excellent results reported seem to support a more aggressive treatment algorithm to reduce the longer-term complications associated with the postthrombotic syndrome, although it is impossible to balance the risks and benefits in this limited series. The primary periprocedural concern remains, reducing (or eliminating) any potential risk to the fetus. The authors have detailed their technical approach in the Methods section that includes specific strategies to reduce the fetal risk, including obstetric monitoring and limiting the radiation exposure. The treatment algorithm in terms of the hierarchy of interventions was not well detailed, but it seemed like they favored the pharmacomechanical approach before catheter-directed thrombolysis, with the open approach reserved for treatment failures or patients unwilling to consent to the percutaneous endovascular approaches. Notably, the experience with catheter-directed tissue plasminogen activator (rt-PA) in this setting is fairly limited, but systemic thrombolysis used has been used during pregnancy for other indications (eg, stroke, pulmonary emboli) without maternal or fetal toxicity. The rt-PA is not believed to cross the placental barrier.

T. S. Huber, MD, PhD

Risk of venous thromboembolism associated with peripherally inserted central catheters: a systematic review and meta-analysis

Chopra V, Anand S, Hickner A, et al (Univ of Michigan Health System, Ann Arbor)

Lancet 382:311-325, 2013

Background.—Peripherally inserted central catheters (PICCs) are associated with an increased risk of venous thromboembolism. However, the size of this risk relative to that associated with other central venous catheters (CVCs) is unknown. We did a systematic review and meta-analysis to compare the risk of venous thromboembolism associated with PICCs versus that associated with other CVCs.

Methods.—We searched several databases, including Medline, Embase, Biosis, Cochrane Central Register of Controlled Trials, Conference Papers Index, and Scopus. Additional studies were identified through hand searches of bibliographies and internet searches, and we contacted study authors to obtain unpublished data. All human studies published in full text, abstract, or poster form were eligible for inclusion. All studies were of adult patients aged at least 18 years who underwent insertion of a PICC. Studies were assessed with the Newcastle–Ottawa risk of bias scale. In studies without a comparison group, the pooled frequency of venous thromboembolism was calculated for patients receiving PICCs. In studies comparing PICCs with other CVCs, summary odds ratios (ORs) were calculated with a random effects meta-analysis.

Findings.—Of the 533 citations identified, 64 studies (12 with a comparison group and 52 without) including 29 503 patients met the eligibility criteria. In the non-comparison studies, the weighted frequency of PICC-related deep vein thrombosis was highest in patients who were critically ill (13·91%, 95% CI 7·68–20·14) and those with cancer (6·67%, 4·69–8·64). Our meta-analysis of 11 studies comparing the risk of deep vein thrombosis related to PICCs with that related to CVCs showed that PICCs were associated with an increased risk of deep vein thrombosis (OR 2·55, 1·54–4·23, $p<0·0001$) but not pulmonary embolism (no events). With the baseline PICC-related deep vein thrombosis rate of 2·7% and pooled OR of 2·55, the number needed to harm relative to CVCs was 26 (95% CI 13–71).

Interpretation.—PICCs are associated with a higher risk of deep vein thrombosis than are CVCs, especially in patients who are critically ill or those with a malignancy. The decision to insert PICCs should be guided by weighing of the risk of thrombosis against the benefit provided by these devices.

▶ The authors have attempted to perform a systematic review and meta-analysis of the literature to determine the incidence of venous thromboembolic events associated with peripherally inserted central catheters (PICCs) and to compare these adverse outcomes with those of central venous catheters. The authors have done an impressive job identifying 64 articles encompassing more than 29 000 patients, although the strength of their observations and conclusions are limited by the quality of the underlying data. Notably, there were no randomized trials, and almost one-third of the studies were published in abstract form alone. The incidence of PICC-associated deep venous thromboses was found to be highest among patients in the intensive care unit (13.9%) and those with cancer (6.8%) and significantly lower in non–intensive care unit patients (3.4%) and those in a mixed ambulatory/inpatient cohort (3.4%). Interestingly, the overall incidence of pulmonary emboli was relatively low (0.5%), accounting for 15% of all thromboembolic events in the group with the highest frequency (intensive care unit patients). Furthermore, the incidence of deep venous thromboses was more than 2-fold higher (odds ratio, 2.55) when the PICCs were compared with central venous catheters. These adverse thromboembolic outcomes should be cause for reflection, despite any limitations in the underlying data. The use of PICCs has expanded, seeming exponentially, in our own institution and has replaced the more traditional central venous lines in many scenarios. They offer many advantages to central venous catheters and can be placed by appropriately trained nonphysicians. However, they should likely not be used as an alternative to central venous catheters in the intensive care unit or as alternative to a peripheral intravenous catheter in uncomplicated floor patients, particularly not for patient comfort alone or to avoid blood draws. Notably, the indications in this study included antibiotic/chemotherapy/blood product administration, central venous access, hemodynamic monitoring, parenteral nutrition, and intravenous hydration. In our own institution, we have instructed the PICC insertion team to contact the primary service when a line is requested in a patient with end-stage renal disease or advanced chronic kidney disease in an attempt to avoid the thrombotic complications and the potential loss of a future dialysis access option. Although the current study documents the incidence of PICC-related thromboembolic events, it provides little guidance about definitive treatment. We have felt compelled to anticoagulate patients with these PICC-related deep venous thromboses but concede that the risk of pulmonary emboli is low, and catheter removal alone may be sufficient.

T. S. Huber, MD, PhD

Carotid

Management of carotid stenosis in women: consensus document

De Rango P, Brown MM, Didier L, et al (Hosp S.M. Misericordia, Perugia, Italy; Natl Hosp for Neurology and Neurosurgery, London, UK; Roger Salengro Hosp, Lille, France; et al)

Neurology 80:2258-2268, 2013

Objective.—Specific guidelines for management of cerebrovascular risk in women are currently lacking. This study aims to provide a consensus expert opinion to help make clinical decisions in women with carotid stenosis.

Methods.—Proposals for the use of carotid endarterectomy (CEA), carotid stenting (CAS), and medical therapy for stroke prevention in women with carotid stenosis were provided by a group of 9 international experts with consensus method.

Results.—Symptomatic women with severe carotid stenosis can be managed by CEA provided that the perioperative risk of the operators is low (<4%). Periprocedural stroke risks may be increased in symptomatic women if revascularization is performed by CAS; however, the choice of CAS vs CEA can be tailored in subgroups best fit for each procedure (e.g., women with restenosis or severe coronary disease, best suited for CAS; women with tortuous vessels or old age, best suited for CEA). There is currently limited evidence to consider medical therapy alone as the best choice for women with neurologically severe asymptomatic carotid stenosis, who should be best managed within randomized trials including a medical arm. Medical management and cardiovascular risk factor control must be implemented in all women with carotid stenosis in periprocedural period and lifelong regardless of whether or not intervention is planned.

Conclusions.—The suggestions provided in this article may constitute a decision-making basis for planning treatment of carotid stenosis in women. Most recommendations are of limited strength; however, it is unlikely that new robust data will emerge soon to induce relevant changes.

▶ The authors have developed a consensus statement for the treatment of carotid artery stenosis in women based on an extensive review of the medical literature, including the seminal randomized trials. The authors are all recognized experts in their respective fields, although they readily concede that the quality of the underlying literature is somewhat limited and that this is unlikely to change in the near future. The analysis is justified based on the fact that women have a higher incidence of stroke than men and the associated outcomes are worse. Furthermore, women have been underrepresented in the seminal, randomized trials for the treatment of carotid artery stenosis. There are several real or perceived differences in the management of carotid stenoses in women. Specifically, they may have a higher incidence of adverse outcome after carotid endarterectomy (CEA) for both symptomatic and asymptomatic stenoses, they may have a higher incidence of adverse outcome with carotid angioplasty and stenting (CAS), the timing for CEA in patients with symptomatic lesions may be more critical, their cardiovascular risk profiles may be different, the characteristics of their carotid plaque and the carotid artery may be different, and there may be differences in their medical treatment or responses to these treatments. It is important to note that many of these identified differences were identified in the earlier randomized CEA trials that are now more than 20 years old. Importantly, there were no gender differences in the periprocedural rates after CEA for symptomatic patients in the more recent Carotid Revascularization Endarterectomy vs Stenting Trial, whereas the higher incidence of adverse periprocedural outcomes associated with CAS in the women were consistent with their symptomatic status (rather than simply gender). The consensus statement does a nice job reviewing the literature and is interesting from an academic standpoint, but the recommendations (ie, the proverbial bottom line) are largely consistent with the results of the well-accepted, randomized carotid trials and are not particularly gender specific. Briefly, CEA is beneficial for both symptomatic women with greater than 50% carotid stenosis provided that the perioperative risk is low (< 4%), CEA is beneficial for asymptomatic women provided that the perioperative stroke risk is low (< 2%), and CAS is appropriate for high-risk symptomatic patients. The statement also emphasizes that the medical therapies designed to reduce the risk of cardiovascular events should be optimized, the interventions should be performed within 2 weeks of the sentinel neurologic event, and a technically perfect procedure should be performed, none of which are particularly surprising or gender specific. The guidelines establish lower thresholds for perioperative adverse events after CEA for both symptomatic (< 4% vs < 6%) and asymptomatic (< 2% vs < 3%) based on the CREST data, albeit somewhat ambitious outside of a clinical trial. It is somewhat discouraging to accept the authors' conclusion that "it is unlikely that new robust data will emerge soon to induce relevant changes" given the general uncertainty surrounding the management of carotid artery stenosis for both men and women.

T. S. Huber, MD, PhD

The risk of carotid artery stenting compared with carotid endarterectomy is greatest in patients treated within 7 days of symptoms

Rantner B, for the Carotid Stenting Trialists' Collaboration (Innsbruck Med Univ, Austria; et al)

J Vasc Surg 57:619-626.e2, 2013

Objective.—Among patients with symptomatic carotid artery stenosis, carotid artery stenting (CAS) is associated with a higher risk of periprocedural stroke or death than carotid endarterectomy (CEA). Uncertainty remains whether the balance of risk changes with time since the most recent ischemic event.

Methods.—We investigated the association of time between the qualifying ischemic event and treatment (0-7 days, 8-14 days, and >14 days) with the risk of stroke or death within 30 days after CAS or CEA in a pooled analysis of data from individual patients randomized in the

Endarterectomy vs Angioplasty in Patients with Symptomatic Severe Carotid Stenosis (EVA-3S) trial, the Stent-Protected Angioplasty versus Carotid Endarterectomy (SPACE) trial, and the International Carotid Stenting Study (ICSS). Data were analyzed with a fixed-effect binomial regression model adjusted for source trial.

Results.—Information on time of qualifying event was available for 2839 patients. In the first 30 days after intervention, any stroke or death occurred significantly more often in the CAS group (110/1434 [7.7%]) compared with the CEA group (54/1405 [3.8%]; crude risk ratio, 2.0; 95% confidence interval, 1.5-2.7). Patients undergoing CEA within the first 7 days of the qualifying event had the lowest periprocedural stroke or death rate (3/106 [2.8%]). Patients treated with CAS in the same period had a 9.4% risk of periprocedural stroke or death (13/138; risk ratio CAS vs CEA: 3.4; 95% confidence interval, 1.01-11.8; adjusted for age, sex, and type of qualifying event). Patients treated between 8 and 14 days showed a periprocedural stroke or death rate of 3.4% (7/208) and 8.1% (19/234), respectively, for CEA and CAS. The latest treatment group had 4% complications in the CEA group (44/1091) and 7.3% in the CAS group (78/1062).

Conclusions.—The increase in risk of CAS compared with CEA appears to be greatest in patients treated within 7 days of symptoms. Early surgery might remain most effective in stroke prevention in patients with symptomatic carotid artery stenosis.

▶ The authors have performed a meta-analysis with data from the 3 European trials (EVA-3S, SPACE, and ICSS) comparing carotid endarterectomy (CEA) and carotid angioplasty/stenting (CAS) for symptomatic patients to determine whether the timing of the procedures impacts outcome. They broke down the time intervals between the symptoms and the procedure into 3 groups, including 0 to 7 days, 8 to14 days, and greater than 14 days. The risk of any stroke or death was significantly greater for CAS for each of the time periods. Notably, the risk was 2.8% for CEA performed within 0 to 7 days, whereas the corresponding value for CAS was 9.4% (risk ratio, 3.79; 95% confidence interval, 1.1—13.1), and these values were consistent in their multivariate model. These findings are particularly relevant given the recent clinical guidelines that advocate carotid revascularization within 2 weeks of the sentinel neurologic event, based on the findings that the highest risk of recurrent events occurs within this time period. However, these data must be interpreted with a mild degree of caution, as the current study was a secondary analysis, albeit a meta-analysis, of 3 excellent randomized trials. Specifically, the timing of the procedure relative to the presenting symptom was not the original study question, and there was likely a fair amount of bias in terms of the timing of the procedure. Notably, only 8% of the procedures were performed within 0 to 7 days and only 15.6% were performed with 8 to 14 days. The timing of the procedure relative to the presenting symptom was not available in 483 patients from the SPACE trial, and, accordingly, these patients were excluded from the analysis. Furthermore, the proportion of the patients with a hemispheric stroke as their presenting event was lowest within the earliest group, suggesting that patients with more severe neurologic events had delayed treatment. There has also been a persistent, annoying criticism of these randomized trials that the higher adverse event rates associated with CAS were caused by the inexperience of the centers/interventionalists, although it is noteworthy that the stroke and death rates in the EVA-3S trial were actually higher among the more experienced providers. The inclusion of the data from the CREST may help overcome some of these limitations although the current data clearly suggest that CEA, rather than CAS, is the optimal treatment for symptomatic carotid stenoses, particularly within the earliest time period.

T. S. Huber, MD, PhD

Access

Fistula First Is Not Always the Best Strategy for the Elderly

DeSilva RN, Patibandla BK, Vin Y, et al (Harvard Med School, Boston, MA)
J Am Soc Nephrol 24:1297-1304, 2013

Whether placing a fistula first is the superior predialysis approach among octogenarians is unknown. We analyzed data from a cohort of 115,425 incident hemodialysis patients ≥67 years old derived from the US Renal Data System with linked Medicare claims, which allowed us to identify the first predialysis vascular access placed rather than the first access used. We used proportional hazard models to evaluate all-cause mortality outcomes based on first vascular access placed, considering the fistula group as the reference. In the study population, 21,436 patients had fistulas as the first predialysis access placed, 3472 had grafts, and 90,517 had catheters. Those patients with a catheter as the first predialysis access placed had significantly inferior survival compared with those patients with a fistula (HR=1.77; 95% CI=1.73 to 1.81; $P<0.001$). However, we did not detect a significant mortality difference between those patients with a graft as the first access placed and those patients with a fistula (HR=1.05; 95% CI=1.00 to 1.11; $P=0.06$). Analyzing mortality stratified by age groups, grafts as the first predialysis access placed had inferior mortality outcomes compared with fistulas for the 67 to ≤79-years age group (HR=1.10; 95% CI=1.02 to 1.17; $P=0.007$), but differences between these groups were not statistically significant for the 80 to ≤89- and the >90-years age groups. In conclusion, fistula first does not seem to be clearly superior to graft placement first in the elderly, because each strategy associates with similar mortality outcomes in octogenarians and nonagenarians.

▶ The authors have attempted to analyze survival among elderly (> 67 years of age) hemodialysis patients based on their incident access configuration in an attempt to determine whether a fistula-first strategy remains appropriate. They linked the US Renal Data System with Medicare claims for their analyses. Importantly, their analyses focused on the initial access configuration rather than the access configuration used at the initiation of dialysis, potentially accounting for any additional access-related morbidity/mortality associated with the first procedure. The authors found that survival was significantly worse if the initial access was a catheter although there were no differences if the initial access was a fistula or a graft. Further analysis by age group found that there was a survival advantage for the fistulas among patients 67 to 79 years of age, but no differences between fistulas and grafts for patients older than 79. Unfortunately, a catheter was the first access type in almost 80% of the cohort (catheter, 78%; fistula, 19%; graft, 3%). The authors reported that patients who had a fistula or a graft as their first predialysis access were more likely to have been seen by nephrologist (fistula, 46%; graft, 43%; catheter, 17%) than those with a catheter. Among the patients whose index access procedure was a fistula, 51% initiated dialysis with a fistula, whereas 43% and 6% initiated dialysis with catheter and graft, respectively. Among those whose index access procedure was a graft, 43% initiated dialysis with a catheter. These results again underscore the adverse sequelae of dialysis catheters given the reduced long-term patient survival, and they identify an important opportunity for continued quality improvement, namely, early referral to a nephrologist for pre–end-stage renal disease care. The results challenge the concept of fistula first, given the absence of a survival benefit for the whole group, particularly among those older than 79 years. Although mature fistulas have repeatedly been found to have improved patency and lower complication rates than grafts, a significant proportion of new fistulas fail to mature, necessitating additional operative procedures and prolonged catheter time as suggested by the current data. Indeed, there has been a gradual evolution from the concept of fistula first to catheter last with an appreciation that the primary goal is a functional, permanent access (either a fistula or a graft) rather than a fistula. I would echo the authors' conclusions that "fistula first should be used in patients who have a high chance for successful fistula, and the remainder should be considered for graft first before hemodialysis initiation." The challenge remains to identify these predictors of success and construct a permanent access in these elderly patients with chronic kidney disease (pre-ESRD), although a modicum of common sense must be exercised, because it is not clear that every octogenarian or nonagenarian is best served with a permanent access (or hemodialysis).

T. S. Huber, MD, PhD

Miscellaneous

Stenting and Medical Therapy for Atherosclerotic Renal-Artery Stenosis

Cooper CJ, the CORAL Investigators (Univ of Toledo, OH; et al)
N Engl J Med 2013 [Epub ahead of print]

Background.—Atherosclerotic renal-artery stenosis is a common problem in the elderly. Despite two randomized trials that did not show a benefit of renal-artery stenting with respect to kidney function, the usefulness of stenting for the prevention of major adverse renal and cardiovascular events is uncertain.

Methods.—We randomly assigned 947 participants who had atherosclerotic renal-artery stenosis and either systolic hypertension while taking two or more antihypertensive drugs or chronic kidney disease to medical therapy plus renal-artery stenting or medical therapy alone. Participants were followed for the occurrence of adverse cardiovascular and renal events (a composite end point of death from cardiovascular or renal causes, myocardial infarction, stroke, hospitalization for congestive heart failure, progressive renal insufficiency, or the need for renal-replacement therapy).

Results.—Over a median follow-up period of 43 months (interquartile range, 31 to 55), the rate of the primary composite end point did not differ significantly between participants who underwent stenting in addition to receiving medical therapy and those who received medical therapy alone (35.1% and 35.8%, respectively; hazard ratio with stenting, 0.94; 95% confidence interval [CI], 0.76 to 1.17; $P = 0.58$). There were also no significant differences between the treatment groups in the rates of the individual components of the primary end point or in all-cause mortality. During follow-up, there was a consistent modest difference in systolic blood pressure favoring the stent group (−2.3 mm Hg; 95% CI, −4.4 to −0.2; $P = 0.03$).

Conclusions.—Renal-artery stenting did not confer a significant benefit with respect to the prevention of clinical events when added to comprehensive, multifactorial medical therapy in people with atherosclerotic renal-artery stenosis and hypertension or chronic kidney disease. (Funded by the National Heart, Lung and Blood Institute and others; ClinicalTrials.gov number, NCT00081731.)

▶ The CORAL Trial was an elegant, randomized, controlled trial comparing renal artery stent placement and medical management with medical management alone for patients with significant renal artery stenosis (at least > 60%) and either hypertension or chronic kidney disease. The primary outcome measure was a composite endpoint encompassing adverse cardiovascular and renal events. Notably, the medical management was protocol driven and included antiplatelet agents, blood pressure control, and glucose control with the antihypertension regimen comprised of an angiotensin II receptor blocker, thiazide diuretic, and a combination calcium channel blocker/statin agent. The authors reported that the renal artery stents did not provide any additional benefit to medical therapy alone in terms of the primary endpoint (Fig 2 in the original article). Furthermore, there were no differences in the primary endpoints for the various, planned subgroup (ie, gender, race, global ischemia, diabetes) analyses. The data appear to provide the final proverbial "nail in the coffin" for renal angioplasty/stent placement in the setting of atherosclerotic renal artery occlusive disease and corroborate the findings of 2 earlier randomized trials (ie, ASTRAL, STAR). I suspect that there may be a role for angioplasty/stent placement in a very small subset of patients with atherosclerotic renal artery disease (eg, poorly controlled hypertension and > 3 antihypertensive agents), but this cohort of patients is likely diminishingly small, and the current trial fails to give us much guidance. Angioplasty may be beneficial for patients with renal artery stenosis secondary to fibromuscular dysplasia, although this subset of patients was specifically excluded from the current trial. The CORAL trial has several limitations, including the fact that the enrollment was somewhat difficult and prolonged. Indeed, the enrollment criteria were expanded after trial initiation. Additionally, the compliance with the medical treatment was quite good and may be better than anticipated outside of a clinical trial. However, the same argument could be put forward about the technical success and conduct of the interventions (ie, excellent outcomes may not be applicable outside of the clinical trial). I trust that these data will finally put an end to any renal artery interventions for atherosclerotic occlusive disease despite the fact that it seems like a very good treatment option, and we should not let our patients be "CORALed" into a renal artery stent as punned by the editorial comments accompanying the publication.

T. S. Huber, MD, PhD

Discontinuation of preoperative clopidogrel is unnecessary in peripheral arterial surgery

Saadeh C, Sfeir J (Notre-Dame de Secours University Hospital, Byblos, Lebanon; Lebanese Univ Hosp, Beirut, Lebanon)

J Vasc Surg 58:1586-1592, 2013

Objective.—The optimal management of preoperative clopidogrel remains controversial, as vascular surgeons are increasingly encountering patients treated with clopidogrel as part of dual antiplatelet therapy. Current practice differs considerably, from cessation of the medication at least 5 days before surgery to proceeding with surgery without delay. The purpose of this prospective, nonrandomized, comparative study was to determine the effect of preoperative exposure to clopidogrel and aspirin on perioperative bleeding complications in patients undergoing open arterial surgery.

Methods.—Data were collected prospectively on 647 consecutive major arterial procedures from 2005 through mid-2012. Patients were classified into two groups: the clopidogrel group consisted of 305 procedures performed in 269 patients who were maintained, after obtaining informed consent, on dual clopidogrel and aspirin up to the time of surgery and the no-clopidogrel group consisted of 342 procedures completed in 298 patients who were taking neither medication together or were taking aspirin alone. The primary composite end point was reoperation for bleeding and bleeding-related death. Secondary end points included blood transfusion requirements, hematoma formation, the procedure duration, as well as hospital and intensive care unit length of stay.

Results.—The patients taking clopidogrel had a higher cardiovascular risk profile and a higher prevalence of prior peripheral and coronary stents ($P < .0001$). Clopidogrel use was common across all operation categories: 59% of carotid endarterectomy patients (104 of 177), 43% of lower extremity bypass patients (147 of 344), and 43% of abdominal aortic bypass patients (54 of 126). The difference in the primary end point between the clopidogrel and no-clopidogrel groups was not statistically significant (0.65% and 0.3%, respectively; $P = .55$). No bleeding-related deaths were observed. Further analysis revealed a similar incidence of stable hematomas. Blood transfusions were mainly required by patients undergoing aortic surgery, at similar rates and volumes in the clopidogrel and no-clopidogrel groups: abdominal aortic bypass cohort (a mean of 1.6 units packed red blood cells needed in 72% vs a mean of 1.6 units in 69%, respectively; $P = .76$); lower extremity bypass cohort (a mean of 1.5 units needed in 15% vs 1.3 units needed in 11%; $P < .004$). The mean operative time and intensive care unit and hospital lengths of stay were not longer in clopidogrel recipients.

Conclusions.—Combined therapy with clopidogrel and aspirin up to the day of surgery is not associated with increased bleeding complications or transfusion requirements. Data from this study do not validate the perceived higher risk of perioperative bleeding in clopidogrel patients and do support the strategy of continued clopidogrel use in patients undergoing peripheral arterial surgery.

▶ The study asks the important question as to whether it is safe to perform open peripheral vascular surgical procedures on patients with dual antiplatelet therapy, a particularly relevant question given the widespread use of drug-eluting coronary stents. The previous data supporting the cessation (or continuation) of clopidogrel are limited for peripheral procedures despite the fairly conclusive evidence for coronary artery bypass procedures. However, it is important to emphasize that most peripheral procedures (with the possible exception of complex aneurysm repairs) are dramatically different from coronary procedures in terms of bleeding risk given the use of cardiopulmonary bypass with the larger obligatory heparin requirement and the impact of the bypass circuit on platelet function. The results of the current prospective trial suggest that dual antiplatelet therapies are not associated with a higher rate of either the primary (reoperation for bleed, bleeding-related death) or secondary (transfusion, hematoma, procedure duration, length of stay) endpoints. Furthermore, the findings were consistent when the procedures were broken down by aortic reconstructions, lower extremity revascularization, and carotid endarterectomy. These results must be interpreted with some caution because the procedures were all performed by a single surgeon, and a variety of potentially nonstandard techniques were implemented at the time of the operation to reduce the bleeding complications including a reduced dose of heparin (35–50 U/kg), topical biological sealants, topical oxidized cellulose, and strict blood pressure control. Indeed, the reoperation rate for bleeding was impressively low (<1%) for all patients, regardless of their antiplatelet therapies. Additionally, the study design was purely observational and fell short of the "gold standard" randomized controlled trial. Lastly, the sample sizes for the relative subgroups (eg, carotid endarterectomy) were small and therefore at risk for a type II error, particularly among the aortic reconstruction patients. Despite these limitations, the study is reassuring for those vascular surgeons who are comfortable operating on patients with dual antiplatelet therapies, and it provides justification for the practice among those who are reluctant. In our own practice, we have continued the patients' clopidogrel, believing that it is easier to manage most bleeding-related complications than those related to thrombosis.

T. S. Huber, MD, PhD

13 General Thoracic Surgery

Intra-Operative Concerns

Subxiphoid pericardial window to exclude occult cardiac injury after penetrating thoracoabdominal trauma

Hommes M, Nicol AJ, van der Stok J, et al (Univ of Cape Town, South Africa; Erasmus Univ Med Centre, Rotterdam, The Netherlands)

Br J Surg 100:1454-1458, 2013

Background.—An occult cardiac injury may be present in patients with an acute abdomen after penetrating thoracoabdominal trauma. This study assessed the use of a subxiphoid pericardial window (SPW) as a diagnostic manoeuvre in this setting.

Methods.—This was a retrospective review of a trauma database (2001–2009). Patients presenting with a penetrating thoracoabdominal injury with an acute abdomen, and in whom there was concern about a potential cardiac injury from the site or tract of the injury, were included.

Results.—Fifty patients with an indication for emergency laparotomy underwent a SPW for a possible cardiac injury. An occult haemopericardium was present at SPW in 14 patients (28 per cent) mandating, median sternotomy. Nine cardiac injuries (18 per cent) were identified including five tangential injuries and four perforations. The specific complication rate relating to the SPW was 2 per cent.

Conclusion.—The SPW is a useful technique at laparotomy to identify cardiac injuries in patients with penetrating thoracoabdominal injuries.

▶ The authors review an 8-year experience of patients presenting at their center with a penetrating thoracoabdominal injury and an acute abdomen in whom there was also concern of a concurrent cardiac injury. Patients presenting in this scenario have a 20% to 30% chance of concurrent cardiac injury if the tract of injury overlies the cardiac silhouette.

Ultrasound scan of the pericardium may have a variable sensitivity and specificity, especially if used when a left hemothorax is present. The authors advocate for a simple subxiphoid pericardial window at the time of laparotomy. Their technique included a 6-cm incision over the xiphoid and using a sponge stick to wipe away the fat pad to reveal the pericardium and allow a 4-cm opening in the pericardium.

For a subxiphoid window, I usually use cautery to separate the fat and reveal the pericardium. Allis clamps on the edge of the diaphragm or pericardium itself can elevate it and facilitate the procedure. A small rake or Army/Navy retractor to elevate the sternum also makes this easier. Because the report is related to penetrating trauma, the authors do not mention irrigation of the pericardium. However, if performing a window for blunt trauma and suspected injury, it is essential to irrigate the pericardium with warm saline and make sure the fluid returns. If it does not, concern over pericardial rupture must be considered to prevent later cardiac herniation, which may prove lethal.

The diagnosis of penetrating cardiac injury can be difficult. Physical examination can be challenging with respect to Beck's triad (hypotension, raised jugular venous pressure, and muffled heart tones) especially in the noisy environments in which these patients are often triaged. The ultrasound scan is very useful and is a readily available test in most trauma centers. However, the results are dependent on operator, machine quality, associated chest wall injuries, underlying lung disease, obesity, pneumothorax, and hemothorax. The reported sensitivity and specificity of subxiphoid window is close to 100% and should be considered if there is persistent concern of concurrent cardiac injury.

C. T. Klodell, Jr, MD

Midodrine: A Novel Therapeutic for Refractory Chylothorax

Liou DZ, Warren H, Maher DP, et al (Cedars-Sinai Med Ctr, Los Angeles, CA)
Chest 144:1055-1057, 2013

Thoracic duct injury is a rare but serious complication following surgery of the neck or chest that leads to uncontrolled chyle leak. Conventional management includes drainage, nutritional modification, or aggressive surgical interventions such as thoracic duct ligation, flap coverage, fibrin glue, or talc pleurodesis; few successful medical therapeutics are available. We report a case of a high-output chylothorax refractory to aggressive medical and surgical interventions. Chyle output decreased substantially after initiating midodrine, an $\alpha 1$-adrenergic agonist that causes vasoconstriction of the lymph system, reducing chyle flow. This case report suggests that midodrine may be a novel therapeutic for refractory chyle leaks.

▶ Thoracic duct injury is a rare but challenging complication that can occur after surgery to the neck or thorax. High-output chylous drainage can lead to metabolic, nutritional, and immunologic derangements.

The initial strategy is usually drainage of the thoracic cavity and nutritional modifications with medium-chain triglyceride diet of total parenteral nutrition. Some successful pharmacologic interventions have also been reported.

Often these less invasive strategies may fail, leading to surgical approaches, including muscle flaps, direct suture of the leak site, talc pleurodesis, or ligation of the thoracic duct at the level of the diaphragm. The ligation of the thoracic duct at the diaphragm has been reported to have an 80% success rate and is considered the most effective approach.

The authors present a case report of persistent chyle leak after several failed surgical attempts. They report the use of the alpha agonist midodrine and achieved successful closure of the leak. The theorized benefit is centered on the alpha-agonist property, which causes smooth muscle contraction and may result in reduced diameter of the lymphatic channels leading to the area of the leak. As the authors point out, midodrine is a readily available oral agent with an alpha-selective adrenergic effect that is usually prescribed for orthostatic or dialysis-induced hypotension. In past editions of the YEAR BOOK, we included other studied remedies for chylothorax, including lymphoscintigraphy. Midodrine may be another arrow in the surgeon's quiver as an additional pharmacologic agent to try for potential chylothorax resolution before proceeding to duct ligation.

C. T. Klodell, Jr, MD

State of the Art of Robotic Thymectomy

Ismail M, Swierzy M, Rückert JC (Universitätsmedizin Berlin - Charitè Campus Mitte, Germany)

World J Surg 37:2740-2746, 2013

Background.—Thymectomy is a widely accepted treatment for most cases of myasthenia gravis and essential for the treatment of thymoma. The development of a minimally invasive procedure for thymectomy resulted in a variety of approaches for surgery on the thymic gland. The use of thoracoscopy-based techniques has continued to increase, including the latest advance in this field, robotic thymectomy.

Methods.—We review the rapid development and actual use of this approach by examining published reports, worldwide registries, and personal communications and by analyzing our database, which is the largest single-center experience and contains 317 thymectomies until 12/2012. The technical modifications of robotic thymectomy are also described.

Results.—Since 2001, approximately 3,500 robotic thymectomies have been registered worldwide. Meanwhile, the results of approximately 500 thymectomy cases have been published. Robotic thymectomy is performed most frequently through a standardized unilateral three-trocar approach. All reports describe promising and satisfactory results for myasthenia gravis. For early-stage thymoma, robotic thymectomy is a technically sound and safe procedure with a very low complication rate and short hospital stay. Oncological outcome without recurrences is promising, but a longer follow-up is needed.

Conclusion.—The unilateral robotic technique can be considered an adequate approach for thymectomy, even with demanding anatomical configurations. Robotic thymectomy has spread worldwide over the last decade because of the promising results in myasthenia gravis and thymoma patients.

▶ Complete thymectomy is essential in treatment of myasthenia gravis (MG) and may be desirable in patients with thymoma. Although stenotomy is considered essential for radical thymectomy by some, many other approaches have been developed in attempts to progressively reduce the invasiveness to the patient. Da Vinci robotic technology has advanced the field of thoracoscopic surgery and may potentially offer advantages beyond thoracoscopic thymectomy, as it allows for advanced visualization potentially leading to more radical thymectomy when compared with thoracoscopic technique.

The authors describe their center's approach to robotic thymectomy and provide a literature search highlighting suggestions for improved technique. The procedure is performed under general anesthetic with a single lung ventilation technique. The patient is positioned at the edge of the table with a 30° anti-decubitus position, and the ipsilateral limb is placed below the level of the table with flexion at the elbow utilizing a beanbag. Most centers perform this procedure with only 3 ports; however, some do utilize a fourth port. The authors advocate for a left-sided approach; however, there is controversy in many centers preferring the right-sided approach. The authors point out that in difficult dissection, they may elect to place a thoracoscope on the contralateral side to further enhance the visualization and safety of the procedure. In general, the camera port of the Da Vinci is placed in the fourth intercostal space at the midaxillary line, and a 30° camera is usually selected. The cephalad port is usually placed in the third intercostal at the anterior axillary line, whereas the more caudal port is usually placed between the midaxillary line and the anterior axillary line in the fifth intercostal space. The authors prefer to do the dissection using an ultrasonic dissector and a bipolar forceps. They use CO_2 insufflation to a pressure of 7 or 8 mm Hg and perform an en bloc resection of all thymic tissue, which is then removed through the 12-mm port site using an endobag. The authors additionally point out a technical pearl in that they routinely open the contralateral pleural cavity to prevent pneumothorax.

We have also utilized many of these same techniques, and the Da Vinci robotic thymectomy is our preferred choice for thymic resection unless contraindications are present. As the authors point out, many centers have selected a thoracic grasper and monopolar cautery as the instruments of choice, although I find the use of the bipolar or ultrasonic dissector quite useful in skeletonizing the innominate vein.

Critics of the robotic procedure have raised concerns about the radicality or completeness of the procedure, the safety of the procedure, its costs, and, not the least of which, the lack of robust data. Few will argue against robotic thymectomy as the surgical technique with the lowest level of invasiveness. The enhanced visualization of the Da Vinci robotic system offers significant advantages over thoracoscopy in my opinion. The instruments are quite intuitive to use, and the wristed tips allow the fulcrum effect of minimally invasive surgery to be avoided. With thymoma patients, the robotic-assisted approach allows for careful attention to the oncologic approach of no-touch dissection.

One interesting finding of the authors is the impressive increase in the number of robotic thymectomies being performed annually, with nearly 1000 robotic thymectomies performed in 2012, according to the manufacturer of the technology. It is estimated by the authors that there must be in excess of 100 centers offering this technique. With this tremendous increase in the number of robotic thymectomies and the number of centers performing robotic thymectomy, care must be placed on defining appropriate credentials and skill certification for this procedure. Although the completion of a robotic thymectomy is relatively straightforward, the technical facility with the equipment should not be overlooked in performing this procedure safely and effectively.

C. T. Klodell, Jr, MD

Complications of Bronchial Stapling in Thoracic Surgery

Yano M, Yokoi K, Numanami H, et al (Nagoya City Univ Graduate School of Med Sciences, Japan; Nagoya Univ Graduate School of Medicine, Japan; Aichi Med Univ, Nagakute, Japan; et al)

World J Surg 38:341-346, 2014

Objective.—The use of staplers for thoracic surgery has been widely accepted and regarded as a safe procedure. However, complications of stapling are occasionally experienced. The aim of this retrospective study was to analyze complications of bronchial stapling.

Methods.—A retrospective multi-institutional review was conducted by the Central Japan Lung Cancer Surgery Study Group, comprising 29 institutions. All instances of bronchial stapling in thoracic surgery were reviewed during the research period.

Results.—Bronchial stapling was performed 2,030 times, using 36 kinds of staplers. The total number of complications related to stapling was 36 (1.8 %); 31 events occurred intraoperatively and five events occurred postoperatively. The intraoperative complications were air leakage ($N = 20$) and stapling failure ($N = 11$), which were caused by stapler-tissue thickness mismatch ($N = 17$), stapler defect ($N = 3$), tissue fragility ($N = 2$), and unknown reasons ($N = 9$). In all 31 cases, intraoperative complications were recovered intraoperatively with additional suturing, and no further complications were observed postoperatively. The postoperative complications were bronchopleural fistula (BPF) ($N = 4$) and bleeding from the chest wall (intercostal artery) ($N = 1$). The rate of BPF was 0.2 % (4 of 2,030). Two of four BPFs induced critical conditions. Postoperative bleeding was caused by the use of Duet TRS™. Both total complications and BPF occurred more frequently in the main bronchus than in the lobar or segmental bronchus. No relationship was seen between the incidence of complications and cartridge colors in lobar bronchial stapling. The compression types of staplers were associated with the incidence of complication.

Conclusions.—Intraoperative and postoperative complications of bronchial stapling were studied. Generally, bronchial stapling in recent thoracic

surgery was safe, but rare postoperative complications may induce critical conditions. Knowledge of potential complications and causes of bronchial stapling may decrease the incidence of stapling complications.

▶ The ubiquitous use of staplers in surgery is undeniable, including their use during thoracic surgery for division of lung tissue, vascular structures, and the bronchus. This is especially true in minimally invasive, thoracoscopic, and robotic thoracic surgery. Although stapler use is essential for the conduct of these minimally invasive procedures, their use also facilitates the conduct and efficiency of open thoracic surgery. There has been conflicting data about the use of the various types of staplers on bronchial tissue. The authors sought to better understand this topic based on a detailed review of their experience stapling bronchial tissue 2030 times with 36 kinds of staplers. Overall complication rate was noted to be 1.8% related to stapling. However, it is critical to understand that if there is a small leak from a sutured anastomosis, additional sutures are added and it is expected. In contrast, any additional adjunctive technique required after stapling was considered a complication.

Staplers are categorized based on the type of compression. Compression can be parallel (such as TA type) or V-shaped (endostapler). Some endostaplers have a modified hinge mechanism and claim parallel compression as part of their mechanism.

In their study, all of the events that happened intraoperatively related to the staplers were easily managed and did not recur or cause postoperative complications. Interestingly, complications occurred more commonly with the parallel compression staplers, but there was no difference between stapler types with respect to development of bronchopleural fistula. Different prior studies have both confirmed and disputed this finding.

Although few surgeons choose primary suturing as the mechanism of bronchial closure during pulmonary surgery, many have strong feelings about the choice of stapler for the bronchial closure. Many surgeons trained to use only the parallel compression type (TA) stapler for bronchial closure and have great trepidation about the use of the hinge compression (endostapler) use on bronchial tissue. Similar to the findings in the author's study, I have routinely used endostaplers on the bronchus for many years. Aside from the advantages of maneuverability and articulation, they facilitate minimally invasive surgery to a greater degree than the parallel compression type stapler. Furthermore, they have the theoretical advantage of placing staples on each side of the cut line so there is never an open bronchus in the surgical field. Although this same feat can be accomplished with 2 parallel staple lines using the other type of stapler, there is often inadequate bronchial length, and it would still require cutting the bronchus with a scalpel. Although some will disagree, I see no advantage to the use of parallel compression staplers in contemporary practice of pulmonary surgery. For those who have trepidation about embracing the hinge type compression stapler, perhaps the work of these authors will prove ameliorative.

C. T. Klodell, Jr, MD

Pre- and Postoperative Management

Outcomes of endovascular repair for blunt thoracic aortic injury

Piffaretti G, Benedetto F, Menegolo M, et al (Circolo Univ Teaching Hosp, Varese, Italy; "G. Martino" Univ Teaching Hosp, Messina, Italy; et al)
J Vasc Surg 58:1483-1489, 2013

Objective.—Consistent long-term follow-up data of thoracic endovascular repair (TEVAR) for acute blunt thoracic aortic injury (BTAI) are largely absent at this time. The late outcomes of TEVAR for BTAI are the focus of this study to evaluate the durability of this type of repair.

Methods.—The records of 46 consecutive cases of TEVAR for BTAI from November 2000 to August 2012 were reviewed. Patient demographics, lesion characteristics, procedure details, and outcomes were recorded. We performed a clinical and body computed tomography angiography follow-up at 1, 6, and 12 months after the intervention; thereafter, it was done on a yearly basis if device-related defects were ruled out.

Results.—There were 35 (76.1%) males. Mean age was 39 ± 18 years (range, 17-92). Indications for intervention were BTAI at the aortic isthmus in 73.9% (n = 34) of the cases, and in the proximal one-half of the descending thoracic aorta in the remaining 26.1% (n = 12). Pseudoaneurysm or free rupture accounted for 44 (95.6%) cases. Primary technical success was obtained in all cases. All patients survived the intervention, open conversion was never required, and no patient required reintervention. In-hospital mortality was 6.5% (n = 3). Mean follow-up was 66 ± 46 months (range, 1-144; median, 72). No patient was lost during this period. All patients who were discharged from the hospital are still alive. Aortic hematoma or hemothorax were completely reabsorbed in 42 (97.7%) cases. Endoleak or modifications of the native aorta were never detected; endograft-related complication was observed in one (2.3%) case only. An asymptomatic collapse was observed at a 36-month follow-up and was managed conservatively.

Conclusions.—Midterm follow-up of TEVAR for acute BTAI is feasible with satisfactory late outcomes. In our experience, TEVAR is a durable and definitive treatment for BTAI.

▶ Thoracic endovascular repair (TEVAR) has been progressively adopted as the treatment of choice for acute blunt thoracic aortic injury. However, it has been hypothesized that, in the long term, TEVAR may be burdened by some critical concerns. There has long been talk of the progressive expansive of the aorta with aging in otherwise healthy individuals as well as device-related complications and the need for prolonged radiation exposure for appropriate surveillance. On the basis of these considerations, there is still some trepidation in confirming TEVAR as the definitive treatment for most blunt aortic injuries. The authors of this study set their aim at reviewing the late outcomes of TEVAR patients in which the TEVAR was implanted for the treatment of acute blunt thoracic aortic injury. In total, they treated 46 patients with a mean age of 39 years. An urgent intervention was required in 30 of their cases. The direct transaortic route was used in all but one patient, and all of the patients were treated with a single endograft. The left subclavian artery was partially or completely covered in 20 patients (43.5%) and was only prophylactically revascularized in one patient.

No patients died from aortic rupture while awaiting repair. The primary technical success was obtained in all cases; all patients survived the intervention. Open conversion was never required in any patient. The mean follow-up was 66 months, and no patients were lost to follow-up during this period. The authors report that the hematoma or hemothorax was completely reabsorbed in 98% of the cases and that there was only one patient with an endograft-related complication, which was a collapse of the endograft at the 36-month follow-up point in an asymptomatic patient.

The most important parts of this study are the length of follow-up and the complete adherence to the radiographic follow-up. Additionally, the absence of significant changes to the native aorta helps ameliorate some of the concerns about the mechanical forces of an endograft on an otherwise healthy aorta. In fact, the recent guidelines of the Society for Vascular Surgery recognize the use of TEVAR for blunt thoracic aortic injuries as being associated with improved outcomes compared with open repair. However, there are concerns related to late outcomes in patients exposed to this technology. In this report and in our own center's experience, TEVAR for the treatment of acute blunt thoracic aortic injuries certainly has very gratifying acute short-term and satisfying mid term results. Again, both in this study and in our own experience it has been found that complete adherence to follow-up is quite feasible. Although the long-term results of TEVAR for blunt trauma aortic injury still await complete elucidation, it would appear that the late complication rate is low, and that the concerns about the changes of the morphology of the aorta exposed to prolonged endograft seem unsubstantiated, at least in this review and in our center's experience.

C. T. Klodell, Jr, MD

Chylothorax Complicating Pulmonary Resection for Lung Cancer: Effective Management and Pleurodesis

Cho HJ, Kim DK, Lee GD, et al (Gachon Univ Gil Med Ctr, Incheon; Univ of Ulsan College of Medicine, Seoul, Korea)
Ann Thorac Surg 97:408-413, 2014

Background.—Chylothorax associated with pulmonary resection for lung cancer, although rare, must be considered as a potential complication during thoracic surgery. In the present study, we investigated the effectiveness of a conservative approach (diet or pleurodesis) to the management of chylothorax.

Methods.—Between January 2000 and December 2010, 3,120 consecutive patients underwent pulmonary resection and mediastinal lymph node dissection at our institution. Among them, 67 patients with confirmed chylothorax were retrospectively reviewed.

Results.—Right-sided chylothorax was more common than left-sided chylothorax ($p = 0.033$). All patients were initially treated with nil per os (NPO; n = 46) or a low long-chain triglyceride (LCT) diet (n = 21). In the NPO group, 24 patients were successfully treated with diet alone and 20 underwent pleurodesis. In the LCT group, 10 patients were successfully treated with diet alone; of the 11 remaining patients, 4 patients improved after NPO. The 7 patients who did not improve with NPO underwent pleurodesis. No significant differences in chest tube output before and after initial treatment, length of stay, or success rate were observed between patients initially treated with NPO and those receiving low LCT. All 32 pleurodeses performed in 27 patients were successful. Two patients underwent surgery without pleurodesis after dietary treatment failure. Postoperative air leakage or drainage for 5 days greater than 21.6 mL/kg were independent risk factors for dietary treatment failure.

Conclusions.—Conservative treatment, including pleurodesis, should be the first choice of treatment for chylothorax complicating pulmonary resection.

▶ Chylothorax after pulmonary resection is fortunately a relatively uncommon problem but one that many of us have seen in clinical practice. Chylothorax is less common after pulmonary surgery than it is after aortic surgery or esophagectomy, and its occurrence may be increased with the magnitude of mediastinal lymphadenectomy. It may have a more favorable prognosis with conservative measures compared with other etiologies, as it is unlikely that the main thoracic duct has been injured during pulmonary resection. In this series, the authors report a relatively high rate of chylothorax (2.1%), which is significantly higher than that in many other series. However, they also point out their aggressive lymph node strategy in all patients. When chylothorax does occur, the initial treatment is complete pleural drainage and nothing by mouth with total parenteral nutrition, a medium change triglyceride diet, or a low-fat diet.

A major strength of the authors' approach is they identify the 50% of patients who do not respond to conservative treatment relatively early and transition them from just dietary modification to potentially pleurodesis. One interesting statistical finding was a correlation of a 5-day chest tube output in excess of 21.6 mL/kg or an average of just more than 300 mL/d in a 70-kg patient being predictive of conservative treatment failure. Additionally, they noted that an ongoing air leak was a risk factor for dietary management failure.

When conservative management has failed, many additional options are available for treatment, including minimally invasive exploration with identification and clipping of the site of the leak or main thoracic duct ligation, pleurodesis, and, in some centers, lymphoscintigraphy and percutaneous thoracic duct embolization. Also recently reported has been the use of pharmacologic agents and α agents such as midodrine. The authors are fairly quick to move to chemical pleurodesis and impressively were able to achieve resolution of the chylothorax in all patients, although they did have several patients who required repeat procedures. However, this may prove to be suboptimal in some patients who may later require repeat surgery on the side that has now had a pleurodesis. Additionally, a major caveat in patients with large-volume leaks of more than 1 L/d, pleurodesis is often not effective. The authors should still be commended for this important contribution in that their study is specific to patients undergoing pulmonary resection, and they have a consistent and algorithmic approach to managing the chylothorax.

Also helpful is that the authors were able to delineate a quantitative amount over which conservative management is more likely to fail to allow the opportunity to rapidly decide if a more aggressive approach is warranted.

C. T. Klodell, Jr, MD

Low-fat diet management strategy for chylothorax after pulmonary resection and lymph node dissection for primary lung cancer

Takuwa T, Yoshida J, Ono S, et al (Natl Cancer Ctr Hosp East, Kashiwa, Chiba, Japan)

J Thorac Cardiovasc Surg 146:571-574, 2013

Objective.—We reviewed our experience of iatrogenic chylothorax after pulmonary resection for primary lung cancer to evaluate a low-fat diet management strategy.

Methods.—From October 2003 to March 2010, 1580 patients underwent lobectomy or greater resection and systematic mediastinal lymph node dissection for primary lung cancer at our institution. Chylothorax was diagnosed on the basis of chylous leakage from the chest tube and was confirmed by presence of triglycerides (>110 mg/dL) in the drainage fluid. We initially treated the patients with chylothorax conservatively with a low-fat diet (fat intake <10 g/day). If chest tube drainage produced >500 mL of chylous fluid during the first 24 hours after the initiation of the low-fat diet, surgical intervention was performed. If chest tube drainage produced >300 mL/day of chylous fluid after 3 days of a low-fat diet, we performed pleurodesis by injecting a preparation of OK-432, a penicillin-treated lyophilized preparation of a *Streptococcus* strain into the thoracic cavity through a chest tube.

Results.—Postoperative chylothorax developed in 37 patients (2.3%), 33 men and 4 women, with a median age of 69 years (range, 44-84). The initial procedures were pneumonectomy in 1 patient and lobectomy in 36 patients. In 23 patients (62%), their condition resolved with the low-fat diet only. A total of 10 patients underwent OK-432 pleurodesis, and 8 of these were cured with continuation of the low-fat diet. These 31 patients who responded to conservative treatment (84%) resumed a normal diet at a median of 10 days (range, 5-27) after the chylothorax diagnosis. The remaining 6 patients (16%) underwent reoperation and were discharged at a median of 18 days (range, 14-33) after the initial surgery.

Conclusions.—A low-fat diet and OK-432 pleurodesis achieved positive results in >80% of patients with chylothorax after pulmonary resection with systematic mediastinal lymph node dissection within 4 weeks after the initial surgery. More than 500 mL of chylous fluid during the first 24 hours after the initiation of the low-fat diet was valid as an indication of the need for surgical intervention.

▶ The authors reviewed their single-center experience with iatrogenic chylothorax after pulmonary resection. The diagnosis was made based on chylous leakage from the chest tube and laboratory confirmation of triglycerides greater than 110 mg/dL in the fluid. The initial treatment was with a low-fat diet ($<$10 g/d) and observation of the chest tube output. Chest tube output in excess of 500 mL over the first 24 hours on the low-fat diet prompted a return to the operating room. Output in excess of 300 mL/d for 3 days prompted a chemical pleurodesis. Lower levels of output were observed. Once the chest tube output remained serous for 24 hours, an ice cream challenge was promptly administered to ensure resolution.

In their series, postoperative chylothorax developed in 2.3% of patients, which is somewhat higher than other series have reported. A low-fat diet and chemical pleurodesis strategy as outlined achieved positive results in greater than 80% of patients. In the small number of patients in the series that required operative exploration, they report identifying a thoracic duct injury in all. They additionally ligated the thoracic duct at the level of the diaphragm as part of the operative routine if exploration was required for chylothorax.

Postoperative chylothorax is relatively rare after pulmonary resection, and as such the management strategies have not been well defined. Some have advocated for strict no oral intake and total parenteral nutrition (TPN). However, TPN is not without its own set of complications. More recently, there have been reports of success with a low-fat diet that are equal to that obtained with TPN. Given that chylothorax has been reported as a complication of neck dissection, cardiac surgery, pulmonary surgery, and esophagectomy, a broad range of practicing surgeons can see this complication. An initial conservative approach to management seems appropriate, reserving reoperation for only the most severe and recalcitrant cases. I have found success with doxycycline chemical pleurodesis with roughly the same treatment algorithm as the authors describe. Other potential interventions include the therapeutic use of lymphoscintigraphy, which we reviewed in last year's Year Book, as well as the α-adrenergic agent, midodrine. Careful consideration of all these tools in our armamentarium is essential to help manage this uncommon but challenging complication.

C. T. Klodell, Jr, MD

Does External Pleural Suction Reduce Prolonged Air Leak After Lung Resection? Results From the AirINTrial After 500 Randomized Cases

Leo F, Duranti L, Girelli L, et al (Centre Hospitalier de Périgueux, France; Fondazione IRCCS Istituto Nazionale dei Tumori, Milano, Italy)

Ann Thorac Surg 96:1234-1239, 2013

Background.—External pleural suction is used after lung resection to promote lung expansion and minimize air leak duration. Published randomized trials failed to prove this advantage but they are limited in number and underpowered in many cases. The aim of the AirINTrial study was to test the hypothesis that external pleural suction may reduce the rate of prolonged air leak in a large, randomized cohort.

Methods.—All candidates for lung resection (with the exception of pneumonectomy) were considered eligible for this single-center study. At the end of operation, patients were stratified by the type of resection (anatomic versus nonanatomic) and randomly allocated into the external suction arm (−15 cm H_2O, group A) or into the no external suction arm (control arm, group B) in a 1:1 ratio. Chest drains were maintained for 3 days and then they were either removed or connected to an Heimlich valve, when an air leak was present. The main endpoint was to compare groups in terms of prolonged air leak (defined as the rate of patients having a chest drain still in place by postoperative day 7).

Results.—Starting on February 2011, 500 patients were randomized over a 21-month period, 250 in group A and 250 in group B. Twenty-one patients in group B (8.4%) required pleural suction owing to large pneumothorax or diffuse subcutaneous emphysema. On postoperative day 7, the chest drain was still in place in 25 patients in group A and in 34 patients in group B (10% and 14%, respectively; $p = 0.2$). Subgroup analysis showed that external pleural suction reduced the prolonged air leak rate in the subgroup of patients who underwent anatomic resection (n = 296, 9.6% in group A and 16.8% in group B; $p = 0.05$).

Conclusions.—Results from the AirINTrial showed that the routine use of external suction reduces the rate of prolonged air leak after anatomic lung resection. More accurate strategies of pleural suction based on the amount of air flow and the degree of lung expansion should be probably established to improve its effectiveness.

▶ The authors present a single-center, 500-patient, randomized trial of external suction compared with no external suction on the chest tube after lung resection. There have been other trials related to this topic, but controversy remains. Some surgeons suggest that applying external suction to the tube(s) promotes full expansion of the lung and obliteration of the air space, thereby forcing apposition of the visceral and parietal pleura and earlier closure of air leaks. Conversely, others suggest that active suction on the chest tubes "pulls air through the leaks," thereby keeping the leaks open longer. Many of the previously published studies suggest that early removal of external suction may lead to earlier closure of air leaks.

In this trial, both groups received external suction at −15 mm Hg until the morning of postoperative day 1. At that time, suction was removed in the control group and maintained in the treatment group. On day 4, the chest tube was connected to a Heimlich valve and then removed if air was absent in the bag connected to the valve. If there was a persistent air leak, the patient was discharged with the valve in place and followed for resolution. The authors used air leak at 7 days as a hard end point, with fewer patients in the external suction group meeting this criteria (10% vs 36%).

Although there are certainly limitations to this study, it exemplifies why controversy remains regarding optimal management. Additionally, it would appear that the rate of air leak in both the treatment and control groups is higher than one would hope. This may be due to a variety of practices among surgeons in handling the fissure and to progression of techniques over time. Most surgeons today would suggest a "fissureless" technique for lobectomy, using only minimal dissection in the fissure to locate the artery and completing the fissures with an endostapler rather than by historical blunt-dissection techniques. Additionally, inspection for any raw area of lung by inflation under saline after the resection may yield a focal target for an aerostatic adjunct. Using these techniques, there is seldom an air leak beyond 48 hours or need for use of a Heimlich valve.

C. T. Klodell, Jr, MD

Optimal Timing of Thoracoscopic Drainage and Decortication for Empyema

Chung JH, Lee SH, Kim KT, et al (Korea Univ Med Ctr, Seoul, South Korea)

Ann Thorac Surg 97:224-229, 2014

Background.—Although video-assisted thoracic surgery (VATS) pleural drainage and decortication have been proven to be effective treatments in the early stages of empyema, the optimal timing of VATS is still not clear. To assess the effectiveness of early VATS drainage and decortication, we reviewed the records of patients who underwent VATS and open decortication for empyema.

Methods.—One hundred twenty-eight patients with empyema were treated with VATS and open decortication over 8 years at Korea University Anam Hospital. The VATS patients (120 patients) were divided into 3 groups based on the interval between the onset of chest symptoms and the time of operation (group 1: <2 weeks; group 2: 2 to 4 weeks; group 3: >4 weeks). Additional 8 open decortication patients with symptom durations greater than 4 weeks were compared with group 3 patients.

Results.—Groups 1 and 2 showed shorter chest tube duration, postoperative hospital stay, surgical procedure time, and fewer prolonged air leaks than group 3. No significant difference was noted between groups 1 and 2; and no difference was noted in the length of postoperative intensive care unit stays or the reintervention and reoperation rates among the 3 groups. In chronic empyema patients, group 3 showed shorter chest tube duration than the open decortication group.

Conclusions.—Patients with symptom durations of less than 4 weeks showed better early results than those with symptom durations greater than 4 weeks. Thus, symptom duration can be considered a reliable preoperative factor in deciding the surgical management of empyema or cases involving loculated pleural effusion.

► Pleural infection, including complicated pleural effusion or empyema, is a well-known potential complication associated with approximately 40% of patients with pneumonia. Most will respond to antibiotics and less-aggressive therapies; however, some will progress to the need for surgical intervention. The overall incidence of empyema appears to be increasing globally across all age ranges. Treatment strategies for initial therapy range from antibiotic treatment alone to drainage with radiographically placed pigtail catheters or chest tubes. However, for more advanced stages of empyema, including those with loculations, often surgical interventions including either minimally invasive video-assisted thoracic surgery (VATS) or open decortications are required.

Many authors have reported the effectiveness of VATS drainage as equivalent to that of open decortication in terms of resolution of empyema as well as potential advantages such as less pain and less postoperative morbidity and mortality.

The authors studied 128 patients who were treated with VATS or open drainage under general anesthesia for empyema. They performed a standard surgical approach to thoracoscopy for the management of the empyema and ultimately left two 28F chest tubes to drain the pleural space. They describe their technique as placing the first port site in the sixth or seventh intercostal site and then digitally taking down the adhesions and placing 2 additional port sites under direct vision. One addition to this technique is that I find it helpful to use sealed trocars similar to those used in laparoscopy, allowing the insufflation of carbon dioxide (CO_2). I have found the addition of CO_2 to a pressure of 10 mm Hg or less helpful in facilitating the dissection of the adhesions and compressing the otherwise diseased lung.

This study summarizes what many surgeons have recognized as the negative impact of delay of treatment for empyema. In evaluating their patients, they divided them into 3 groups according to the duration between symptom onset and the surgical procedure. Those 3 groups were segregated as less than 2 weeks, 2 to 4 weeks, and more than 4 weeks. Interestingly, even in the later stages, their data suggest that the VATS decortication can be successful. Additionally, the shorter duration between symptom onset and intervention independently predicted shorter chest tube duration and hospital stay. Patients operated on within 4 weeks suffered significantly fewer prolonged air leaks and a less prolonged recovery. Also noted in their study is the association between a higher presenting white blood cell count and negative outcomes. As a second step in their study, they compared a small group of open decortication patients with those that had late-stage VATS decortication. The only significant difference was noted to be longer chest tube duration in the open group, but essentially all other measured endpoints favored the VATS group.

This report reinforces the negative impact of delay in surgical therapy for empyema. This study suggests that patients and surgeons alike would benefit from education of primary care and referring physician so that earlier intervention can be more easily accomplished.

C. T. Klodell, Jr, MD

Miscellaneous

Randomized clinical trial of pigtail catheter *versus* chest tube in injured patients with uncomplicated traumatic pneumothorax

Kulvatunyou N, Erickson L, Vijayasekaran A, et al (Univ of Arizona, Tucson)
Br J Surg 101:17-22, 2014

Background.—Small pigtail catheters appear to work as well as the traditional large-bore chest tubes in patients with traumatic pneumothorax, but it is not known whether the smaller pigtail catheters are associated with less tube-site pain. This study was conducted to compare tube-site pain following pigtail catheter or chest tube insertion in patients with uncomplicated traumatic pneumothorax.

Methods.—This prospective randomized trial compared 14-Fr pigtail catheters and 28-Fr chest tubes in patients with traumatic pneumothorax presenting to a level I trauma centre from July 2010 to February 2012. Patients who required emergency tube placement, those who refused and those who could not respond to pain assessment were excluded. Primary outcomes were tube-site pain, as assessed by a numerical rating scale, and total pain medication use. Secondary outcomes included the success rate of pneumothorax resolution and insertion-related complications.

Results.—Forty patients were enrolled. Baseline characteristics of 20 patients in the pigtail catheter group were similar to those of 20 patients in the chest tube group. No patient had a flail chest or haemothorax. Pain scores related to chest wall trauma were similar in the two groups. Patients with a pigtail catheter had significantly lower mean(s.d.) tube-site pain scores than those with a chest tube, at baseline after tube insertion (3·2(0·6) *versus* 7·7(0·6); $P < 0·001$), on day 1 (1·9(0·5) *versus* 6·2(0·7); $P < 0·001$) and day 2 (2·1(1.1) *versus* 5·5(1·0); $P = 0·040$). The decreased use of pain medication associated with pigtail catheter was not significantly different. The duration of tube insertion, success rate and insertion-related complications were all similar in the two groups.

Conclusion.—For patients with a simple, uncomplicated traumatic pneumothorax, use of a 14-Fr pigtail catheter is associated with reduced pain at the site of insertion, with no other clinically important differences noted compared with chest tubes. Registration number: NCT01537289 (http://clinicaltrials.gov).

▶ Fewer than 10% of blunt injuries and 15% to 30% of penetrating thoracic injuries require surgical management. Most can be managed with tube thoracostomy alone to expand the lung (pneumothorax) or to drain the blood (hemothorax). The standard size used for such indications classically has been between a 32F and a 40F chest tube. These large tubes are usually inserted by a cut down technique and can be relatively traumatic during insertion, causing ongoing pain and discomfort. In contrast, pigtail catheters have been adapted for drainage, utilizing their size and Seldinger technique of insertion in hopes of decreasing both pain and discomfort. Although it is known that pigtail catheters have similar efficacy as chest tubes, the effect of tube size on insertion-related pain and subsequent site pain is not known. To that end, the authors designed this study to test the hypothesis that pigtail catheters would be associated with less tube-site pain than other chest tubes. Their eligibility criteria included an age of at least 18 years, traumatic pneumothorax requiring chest tube insertion, and a patient who was both willing to participate and conscious and able to report pain. If the patient was later noted to have a hemothorax, the patient was not enrolled in the study. Patients were randomly assigned via a sealed envelope into either the pigtail catheter or the open chest tube group, and both pigtail and chest tube were inserted at the bedside by the surgeon or a resident under the supervision of the surgeon.

The pigtail was inserted using a modified Seldinger technique, whereas the larger chest tubes were inserted using a cut down technique. In both situations, the patients did receive both local anesthetics and systemic narcotics for analgesia. Their pain was measured on a numeric rating scale, as was the total pain medication usage monitored over the first 24 hours. The primary outcomes were tube site pain after tube insertion on days 1, 2, and 3 as well as total intravenous pain medication usage. Secondary outcomes were the success rate of pneumothorax resolution and tube insertion-related complications.

The results of this randomized, prospective, 40-patient study included the fact that tube site pain was significantly lower after the pigtail insertion at baseline and subsequent time points. In fact, the 14F pigtail catheters were associated with a greater than 50% reduction in tube site pain when compared with the 28F chest tubes.

Although there are likely several reasons to explain the difference, including the tube caliber, there may be an impact of reduced tissue trauma. One major weakness of this study is that the open cut down technique was used for the 28F chest tube potentially causing some biasing of results based on the technique of insertion. Commercially available Seldinger type chest tubes are available in 28F and would have perhaps been a better comparison of the tube size impact rather than the technique impact. In fact, prior studies have noted that when comparing 28F to 32F chest tubes with 36F to 40F chest tubes, there was no difference in tube-site pain when they were all placed by cut down technique. However, the strength of this study is its prospective and randomized design and clearly showing that a small-caliber pigtail catheter placed by Seldinger technique can be effective in resolving the traumatic pneumothorax and provide excellent patient comfort.

C. T. Klodell, Jr, MD

Traumatic tricuspid valve rupture presenting as third-degree atrioventricular block

Theodoropoulos I, Cheeyandira A, Tortella BJ (Drexel Univ College of Medicine, Philadelphia, PA; Hahnemann Univ Hosp, Philadelphia, PA)
J Emerg Med 45:175-177, 2013

Background.—Cardiac valve injury after blunt chest trauma is extremely rare, and the tricuspid valve is most commonly affected because of the anterior location of the right ventricle. Tricuspid valve insufficiency can range from a subclinical presentation to acute cardiac failure.

Objective.—Diagnosis is difficult in trauma patients because hypotension is usually attributed to hemorrhage and anatomical cardiac injuries might be overlooked.

> *Case Report.*—This is a case of a 70-year-old patient with a history of rheumatic heart disease who suffered a complete rupture of her papillary muscles leading to tricuspid insufficiency after a motor vehicle collision. She presented with third-degree atrioventricular block.

Conclusions.—Consideration of screening for anatomical heart injuries in blunt trauma patients with new onset dysrhythmias is recommended to explain hypotension not attributable to hemorrhage.

▶ With the high volume of thoracic blunt trauma seen in the United States, even an uncommon injury such as traumatic tricuspid insufficiency can be seen. Although still relatively rare, this injury has been reported with increasing frequency in recent years. The acute presentation can range from fulminant acute right heart failure to minimal regurgitation diagnosed years after the event. The diagnosis can be especially difficult in trauma patients, as there are many causes for hypotension often present.

Blunt cardiac injury itself is most frequently associated with motor vehicle collisions, with a cardiac contusion being the most common. Tricuspid valve insufficiency after blunt trauma is extremely rare, with a previous report finding only one such injury in more than 6000 admissions.

The tricuspid valve is the most commonly affected heart valve, with about 200 cases reported in the literature. Anatomically, this makes sense given the immediate retrosternal position of the right ventricle and the relative fragility of the tricuspid valve and subvalvular apparatus compared with the other heart valves. It is theoretically possible that when force is applied to the heart during systole, when the atrial ventricular valves are closed there may be sufficient force to rupture the valvular apparatus or valve itself. Chordal rupture is the most frequently reported injury, followed by rupture of the anterior papillary muscle or the leaflet itself. Valve function may be only minimally altered by rupture of 1 or 2 chordae, leading to delayed presentation. However, rupture of the papillary muscle leads to a flail segment of the leaflet and severe insufficiency acutely. Patients with otherwise normal hearts before their injury have relatively normal right atrial size and poorly tolerate this now acute high-volume regurgitant fraction.

Any new onset dysrhythmias associated with trauma may also be a warning sign of associated cardiac injury. This may range from sinus tachycardia to atrial fibrillation or, as the authors present, third-degree atrioventricular block. Anatomically, it would make sense for atrial ventricular block to be an associated finding with tricuspid valve injury given the proximity of the tricuspid valve annulus to the atrial ventricular node. The atrial ventricular node is located very near the septal leaflet of the tricuspid valve and, depending on the mechanism of injury, could easily be injured. Because of the relatively uncommon occurrence of this injury, we must all remain vigilant to ensure this diagnosis is not missed. Cardiac ultrasound scan is often the preferred screening method. However, transthoracic echocardiography may be difficult to obtain appropriate windows given concomitant chest wall injuries and mechanical ventilation in these multiply injured patients. For these reasons, coupled with a high index of suspension should be a low threshold to request transesophageal echocardiography. Operative repair or replacement of the valve will be required if the concomitant injuries permit. Consideration will have to be given to any associated head injuries especially, as cardiopulmonary bypass will be required with full heparinization. With this caveat, surgical correction of traumatic valvular insufficiency should be relatively straightforward if the concomitant injuries are stable.

C. T. Klodell, Jr, MD

Outcomes of Cholecystectomy in US Heart Transplant Recipients

Kilic A, Sheer A, Shah AS, et al (The Johns Hopkins Hosp, Baltimore, MD)
Ann Surg 258:312-317, 2013

Objective.—The aim of this study was to evaluate outcomes and predictors of in-hospital mortality after cholecystectomy in heart transplant (HTx) recipients.

Background.—There is a paucity of data on outcomes after cholecystectomy in HTx recipients.

Methods.—The Nationwide Inpatient Sample (NIS) database was used to identify HTx recipients who underwent cholecystectomy between 1998 and 2008. Multivariate logistic regression analysis was constructed using clinically relevant covariates (age, gender, Charlson comorbidity index, race, admission acuity, complicated gallstone disease, hospital teaching status, and open versus laparoscopic approach) to identify predictors of in-hospital mortality.

Results.—A total of 1687 HTx recipients underwent cholecystectomy (open $n = 420$; laparoscopic $n = 1267$) during the study period. Mean age was 57.1 ± 12.5 years, and there were 1230 (72.9%) males. The majority of patients had acute cholecystitis ($n = 1218$; 72.2%) and were admitted urgently/emergently ($n = 1028$; 60.9%). Overall inpatient mortality occurred in 37 (2.2%) patients, with a higher mortality rate in open cholecystectomy compared with laparoscopic (6.2% vs. 0.9%; $P = 0.009$), and in urgent/emergent versus elective cases (3.6% vs. 0%; $P = 0.04$). Open or urgent/emergent cholecystectomies also had higher overall complication and respiratory failure rates as compared with laparoscopic or elective cases. Predictors of inpatient mortality in multivariable analysis included urgent/emergent admission, open cholecystectomy, and complicated gallstone disease (each $P < 0.05$).

Conclusions.—This is the largest reported study to date of cholecystectomy in HTx recipients. HTx patients appear to be at increased risk of inpatient mortality and morbidity after cholecystectomy as compared with the general population, and this rate is particularly high in those with a nonelective admission who undergo open cholecystectomy for complicated gallstone disease. Therefore, strong consideration should be given to prophylactic cholecystectomy in HTx recipients with asymptomatic and uncomplicated gallstone disease.

► The authors report on a decade-long national inpatient sample of US heart transplant recipients who underwent cholecystectomy. Logistic regression analysis is used to define the predictors of in-hospital mortality. Most of the patients had acute cholecystitis, and were admitted urgently. Predictors of mortality included urgent/emergent status, open cholecystectomy, and complicated gallstone disease.

There continues to be a plateau in heart transplantation rate at approximately 2500 recipients annually. It is well known that heart transplant recipients are at increased risk of gallstone formation, likely related to weight changes, immunosuppressant drugs, and the presence of diabetes and coronary artery disease. Some controversy remains across the country as to the best management of potential heart transplant recipients with asymptomatic cholelithiasis. Some groups have advocated treating these patients like the general population, with expectant management, whereas others advocate for cholecystectomy, given the increased risks of complications should cholecystitis develop after transplantation.

In their review, the overall mortality rate after cholecystectomy was 2.2%, although the mortality rate was higher after open vs laparoscopic approaches (6.2% vs 0.9%), as was the major complication rate (17.1% open vs 6.5% laparoscopic). All patients with inpatient mortality also had complicated gallstone disease.

Their analysis of the sample suggests the annual rate of cholecystectomy in heart transplant recipients to be 7.7%, which is much higher than that of the general population.

The issue of how to manage symptomatic cholelithiasis or complicated gallstone disease is straightforward and agreed upon. However, the question of the potential transplant patient with asymptomatic cholelithiasis remains. The author's conclusion that all heart transplant candidates with gallstones should undergo cholecystectomy irrespective of symptoms seems reasonable. This strategy would eliminate the need for multiple ultrasound scans and minimize the risk of developing severe biliary complications. It would also eliminate much of the impact of operating on these patients while immunosuppressed, with the tradeoff that their cardiac function is poorer than it will be after transplantation.

This is the largest study to date examining the outcome of cholecystectomy in heart transplant patients. Although the overall mortality rate is relatively low (2.2%), the data suggest that cholecystectomy may be warranted in all stable potential heart transplant candidates.

C. T. Klodell, MD

Operative Management of Rib Fractures in the Setting of Flail Chest: A Systematic Review and Meta-Analysis

Leinicke JA, Elmore L, Freeman BD, et al (Washington Univ School of Medicine, St Louis, MO)

Ann Surg 258:914-921, 2013

Objective.—To perform a systematic review and meta-analysis of studies comparing operative to nonoperative therapy in adult FC patients. Outcomes were duration of mechanical ventilation (DMV), intensive care unit length of stay (ICULOS), hospital length of stay (HLOS), mortality, incidence of pneumonia, and tracheostomy.

Background.—Flail chest (FC) results in paradoxical chest wall movement, altered respiratory mechanics, and frequent respiratory failure. Despite advances in ventilatory management, FC remains associated with significant morbidity and mortality. Operative fixation of the flail segment has been advocated as an adjunct to supportive care, but no definitive clinical trial exists to delineate the role of surgery.

Methods.—A comprehensive search of 5 electronic databases was performed to identify randomized controlled trials and observational studies (cohort or case-control). Pooled effect size (ES) or relative risk (RR) was calculated using a fixed or random effects model, as appropriate.

Results.—Nine studies with a total of 538 patients met inclusion criteria. Compared with control treatment, operative management of FC was associated with shorter DMV [pooled ES: −4.52 days; 95% confidence interval (CI): −5.54 to −3.50], ICULOS (−3.40 days; 95% CI: −6.01 to −0.79), HLOS (−3.82 days; 95% CI: −7.12 to −0.54), and decreased mortality (pooled RR: 0.44; 95% CI: 0.28–0.69), pneumonia (0.45; 95% CI: 0.30–0.69), and tracheostomy (0.25; 95% CI: 0.13–0.47).

Conclusions.—As compared with nonoperative therapy, operative fixation of FC is associated with reductions in DMV, LOS, mortality, and complications associated with prolonged MV. These findings support the need for an adequately powered clinical study to further define the role of this intervention.

► Flail chest (defined as fracture of 3 or more sequential ribs in 2 or more locations) results in paradoxical movement of the chest wall and leads to altered respiratory mechanics and potentially respiratory failure. Patients with a flail chest often have a prolonged hospitalization, prolonged ventilator support, and intensive care unit (ICU) stays, which may be associated with significant morbidity, mortality, and health care costs.

The standard treatment has been pulmonary toilet, excellent pain control, and ventilator support if required. Various studies reported on the impact of operative fixation of the flail chest and the impact on outcome and other variables. These studies have resulted in conflicting results as to the risks and benefits of operative fixation of the flail chest.

The authors undertook a meta-analysis to compare operative and nonoperative management of flail chest. The primary outcome was duration of mechanical ventilation, with secondary outcomes of ICU length of stay, hospital length of stay, mortality, incidence of pneumonia, and rate of tracheostomy.

Initially identifying 1407 studies, ultimately 9 studies met inclusion criteria. These included 2 randomized controlled trials, 4 cohort studies, and 3 case-control studies. These studies involved a total of 538 patients receiving either operative fixation (n = 219) or nonoperative therapy (n = 319).

In their analysis, operative management was associated with reductions in duration of mechanical ventilation, ICU length of stay, hospital length of stay, mortality, pneumonia, and the rate of tracheostomy.

In a recent survey of opinions, only 33% of responding surgeons felt operative fixation was indicated after 7 days of ventilator support. This study suggests that operative fixation of flail chest has a beneficial effect and perhaps should be considered sooner in the course. Theoretically, the earlier the flail segment is repaired the more mitigation of the deleterious consequences that might be gained. Conversely, intervention performed later in the course may yield diminishing returns.

Although meta-analysis is not intended to guide clinical practice, this study confirms the anecdotal experience of many trauma surgeons. It seems prudent to consider early fixation for flail chest. Moreover, I am often referred patients months after flail chest with either chronic pain or problematic motion of the chest wall with poor healing. The operative fixation of poorly healed rib fractures is perhaps more challenging than repair at the time of the initial injury, which may be another factor to consider when selecting therapeutic options for flail chest.

C. T. Klodell, Jr, MD

Hemorrhagic Complications of Thoracentesis and Small-Bore Chest Tube Placement in Patients Taking Clopidogrel

Mahmood K, Shofer SL, Moser BK, et al (Duke Univ Med Ctr, Durham, NC)
Ann Am Thorac Soc 11:73-79, 2014

Rationale.—Clopidogrel is a commonly used antiplatelet medication. The risk of local hemorrhage associated with use of this drug during routine thoracentesis or small-bore chest tube placement is not well established.

Objectives.—We conducted a prospective cohort study to assess the risk of hemothorax in patients taking clopidogrel while undergoing either pleural procedure.

Methods.—Twenty-five consecutive adult patients who were taking clopidogrel at the time they were offered thoracentesis or small-bore (14 Fr) chest tube placement consented to continue taking the drug through their procedure. A control group consisted of 50 patients undergoing these pleural procedures who were not taking clopidogrel at the time they consented to undergo either procedure. All of the pleural procedures were performed under ultrasound guidance by an interventional pulmonologist or a fellow under direct faculty supervision. Hospitalized patients were screened for hemothorax by observing for a post-procedure drop in blood hemoglobin content of 2 g/dl or reaccumulation of their pleural effusion within 24 hours of the procedure. Outpatients were called within 2 weeks after their procedure to determine whether they had any symptoms suggestive of hemothorax.

Measurements and Main Results.—There was one case of hemothorax after thoracentesis in the clopidogrel group versus none in the control group. The one patient with hemothorax required transfusion with 2 units of packed red blood cells and small-bore chest tube placement, and clopidogrel was withheld. There were no other clinically apparent complications of either procedure.

Conclusions.—Considered in combination with other small previously published studies, this single-center, nonrandomized, controlled prospective cohort study suggests that the rate of clinically consequential hemorrhage after ultrasound-guided thoracentesis or chest tube placement in patients taking clopidogrel is sufficiently low to warrant a large, randomized clinical trial designed to determine the safety of performing these procedures without interrupting clopidogrel therapy.

▶ Clopidogrel is an irreversible inhibiter of the platelet adenosine diphosphate (ADP) receptor. It is widely used in the management of coronary artery disease and cerebrovascular disease, with a particular indication for preventing thrombosis of endovascular stents. More importantly, premature discontinuation of clopidogrel carries an increased risk for stent thrombosis and is associated with increased mortality. This is particularly apparent when the clopidogrel is indicated for drug-eluding stents placed into coronary circulation, in which case, abrupt withdrawal can lead to a higher incidence of stent thrombosis, myocardial infarction, and death. The use of clopidogrel is usually considered a contraindication for elective surgery procedures because of increased risk for sign hemorrhage. The authors conducted a prospective cohort study to assess the risks of bleeding complications with thoracentesis and small-bore chest tube placement in patients taking clopidogrel and compared their risks with a simultaneously selected control group not using clopidogrel at the time of their procedure.

In all patients, they used ultrasound scan to select the best access site, although it was usually in the midaxillary or midscapular line. In total, they enrolled 25 patients in the clopidogrel group and 50 in the control group. Most clopidogrel patients were also receiving aspirin therapy. One patient in the 25 patients on clopidogrel did develop a hemothorax that was managed with drainage, whereas none of the patients not taking the clopidogrel developed this complication.

Thoracentesis and chest tube placement are relatively safe procedures when performed correctly by experienced clinicians. Hemothorax is a recognized complication that occurs in approximately 1% of patients; however, in this study, one patient of 25 (4%) developed hemothorax while taking clopidogrel despite an ultrasound-guided procedure.

The strength of the study is the prospective design with rigorous screening for postprocedure bleeding, and a major limitation is the telephone follow-up they used to determine if the patient had any symptoms suggestive of a hemothorax. Routine outpatient radiographs were not routinely obtained on patients unless they developed shortness of breath or pain.

This study does highlight that the procedures can be performed safely on patients on clopidogrel with a slightly higher incidence of complications. However, it is important to highlight the deleterious consequences of the sudden cessation of clopidogrel especially in patients with drug-eluding stents. Similar studies have verified that general thoracic surgeries, such as pulmonary surgery, can be performed while on clopidogrel if required. When considering cessation of therapy in a patient with coronary stents, many factors should be considered, such as the type of stent and duration of implant. If there is any question as to the appropriateness of therapy, consultation with an interventional cardiologist can prove helpful.

C. T. Klodell, Jr, MD

Commercial Air Travel After Pneumothorax: A Review of the Literature

Bunch A, Duchateau F-X, Verner L, et al (Univ of Virginia Health System, Charlottesville; Allianz Global Assistance, Paris, France)

Air Med J 32:268-274, 2013

Because of the physiological stresses of commercial air travel, the presence of a pneumothorax has long been felt to be an absolute contraindication to flight. Additionally, most medical societies recommend that patients wait at least 2 weeks after radiographic resolution of the pneumothorax before they attempt to travel in a nonurgent fashion via commercial air transport. This review sought to survey the current body of literature on this topic to determine if a medical consensus exists; furthermore, this review considered the scientific support, if any, supporting these recommendations. In this review, we found a paucity of data on the issue and noted only a handful of prospective and retrospective studies; thus, true evidence-based recommendations are difficult to develop at this time. We have made recommendations, when possible, addressing the nonurgent commercial air travel for the patient with a recent pneumothorax. However, more scientific research is necessary in order to reach an evidence-based conclusion on pneumothoraces and flying.

► The authors review various expert opinion and literature to answer a few important questions related to nonurgent air travel after pneumothorax. The management strategies for pneumothorax are well established, although there is controversy regarding the waiting period before patients can fly on commercial flights after pneumothorax.

It is important to realize that commercial flights operate at altitudes between 28 000 and 48 000 feet usually, but do not pressurize to sea level in the cabin. For structural and fuel efficiency reasons, the cabin is often only pressurized to the equivalent of 7500 feet. This fact raises the concern that a patient with a stable or asymptomatic pneumothorax could suffer expansion and become symptomatic or even develop a tension pneumothorax. It is estimated that a pneumothorax could expand by as much as 30% under these circumstances.

The current guidelines are based primarily on expert opinion, as the literature is sparse on this topic. Most experts recommend a 14-day waiting period from the time of radiographic resolution of the pneumothorax until flying. Some experts suggest a 7-day waiting period may be appropriate for a spontaneous pneumothorax, but advocate for the full 14 days for traumatic pneumothorax.

In situations in which the flight is necessary for various reasons, some experts recommend the use of Heimlich valve and allowing the patient to fly with the chest tube in place. There are some that suggest a medical accompaniment should be considered.

Although based on more consensus opinion than literature, these would seem to be reasonable guidelines to follow clinically. Although not specifically mentioned, I have always held to the 14-day waiting period after pleurodesis for spontaneous pneumothorax as well.

C. T. Klodell, Jr, MD

Slipping Rib Syndrome in an Adolescent: An Elusive Diagnosis

Turcios NL (Robert Wood Johnson Univ Hosp, New Brunswick, NJ)
Clin Pediatr 52:879-881, 2013

Background.—Slipping rib syndrome is not common but is a recognized cause of recurrent pain in the lower chest or upper abdomen in adolescents. Weakness of the sternocostal, costochondral, and/or costovertebral/costotransverse ligaments permits the rib to become hypermobile. The tenth rib is affected most often, and the condition is usually unilateral but can be bilateral. Intermittent pain under the rib cage or in the upper abdomen may radiate from the costochondral area to the chest or back. The patient may report a history of trauma, but this is not always present. The pain can be sharp, intense, and last for several minutes or minor, moderately severe, or sufficient to limit activities. Sometimes a slipping or popping sensation is felt. Many laboratory and radiological tests or even laparoscopic investigations may be undertaken without making a diagnosis. Certain postures and movements result in pain, including lying or turning in bed, sitting or rising from a chair, driving, stretching, reaching, bending or twisting the trunk, coughing, walking, or lifting. Many of these signs were present in the reported case.

> *Case Report.*—Girl, 15, complained of lower chest pain that began about 3 years previously. When she lay down or turned in bed, bent or twisted her trunk area, or did deep breathing, she experienced sharp, intense, intermittent bilateral lower chest pain that radiated to the mid-lower sternum and back. One to 2 months before her visit the pain increased in intensity and frequency and interfered with sleeping and exercising. She had no history of shortness of breath, dizziness, fainting, or trauma to the chest or abdomen and

had already undergone several chest x-rays and doctor visits to assess the problem.

Physical examination revealed direct bilateral tenderness over the lower costal cartilages and a positive "hooking" maneuver bilaterally that produced a bilateral clicking sound, confirming the diagnosis of bilateral slipping rib syndrome. At surgery, the lower ribs were capped in cartilage and not connected to either the sternum or adjacent ribs above and below them. The impingement of "floating" anterior ends on the intercostal nerves caused pain, so the costal cartilages were resected. The patient was pain free 3 months after surgery.

Analysis.—The differential diagnosis of slipping rib syndrome includes conditions such as cholecystitis, esophagitis, gastric ulcer, hepatosplenic problems, stress fracture, inflammation of the chondral cartilage, and pleuritic chest pain. The ability to relate the pain to certain movements or postures, a history of recent trauma, and reproduction of the symptoms with the hooking maneuver establish the diagnosis. Treatment for mild cases consists of simple reassurance, use of ice packs and/or mild pain medication to relieve symptoms coupled with temporary reduction in physical activity. Temporary relief of moderately severe pain can be obtained using a intercostal block with local anesthetics and steroids. If conservative management fails or daily activities are restricted, resection of the anterior end of the rib and costal cartilage is often successful. Intercostal nerves are preserved to avoid neuropathic pain from developing. The outcome varies.

Conclusions.—The signs and symptoms of slipping rib syndrome should be familiar to all clinicians who treat pediatric patients. With early and proper diagnosis, based on history and the hooking maneuver, patients can avoid extensive diagnostic workup and possibly months or years of chronic pain and discomfort.

▶ Slipping rib syndrome is a relatively uncommon but recognized cause of upper abdominal and lower chest pain in both adolescence and adults. The authors' present a case study of a 15-year-old girl who presented with bilateral slipping rib syndrome and review the disease, its differential diagnosis, diagnosis, and options for treatment. These patients present with what can be sharp and intense pain or what can be just a minor nuisance that is noted during exercise. They will usually describe a popping or cracking, and it's easy to understand how this mimics many types of visceral pain. This finding often leads to many laboratory and radiologic tests and multiple physician visits. It is not uncommon for these patients to be seen at some time during the workup by a general surgeon for consideration of abdominal pain. The pain often is precipitated by certain postures or movements such as lying or turning in bed, sitting or standing from a chair, driving, stretching, reaching, bending or twisting the trunk, coughing, walking, or lifting.

The differential diagnosis of slipping rib syndrome includes myriad conditions but often can masquerade as cholecystitis, esophagitis, gastric ulcer, or hepatosplenic abnormalities. Most often, it is initially diagnosed as costochondritis or pleuritic chest pain. An important question is to ask the patient about association between certain movements or postures and pain intensity, as these are unlikely to be related to the other conditions on the differential.

It is important to remember in anatomy that ribs 1 through 7 attach directly to the sternum, whereas ribs 8, 9, and 10 are attached anteriorly by a cartilaginous cap in children and a fibrous band in adults. Most often, it is the 10th rib that has a loose connection and is affected with the slipping rib syndrome. The rib basically intermittently slips out of place causing stretching of the ligamentous support and pain. Occasionally, there is a fingerlike projection of the cartilaginous structure that passes essentially deep to the costal margin and can cause persistent irritation. The diagnosis is facilitated by what is called the hooking maneuver as originally described by Heinz and Zavala. This technique involves placing the fingers under the costal margin of the patient on the side in question and pulling outward and upward. A positive test result is diagnostic and causes pain and a click of the loose rib.

If the pain is only minor, a conservative approach of nonsteroidal anti-inflammatory drugs may be appropriate. For more severe pain, intercostal blocks with local anesthetics and even steroids may be helpful. If these conservative measures fail, then surgical intervention with resection of the anterior edge rib and the costal cartilage may be performed, which in my experience has yielded excellent outcomes. It is important during this procedure to preserve the intercostal nerves to ensure that there is no postprocedure neuropathic pain. These procedures can almost always be done in the outpatient setting, but I find are best done in the operating room with monitored anesthesia care or general anesthetic.

Although I have usually not included case studies in the YEAR BOOK, this one provides a review of a very important condition. I see 1 to 2 cases of slipping rib syndrome each year. Often the patients have sought medical attention for months to years and have seen many physicians. As the authors point out, it is not uncommon for the patients to have been seen by a general surgeon, and some have undergone diagnostic laparoscopy in search of an etiology of the upper abdominal pain. I hope this review helps remind us of the seldom-seen, important-to-diagnose, slipping rib syndrome and the relatively easy treatment algorithm.

C. T. Klodell, Jr, MD

Arterial Thoracic Outlet Syndrome: A 32-Year Experience

Marine L, Valdes F, Mertens R, et al (Pontificia Universidad Católica de Chile, Santiago)

Ann Vasc Surg 27:1007-1013, 2013

Background.—Clinical manifestations of thoracic outlet syndrome (TOS) differ depending on the compromised anatomic structure. Arterial

TOS is the least common (1-5% of all cases of TOS), yet the most threatening, due to the risk of limb loss.

Methods.—We conducted a retrospective review of consecutive patients treated for arterial TOS between January 1979 and June 2012. Medical records and diagnostic images were reviewed, and follow-up was obtained.

Results.—Nineteen procedures were performed in 18 patients for symptomatic arterial TOS. The average age was 34 years (range 16–69 years), and 12 patients were female (63.2%). Surgical indications were upper limb critical ischemia in 8 (acute in 5 cases and acute-on-chronic in 3 cases) and claudication in 11. Imaging studies revealed a subclavian aneurysm in 7 patients, stenosis in 4 patients, and 2 patients with subclavian artery occlusion. The 6 remaining cases had symptoms caused by arterial compression in dynamic studies without arterial wall damage at rest. All limbs underwent surgery with outlet decompression; in addition, 13 underwent arterial reconstruction, and 7 were treated for distal embolic complications. There were no deaths, amputations, or early reoperations; 1 patient was readmitted 2 weeks after surgery for chylothorax, which resolved with conservative measures. During a mean follow-up of 155.8 ± 103.1 months, 1 patient underwent successful reintervention at 4 months for bypass occlusion.

Conclusions.—Arterial TOS is an infrequent but relevant manifestation of TOS. An accurate and early diagnosis allows for timely surgery and adequate results, as shown in this group of patients.

▶ Thoracic outlet syndrome (TOS) is a constellation of signs and symptoms related to compression of either vascular or neural structures of the upper limb at the point where they cross the neck and thorax through a compact anatomic space surround by bone, ligaments, and muscle. The 3 forms TOS depend on the structure compressed including the brachial plexus roots, the subclavian vein or artery, or neural structures. Neurogenic TOC is the most frequent clinical expression of this disease process. Arterial TOS is the least common but may be the most severe because damage to the arterial wall leads to stenosis or aneurysm, eventually causing limb-threatening ischemia.

The authors performed a retrospective study of consecutive patients who were treated for TOS of the arterial subtype over a 32-year period. During the study period, 82 TOS patients were treated using decompressive surgeries in 90 limbs. Neurogenic TOS predominated as expected with nearly 56% of the cases; venous TOS made up 23% of the cases, and arterial TOS constituted 21% of cases. The authors attribute the high percentage of arterial TOS to being an arterial referral center for the region. The mean age of the arterial TOS patients was 34 years, and all patients complained of ischemic pain at presentation or intermittent claudication in the extremity. The imaging studies confirmed a cervical rib in 9 of the cases, and in 7 of the cases, the subclavian aneurysm presented with a distal embolization. Of those 7, 6 presented with critical ischemia.

The authors' surgical treatment consisted of at least 2 types of repairs: outlet decompression and subsequent arterial reconstruction. The decompression was achieved through a supraclavicular approach and a transaxillary approach in almost equal proportions. The authors should be congratulated in that they report no hospital mortality, no cases of amputation or early reintervention, and clinical success in all patients.

It is believed that TOS occurs because a subclavian artery is repeatedly compressed in the scalene triangle at the level of the first rib and at the costoclavicular space, damaging its wall. Although its incidence is relatively low, representing 5% of all TOS cases, it may have the most devastating consequences if overlooked. The repetitive trauma and chronic compression of that artery damages its wall, leading to stenosis, poststenotic dilation, and thrombosis. As represented in this study, cervical ribs are found in approximately half of the cases. Similarly, the presence of Adson sign (disappearance of the radial pulse when raising the arm, with contralateral cervical rotation, hyperextension, and deep inhalation) is reported in 10% to 20% of the asymptomatic population. Given that Adson sign may be positive in the asymptomatic population, it is critical to reinforce the clinical diagnosis with Doppler ultrasound and more commonly either computed tomography scan or magnetic resonance angiogram. Treatment should be strongly considered for all asymptomatic TOS patients with a proven arterial lesion or in symptomatic patients.

It is always recommended to resect a first rib even if a cervical rib is resected at the same time to decrease the likelihood of either concomitant or subsequent development of neurogenic TOS, which may occur in up to 30% of patients. Additional considerations in current clinical practice involve the use of endovascular treatment for aneurysm of the subclavian artery in TOS with subsequent decompression surgery to prevent stent fracture or restenosis following the procedure. Like so many fields of surgery, the best contemporary treatment for arterial TOS continues to evolve.

C. T. Klodell, Jr, MD

Benign Esophageal Disease

Esophagography After Pneumomediastinum Without CT Findings of Esophageal Perforation: Is It Necessary?

Wu C-H, Chen C-M, Chen C-C, et al (Chang Gung Univ, Gueishan, Taoyuan, Taiwan)

AJR Am J Roentgenol 201:977-984, 2013

Objective.—The purpose of our study was to determine the necessity of fluoroscopic esophagography in patients with pneumomediastinum on CT but without CT findings of esophageal perforation.

Materials and Methods.—From January 1, 2006, through December 31, 2010, there were 4305 fluoroscopic esophagography examinations including 533 with CT identified from a search of our PACS. Patients with pneumomediastinum on CT who were subsequently referred for emergent fluoroscopic esophagography to exclude esophageal perforation were enrolled. Fluoroscopic esophagography examinations performed within 3 days of CT were included. Patients with a history of esophageal disease were excluded. As a result, 103 patients were enrolled in the study; patients were divided into groups on the basis of whether there was additional clinical history of esophageal damage (trauma group) or not (nontrauma group). Images were reviewed by two board-certified radiologists blinded to the clinical data and radiologic reports for the presence or absence of esophageal perforation. A positive result on CT was defined as esophageal injury or periesophageal infiltration that coexisted with periesophageal air. A positive fluoroscopic esophagography result was defined as oral contrast medium leakage from the esophagus.

Results.—Esophageal perforation was diagnosed in 15 of the 103 patients. The CT findings were significantly correlated with esophageal perforation ($p < 0.001$ in the trauma group, and $p = 0.001$ in the nontrauma group). The respective sensitivity and negative predictive value (NPV) of CT versus fluoroscopic esophagography in the trauma group were 100% versus 66.7% and 100% versus 87.9%; in the nontrauma group, the sensitivity and NPV were 100% for CT and fluoroscopic esophagography. Thus, the sensitivity and NPV of CT were either superior or equal to those of fluoroscopic esophagography.

Conclusion.—The results of our study suggest that performing fluoroscopic esophagography in patients with pneumomediastinum is unnecessary when CT is negative for esophageal perforation.

▶ The authors set out to determine the necessity of fluoroscopic esophagography in patients with pneumomediastinum on computed tomography (CT), but without CT findings of esophageal perforation. Pneumomediastinum is a relatively common presentation in the emergency department and infrequently is the result of esophageal perforation. However, the consequences of a neglected esophageal perforation may be severe. Esophageal perforation is a life-threatening condition with a mortality rate of approximately 20%. When perforation of the esophagus is suspected, fluoroscopic esophagography is often the method of choice for diagnosis. The potential risks and logistical issues with this procedure include the need to transport to the fluoroscopy suite, multiple additional medical personnel required, and the risk of a false-negative result. There is also cause for concern related to potential aspiration of the contrast medium and deleterious consequences. In contrast, CT may be equally efficacious and does not suffer from many of these limitations. The authors point out that any leakage or periesophageal air is easily seen on CT scan and readily available to critically ill patients without delay or need for additional personnel.

The authors identified 103 patients who had a CT followed by esophagography for suspected perforation. Of these patients, 86 had contrasted CT scans and the remainder noncontrasted. Interestingly, the presence, or absence, of contrast did not correlate with the diagnostic yield or interobserver agreement. Esophageal perforation occurred most frequently in the distal cervical esophagus followed by thoracic and abdominal segments. The correlation between CT and esophagography findings was excellent, and, importantly, no perforations were missed by CT scan. Hence, the sensitivity and negative predictive value of CT scan for esophageal perforation in this series was 100%. Thoracic CT can access any periesophageal inflammation. Given the reportedly high sensitivity and negative predictive value in detecting aerodigestive tract perforations in patients with pneumomediastinum, it would seem reasonable to utilize this as the primary diagnostic modality and reserve esophagography for only select cases.

C. T. Klodell, Jr, MD

Tumor Biology and Prognostic Variables

Does the Mode of Surgical Resection Affect the Prognosis/Recurrence in Patients With Thymoma?

Nakagawa K, Asamura H, Sakurai H, et al (Natl Cancer Ctr Hosp, Tokyo, Japan)
J Surg Oncol 109:179-183, 2014

Background.—Among the various controversies in the treatment strategies for patients with thymoma, the optimal mode of resection needs to be defined. To explore whether or not the mode of resection affects the prognosis/recurrence in patients with thymoma, we evaluated the treatment outcome of patients with resected thymoma.

Methods.—One hundred seventy-three nonmyasthenic patients with stage I or II resected thymoma were studied. Patients were divided into two groups: a thymomectomy (resection of thymoma without total thymectomy) group (n = 100) and a thymothymomectomy (resection of thymoma with total thymectomy) group (n = 73). The differences in the clinicopathological characteristics and prognosis between the two groups were examined.

Results.—Myasthenia gravis developed postoperatively in three patients (3%) in the thymomectomy group and in 6 (8%) in the thymothymomectomy group. The 5- and 10-year overall survival rates in the thymomectomy group were 96.7% and 92.2%, and those in the thymothymomectomy group were 94.0% and 86.2%, respectively ($P = 0.755$). Two patients (2%) in the thymomectomy group and 4 (5%) in the thymothymomectomy group experienced recurrence.

Conclusions.—There was no difference in prognosis/recurrence between the two groups. Thymothymomectomy might not always be necessary for nonmyasthenic patients with stage I or II thymoma.

▶ Surgical resection is considered the definitive treatment for thymoma. The extent of resection remains controversial, but recent guidelines and reviews have recommended a complete en bloc resection of the tumor with the entire thymus gland (thymothymomectomy), primarily via a median sternotomy. The surgical methods are the standard treatment for thymoma with myasthenia gravis (MG), but the usefulness and necessity of these same surgical methods for thymoma without MG has not been fully evaluated. A recent comparative study reviewed the surgical results of early-stage nonmyasthenic thymoma treated by thymomectomy with and without extended thymectomy and concluded that perhaps extensive resection was not warranted or beneficial in nonmyasthenic thymoma patients.

The authors reviewed 173 nonmyasthenic patients who had either stage 1 or stage 2 thymomas. Although the original descriptions of the thymic resections were all via median sternotomies, over the past 10 to 15 years, the evolution of minimally invasive thoracoscopic and even mini thoracotomy approaches have become standard for many patients with thymoma. In this particular study, the authors noted that the clinicopathologic backgrounds of the 2 groups are not statistically significantly different, and both groups had a relatively equal predominance of median sternotomy with lesser numbers of anterolateral thoracotomy and video-assisted thoracoscopy.

This study suggests that complete resection of the entire thymus gland through median sternotomy as historically recommended may not be necessary for stage 1 and 2 thymomas. The authors acknowledge several criticisms of this philosophy. First, there is concern that MG may occur after resection of less than the entire thymus in patients with thymoma. However, the authors note that the occurrence of postoperative MG was equal to or even slightly less in the group that had a more local resection in stage 1 and 2. The second criticism raised is the likelihood of increased risk of local recurrence in the remnant thymus gland. However, in several previous reports, the local recurrence rate after a resection of a thymoma was less than 5%, and in this study, only 1 patient (1%) in the thymomectomy group experienced a local recurrence. Given that the thymoma is often indolent in nature when the tumor is completely encapsulated, it seems possible to achieve curative resection with only a partial thymus gland incision.

Although I believe that total thymus resection is preferable when technically feasible, this manuscript does solidify the position that the more minimally invasive approaches are appropriate for patients with stage 1 or 2 thymoma. In our center, I have transitioned almost completely to the use of the Da Vinci robot for the resection of thymus tissue. Historically, I primarily used video-assisted thoracoscopic surgery and reserved median sternotomy for the largest of tumors. However, with increasing experience with the robotic approach, it has anecdotally seemed that added visualization and the ability to more completely resect the thymus gland seemed advantageous. The patients are often in the hospital only 1 or 2 days and can often return to full activity within a week. I applaud the authors' efforts to critically review the impact of complete thymic removal on outcomes in patients with stage 1 and 2 thymoma and think this further solidifies minimally invasive approaches as the treatment of choice in the early stages of this disease process.

C. T. Klodell, Jr, MD

Staging of Non-small Cell Lung Cancer

A National Study of Nodal Upstaging After Thoracoscopic Versus Open Lobectomy for Clinical Stage I Lung Cancer

Licht PB, Jørgensen OD, Ladegaard L, et al (Odense Univ Hosp, Denmark)
Ann Thorac Surg 96:943-950, 2013

Background.—Nodal upstaging after surgical intervention for non-small cell lung cancer (NSCLC) occurs when unsuspected lymph node metastases are found during the final evaluation of surgical specimens. Recent data from The Society of Thoracic Surgery (STS) database demonstrated significantly lower nodal upstaging after thoracoscopic (VATS) lobectomy than after thoracotomy. STS data, however, may be biased from voluntary reporting, and survival was not investigated. We used a complete national registry to compare nodal upstaging and survival after lobectomy by VATS or thoracotomy.

Methods.—The Danish Lung Cancer Registry was used to identify patients who underwent lobectomy for clinical stage I NSCLC from 2007 to 2011. Patient demographics, comorbidity, preoperative staging, surgical approach, number of lymph nodes harvested, final pathology, and survival were evaluated. Nodal upstaging was identified by comparing cT N M with pT N M.

Results.—Lobectomy for clinical stage I NSCLC was performed in 1,513 patients: 717 (47%) by VATS and 796 (53%) by thoracotomy. Nodal upstaging occurred in 281 patients (18.6%) and was significantly higher after thoracotomy for N1 upstaging (13.1% vs 8.1%; $p < 0.001$) and N2 upstaging (11.5% vs 3.8%; $p < 0.001$). Overall unadjusted survival was significantly higher after VATS, but after adjusting for differences in sex, age, comorbidity, and pT N M by Cox regression analysis, we found no difference between VATS and thoracotomy (hazard ratio, 0.98; 95% confidence interval, 0.80 to 1.22, $p = 0.88$).

Conclusions.—National data confirm that nodal upstaging was lower after VATS than after open lobectomy for clinical stage I NSCLC. Multivariate survival analysis, however, showed no difference in survival, indicating that differences in nodal upstaging result from patient selection for reasons not captured in our registry.

► Nodal upstaging after surgical intervention for non–small cell lung cancer (NSCLC) occurs when unsuspected lymph node metastases are found during the final histopathologic evaluation of surgical specimens. It is critical information for determining prognosis, influencing the need for adjuvant therapy and, consequently, survival. The detection of unsuspected lymph node metastases is directly dependent on removal or sampling of lymph nodes basins, which is therefore dependent on the completeness of lymph node dissection. A recent study by the Society of Thoracic Surgeons shows a significantly lower rate of nodal upstaging after thoracoscopic lobectomy rather than traditional open lobectomy, prompting the authors to look at their nationwide data set.

The authors' study covers 5 years and 1513 patients, which were relatively equally divided among men and women. All patients underwent standard anatomic lobectomy for stage I NSCLC, with a thoracoscopic approach used in 47% of the surgeries. The number of lymph node basins dissected was not statistically different between the thoracoscopic and open approaches. Nodal upstaging was noted to occur more frequently after thoracotomy than thoracoscopic removal of the lung.

Thoracoscopy is generally assumed to be less traumatic than thoracotomy with reduced postoperative pain, better pulmonary function, and shorter hospital stay and is more frequently sought by patients in this current era. However, adequately powered studies comparing thoracoscopy with open thoracotomy are lacking in the literature. This study suggests that there is a higher rate of nodal upstaging after thoracotomy than thoracoscopy. Certainly, it is reasonable to question if thoracoscopy is an adequate oncologic approach when upstaging is so much lower than that of thoracotomy both in this study and the Society of Thoracic Surgeons database.

A significant weakness of this study is that although their database does tell the number of basins, it does not tell the total number of lymph nodes removed; therefore, there may be a difference in the amount of lymph node tissue harvested between the 2 techniques. However, if this were the case, you would expect a survival difference between 2 groups. Another important criticism of the study would be the retrospective nature of the study as well as the relatively infrequent use of the positron emission tomography scanning and that the approach was selected based on surgeon preference, which may have some intangible factors. With this type of selection bias, it would not be surprising to find a higher degree nodal upstaging in the open group. This study and the earlier Society of Thoracic Surgeons study continue to fuel the debate about the need for a randomized prospective trial of the open and thoracoscopic techniques. Although this trial may be feasible in Europe, my suspicion is it will be difficult to accomplish such a trial in the United States.

C. T. Klodell, Jr, MD

Article Index

Chapter 1: General Considerations

Chapter 2: Trauma

Chapter 3: Burns

Chapter 4: Critical Care

Chapter 5: Wound Healing

Chapter 6: Transplantation

Chapter 7: Surgical Infections

Chapter 8: Endocrine

Chapter 9: Nutrition

Chapter 10: Gastrointestinal

Chapter 12: Vascular Surgery

Chapter 13: General Thoracic Surgery

Author Index

K

L

M

N

O

P

R

S

T

U

V

W

X

Y

Z

FSC
www.fsc.org
MIX
Papier | Fördert gute Waldnutzung
FSC® C083411

Kolibri 360 GmbH
Ferdinand-Jühlke-Straße 7
99095 Erfurt, Deutschland
produktsicherheit@kolibri360.de